NU
AND
NEUROSCIENCES

NURSING AND THE NEUROSCIENCES

Edited by

DOUGLAS ALLAN RGN RMN RCT Neuro Cert

Clinical Nurse Teacher, Glasgow South College of Nursing and Midwifery,
Southern General Hospital, Glasgow

Churchill Livingstone ▦

EDINBURGH LONDON MELBOURNE AND NEW YORK 1988

CHURCHILL LIVINGSTONE
Medical Division of Longman Group UK Limited

Distributed in the United States of America by
Churchill Livingstone Inc., 1560 Broadway, New York,
N.Y. 10036, and by associated companies, branches
and representatives throughout the world.

First published 1988

ISBN 0-443-03550-4

British Library Cataloguing in Publication Data
Nursing and the neurosciences.
  1. Neurological nursing
  I. Allan, Douglas
  616.8'024613   RC350.5

Library of Congress Cataloging in Publication Data
Nursing and the neurosciences.
  Includes index.
  1. Neurological nursing. I. Allan, Douglas,
1953–   [DNLM: 1. Nervous System Diseases —
nursing. 2. Neurosurgery — nursing.   WY 160 N9742]
RC350.5.N85   1988   616.8'024613   87-29912

Produced by Longman Singapore Publishers (Pte) Ltd.
Printed in Singapore.

Preface

This text represents a watershed in the history of neuroscience nursing within the UK. This is the first high level neuroscience nursing textbook specifically written for the British nurse. It encompasses both neurosurgical and neuromedical nursing practice along with sections devoted to neurological trauma and specific neuropaediatric problems. Information is also provided on nervous system physiology and pain relief from a neurosurgical viewpoint.

It is hoped that this text will satisfy the needs of the practising neuroscience nurse and post-basic students. It is always difficult to produce the first edition of a new text and especially to decide what to include or to leave out. Comments on our efforts are warmly welcomed as this is the only way we can move forward and build on our body of knowledge for the benefit of neuroscience nursing in the future.

As one would expect, a project of this nature relies upon the goodwill and nature of many individuals. My wife, Morag, and son and daughter, Ross and Sarah, have by now learned to live with and tolerate a nurse author. Their patience and understanding are immeasurable. The contributors have provided a valuable input of their expertise and time and I am extremely grateful to them for this. Many colleagues and friends from the world of neuroscience, orthopaedic and paediatric nursing, both within the UK and abroad, have offered useful help and criticism from the planning stages right through to the final draft.

I am grateful for the help provided by my colleagues at the Institute of Neurological Sciences, Glasgow, and Robin Johnstone, Consultant Neurosurgeon, deserves a particular mention for the valuable advice which he provided for one of the contributors. The British Society of Neuromedical and Neurosurgical Nurses has, and continues to provide, a forum whereby neuroscience nurses have the opportunity to meet together and exchange views. Much of the expertise within these pages originated from such meetings. No writing project would survive without the valuable help from library services; I am particularly indebted to the librarians of the Glasgow South College of Nursing and Midwifery, Southern General Hospital, Glasgow. Their ability to find obscure references never ceases to amaze me and the quality of advice they offer on various matters is exemplary. The staff at Churchill Livingstone have guided the final manuscript through the difficult process of preparation for publication; I thank them for their support.

Glasgow 1988   Douglas Allan

Contributors

Douglas Allan
RGN RMN RCT Neuro Cert
Clinical Nurse Teacher, Glasgow South College of Nursing and Midwifery, Southern General Hospital, Glasgow

Morag Allan
RGN RSCN NNEB
Staff Nurse, Royal Hospital for Sick Children, Glasgow

Patricia Ann Cooksley
SRN CMBI Dip Nurs (Lond Univ)
Ward Sister, Neuromedical Subregional Unit, Plymouth General Hospital, Plymouth

Jane M. Davies
BN SRN NDNC
Formerly Sister, Recovery Unit, The National Hospital for Nervous Diseases, London

Norma Johnston Grant
RGN CCNS Cert in Neuromedical and Neurosurgical Nursing
Ward Sister, Neurosurgery, Institute of Neurological Sciences, Southern General Hospital, Glasgow

C. A. Greenway
SRN
Staff Nurse, Neurology Department, Freedom Fields Hospital, Plymouth

Elizabeth Jamieson
RGN ONC RCNT
Clinical Teacher, Department of Health and Nursing Studies, College of Technology, Glasgow

Margot E. Virginia Lindsay
BA(Hons) SRN
Staff Nurse, National Hospital for Nervous Diseases, London

Catherine McFarlane
RGN SCM ONC
Ward Sister, Department of Orthopaedics, Western Infirmary, Glasgow

A. F. McGuire
RGN ONC
Ward Sister, Gartnavel General Hospital, Glasgow

Lesley Pemberton
SRN FETC RCNT Pt 1
Midwifery Teacher's Cert Dip N (Lond)
Nurse Tutor, Oldham School of Nursing; Member of the British Society of Neuromedical and Neurosurgical Nurses; Member of the RCN Oncology Nurses' Society

Contents

1

Anatomy and physiology of the nervous system

The human nervous system is a highly complex and vital part of the body. It is responsible for communication, control, behaviour and intellectual attainments. New information is being sought — and found — even at present, about the nervous system. Although much remains to be discovered, there is a lot of fascinating information to be learned from our present knowledge.

In this chapter, the aim is to describe some aspects of the nervous system in relation to its normal structure and function. The nurse may then understand some of the abnormalities and disturbances which can arise.

In general the system can be described, quite simply, in two parts: the *central nervous system*, which consists of the brain and the spinal cord, and the *peripheral nervous system*, which consists of the cranial and spinal nerves (peripheral nerves). The *autonomic nervous system* is sometimes included in the peripheral system, but is part of both the central and peripheral systems.

Millions of neurones (nerve cells and nerve fibres) make up the functional parts of the nervous system. These are surrounded and supported by interstitial cells, or neuroglia.

NERVOUS SYSTEM CELLS

Neuroglia

Neuroglia are ancillary cell[s of the nervous] system. They are not invol[ved...]

transmission of nerve impulses, but they have important functions. Some of the neuroglial cells are closely linked with nerve cells, and there is evidence of a degree of interdependence between the two types of cells.

Four types of neuroglial cells have been identified — *astrocytes, oligodendrocytes, microglia* and *ependyma*. The first two are also known as *macroglia*. In the embryo, the macroglial and ependymal cells develop from the ectodermal tissue. The microglial cells develop, at a later stage, from the mesodermal tissue; they are cells which have invaded the nervous system.

Astrocytes are the most numerous of the neuroglial cells, and are scattered throughout the central nervous system. Their name is derived from the star-shaped appearance of the cells, which have many processes projecting from the cell bodies. These processes are often attached to capillaries and larger blood vessels. Some are attached to neurones and, near the surface of the brain, to the pia mater (a thin membrane which adheres to the surface of the brain and spinal cord). Astrocytes also form a layer, intertwined with ependymal cells, in the ventricles of the brain.

Because of their attachment to blood vessels and neurones, the astrocytes provide a structural and supporting framework. It is thought that they may also have a role in transporting chemicals between capillaries and nerve cells. More importantly, they may prevent some substances from passing into the brain from the bloodstream, forming part of the 'blood-brain barrier'.

Oligodendrocytes are situated adjacent to nerve cells and, in greater numbers, around nerve fibres. They are named oligodendrocytes because they have only a few short processes (dendrites) projecting from their cell bodies. The large numbers of these cells which surround nerve fibres indicate that they are responsible for forming the fatty covering (myelin sheath) of these fibres in the central nervous system. The membrane of the oligodrocyte is wrapped around a nerve fibre mber of layers, which varies in different sites. In some areas, numerous nerve fibres may be surrounded by one single oligodendrocyte — these are known as unmyelinated fibres. Oligodendrocytes which lie close to nerve cells probably help them to thrive and grow.

Microglia, as the name suggests, are small cells which are scattered throughout the central nervous system in small numbers. When nervous tissue is damaged, they enlarge and display phagocytic properties. Their role in ingesting and digesting tissue debris indicates that they are scavenger cells, belonging to the reticuloendothelial system.

Ependyma are cells which line the ventricles of the brain and the central canal of the spinal cord. They form a single layer of epithelial cells, some of which are flattened and some cuboidal or columnar. Most of the ependymal cells which line the ventricles are ciliated, whereas, in other areas, ciliated cells are spaced among unciliated cells. As mentioned in the section on astrocytes, some of the ependyma are intertwined with astrocytes to form an internal membrane in the ventricles. The function of this membrane is not understood.

NEURONES

Neurones are considered to be the functional units of the nervous system. Each one consists of a cell body and projecting processes, and is responsible for the transmission of nerve impulses. Neurones may be classified according to their function in three ways:

1. Sensory neurones, which transmit impulses to the brain and spinal cord
2. Motor neurones, which transmit impulses from the brain and spinal cord to muscles and glands
3. Intermediate neurones, which transmit impulses from sensory to motor neurones.

The size and shape of neurones varies, according to their location and function. Three main types of neurones (see Fig. 1.1) are described as:

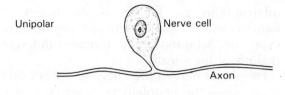

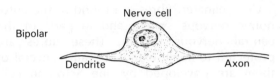

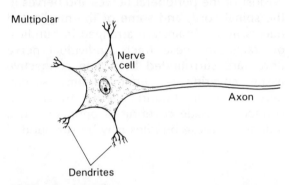

Fig. 1.1 Types of neurones.

Unipolar — cells with one projecting process
Bipolar — cells with two distinct processes
Multipolar — cells with a number of processes.

Structure of neurones

Cell bodies

The size of the cell bodies varies from 5 micrometres to 135 micrometres in diameter. They appear grey in colour and are thus referred to as 'grey matter'. Each cell is enclosed in a semi-permeable membrane, composed of lipid and protein molecules and an external glycoprotein coat. This membrane also extends along the surfaces of the cell processes.

Within the cell body is a nucleus, cytoplasm and various organelles.

The nucleus is usually spherical and centrally situated, and is surrounded by a nuclear membrane. There is a prominent nucleolus, which synthesises ribonucleic acid. Like other cells of the body, the cytoplasmic organelles are mitochondria, Golgi apparatus, centrosome and microtubules. Three additional structures, which are peculiar to nerve cells, are also present in the cytoplasm — neurofibrils, neurofilaments and Nissl material (or Nissl's granules).

Neurofilaments have been identified on electron microscopy, and it is thought that they make up the neurofibrils, although this is not certain. These two structures are probably responsible for the rapid transport of essential substances and nerve impulses through the cell. Nissl material can be identified when nerve cells are stained with basic dyes, and large nerve cells contain more than small nerve cells. Motor neurones contain coarse clumps of Nissl material, but it is more finely distributed in sensory neurones. This granular substance contains ribosomes, which are responsible for synthesising proteins.

Some pigment granules are also found in the cytoplasm of nerve cells. The amount of pigment — lipofuscin, which is a yellowish-brown colour — increases with age, but its significance is not known. A few groups of nerve cells, such as the substantia nigra, contain another pigment — melanin — which is probably a by-product of chemical reactions involving tyrosine and dopamine. Again, the significance is not known.

Nerve processes

The nerve processes are thread-like extensions of the cell bodies, which are known as dendrites and axons.

Dendrites are short, branching processes which act as cell receptors. Most of the neurones in the central nervous system have several dendrites, i.e. they are multipolar. The distal ends of dendrites form synapses (connections), which pick up impulses from other nerves or tissues and transmit them into the cell body.

Axons, or nerve fibres, conduct impulses away from the cell body. Each cell has only one axon, but these vary in length and diameter from one type of cell to another. The axons terminate in small, branching filaments, or fibrils, which form a synapse with other neurones or with muscles. Some axons give off collateral branches along their length. The axons consist of a membrane — axolemma — which contains cytoplasm — axoplasm — within. All of the axons in the peripheral nervous system, and some in the central nervous system, are surrounded by a myelin sheath (Fig. 1.2). Concentric rings of fatty material are wrapped around the axon, forming this sheath, helping to protect and insulate it. The term 'white matter' comes from the high fat content of the myelin sheath which gives it a creamy white colour. Myelin sheaths are formed by oligodendrocytes in the central nervous system and by Schwann cells in the peripheral nervous system. About every 100 micrometres to 1 millimetre along the axon, the myelin sheath is segmented. These interruptions are known as the nodes of Ranvier, and are due to different oligodendrocytes or Schwann cells forming different regions of the sheath.

Peripheral nerve fibres have an extra outer covering — the neurilemma — which is also formed by Schwann cells (Fig. 1.2). It adds extra protection to the nerve fibres and is thought to play a part in the regeneration of injured peripheral nerves.

Unmyelinated fibres are found in the autonomic nervous system and in parts of the central nervous system. These fibres are protected to some extent, because several of them are enveloped by one Schwann cell. They appear greyish in colour and, like cell bodies, are referred to as 'grey matter'.

Most of the peripheral nerves and nerves in the spinal cord, and some of the myelinated nerves in the brain, are arranged in bundles, or tracts. In these tracts, individual nerve fibres are surrounded by a fine connective tissue covering — endoneurium; several nerve fibres are bound together by another connective tissue covering — perineurium; a number of these bundles may be surrounded

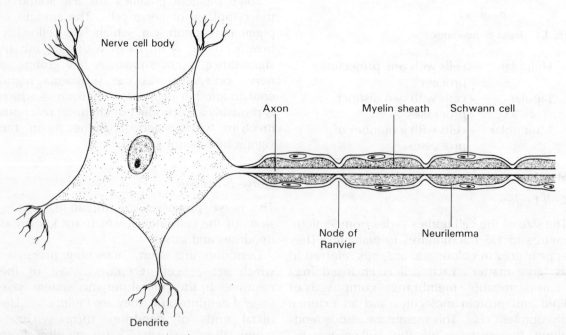

Fig. 1.2 Axon-myelin sheath and neurilemma.

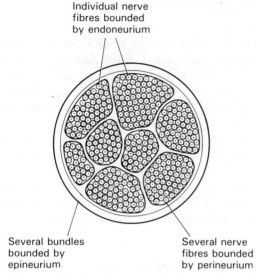

Fig. 1.3 Nerve tracts.

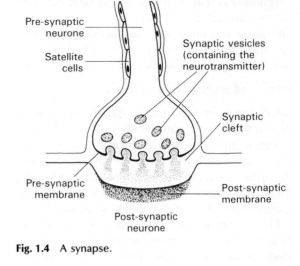

Fig. 1.4 A synapse.

by yet another connective tissue covering — epineurium (Fig. 1.3).

Conduction of nerve impulses

A nerve impulse is initiated by a stimulus, such as a change in temperature, pressure or chemical environment. The impulse is a self-propagating wave of electrical charge along the membrane of the neurone. In the resting state, sodium ions are continually pumped out of the neurone. These ions are positively charged. With adequate stimulation, the permeability of the membrane changes, allowing an influx of sodium ions. This results in a positive electrical charge — action potential — which travels along the length of the neurone, whilst each preceding area of the membrane quickly returns to a negative state. These positive-negative changes occur in rapid succession, spreading to the end of the axon. Speed of transmission is increased by the impulse jumping from one node of Ranvier to the next in myelinated fibres, which is known as saltatory conduction. Generally, the larger the diameter of the axon, the faster is the speed of transmission.

Synapses

The junctions between one neurone and another, and between neurones and muscles or glands, are known as synapses (Fig. 1.4). Nerve impulses are transmitted across the gap between the adjacent tissues by chemical transmitters (neurotransmitters). The chemical is stored in vesicles in the expanded end of the axon and is released when the nerve impulse reaches this point. Several chemical transmitters have been identified, the most common ones being acetylcholine and nor-adrenaline. Many of these neurotransmitters are excitory, resulting in the nerve impulse being transmitted to the adjacent tissue, but some have an inhibiting effect and prevent the transmission of impulses from neurones situated nearby.

Synapses vary from the simple arrangement of an adjacent axon and dendrite to more complex structures. The area receiving stimulation from the neurone has a specially constructed membrane which is able to receive the neurotransmitter. This then brings about changes in the tissue, e.g., causing muscle contraction. Neurotransmitters are either destroyed by enzymes or reabsorbed into the axon after use. For example, acetylcholine is destroyed by cholinesterase, nor-adrenaline is reabsorbed into the axon. Certain drugs can affect the transmission of nerve impulses by blocking the action of these chemical transmitters.

Injury and regeneration of neurones

Nerve cells are extremely sensitive to their environment and can be damaged by lack of oxygen, poisons, infective agents or trauma. The main nutrients which nerve cells require in order to develop and function normally include glucose, sodium, calcium, potassium, magnesium, iron and B group vitamins.

Degeneration of neurones is known as neuropathy, and may either be in the form of *demyelination* (degeneration of Schwann cells) or *Wallerian degeneration* (damage to the axon). Damage to the axon usually results in changes to the cell body. The changes vary according to the type of neurone, but typical aspects of neuronal response to injury are described below.

Changes in the cell body

The first signs of reaction are seen within 24 to 48 hours after injury to the axon. Fragmentation of the Golgi apparatus occurs, which may lead to damage of the cell membrane. The Nissl's granules break up — this process is known as *chromatolysis* — the nucleus is displaced from its central position and the cell body swells (cellular oedema). This reaction reaches its peak around 10 to 20 days after injury and is more severe the closer the damage is to the cell body. In some cases, the nucleus may be pushed out of the cell and the cell dies. Otherwise, signs of recovery occur even while the aforementioned changes are taking place. The nucleus enlarges and there is increased ribonucleic acid and protein synthesis, which is necessary for regeneration of the axon. The recovery period may take several months with gradual restoration of the ribonucleic acid and protein contents. Cells can recover even if the axon does not regenerate, but they tend to be smaller than normal.

Changes in the axon

The axon relies on proteins from the cell body, and is unable to survive for long if it is completely separated. Most damage occurs in the part of the axon farthest away from the cell body, and from the site of injury back to the previous node of Ranvier. Within the first day, the axon becomes swollen and irregular, and begins to fragment by the 3rd to 5th day. The myelin sheath disintegrates into fat droplets, which eventually disappear over a few weeks. Schwann cells undergo mitosis and probably play a part in phagocytosis, assisting in the removal of the myelin droplets.

Regeneration of nerve fibres

Peripheral nerves. In the first few days, the Schwann cells proliferate and fill the gap in the endoneurial sheath. This forms a bridge through which new fibrils (numerous branches of regenerating nerve fibres) can cross. Rate of growth of the fibrils is slow — 2 to 4 millimetres per day — and one fibril will mature into a new axon, connecting with the distal uninjured segment. However, the process is not always satisfactory. Some fibrils grow into adjacent tissue, rather than crossing the endoneurial tube, and may form swellings — neuroma — which can be a source of pain. Motor and sensory fibres may become 'crossed' and remain functionless. Sensory fibres may not make contact with skin receptors, resulting in a residual loss of sensation. If a fibre is crushed, rather than completely severed, regeneration is more likely to be almost perfect.

In the process of regeneration, a new myelin sheath is laid down by Schwann cells. Regeneration can be assisted by surgical intervention. Suturing of the outer connective tissue sheaths of injured nerves, within a month of injury, increases the chances of restoration of function. However, this is unlikely to occur if the suturing is postponed beyond 6 months.

Central nervous system. Degeneration of cell bodies and axons in the central nervous system follows the same pattern as in the peripheral system. Microglial cells act as macrophages to remove debris and scar tissue is formed by astrocytes. In the past, it has generally been accepted that regeneration of axons does not occur in the central nervous system. Although there is some regeneration, most of the fibres degenerate within 2 to 3 weeks, because oligodendrocytes do not possess the same properties as Schwann cells for forming new endoneurial sheaths. However, research has been done on chemicals which reduce glial reactions and 'nerve growth factor' which improves the growth of axons; thyroid hormone is also known to improve axon regeneration by stimulating protein synthesis. Spinal cord reconstruction, in paraplegic patients, has recently been attempted in selected people, with a reported success rate of 60%. For this procedure, carried out about 1 year after the initial injury, nerve fibres are taken from the leg and implanted into the damaged section of the spinal cord and surrounded by Schwann cell cultures.

CENTRAL NERVOUS SYSTEM

The brain and the spinal cord develop from ectodermal tissue in the embryo. By about the 16th day of development, a structure known as the *neural plate* appears in the midline of the embryo. This develops into the *neural tube* by about the 3rd week of life. The upper end of the neural tube develops into the brain and the remainder into the spinal cord, while the canal within the tube becomes the ventricles of the brain and the central canal of the spinal cord.

BRAIN

Initially, the brain develops as three vesicles — the *forebrain* (prosencephalon), *midbrain* (mesencephalon) and *hindbrain* (rhombencephalon). Secondary brain vesicles develop about 1 week later — 5th week of life — forming the *diencephalon* and *telencephalon* of the forebrain and the *metencephalon* and *myelencephalon* of the hindbrain. The midbrain remains unchanged. When describing the mature brain, the following terms are used :

telencephalon — consisting of the cerebral hemispheres (cerebral cortex, olfactory system, corpus striatum and connecting nerve fibres)

diencephalon — consisting of the thalamus, subthalamus, epithalamus and hypothalamus

mesencephalon — known as the midbrain

metencephalon — known as pons varolii and cerebellum

myelencephalon — known as medulla oblongata.

The diencephalon and telencephalon are known as the cerebrum; the midbrain, pons and medulla form the brain stem.

The brain reaches its full size by the age of 18 years and, in the adult, is one of the largest organs of the body. It weighs, on average, 1350 g in the male and 1275 g in the female — variations exist according to age and stature. Many millions of neurones are contained within the brain, but research, so far, indicates that a significant number do not appear to have any specific functions. Recent research has shown that some people with very sparse brain tissue have normal physical and mental development.

The three main areas of the brain — cerebrum, brain stem and cerebellum — are described in more detail below.

Cerebrum

As already noted, the cerebrum consists of the two cerebral hemispheres (telencephalon) and a central core (diencephalon).

Cerebral hemispheres

The surface, or cortex, of the cerebrum consists of grey matter and makes up about 40% of the weight of the brain. It consists of layers of nerve cells and nerve fibres, varying in thickness from 4.5 to 1.5 millimetres. The cortex has a convoluted appearance, which gives a greater surface area to the cerebral hemispheres. The folds of the convolutions — *gyri* — have fissures — *sulci* — in between them. Some of these gyri and sulci are used as identification marks of specific areas of the hemispheres.

Each cerebral hemisphere consists of four lobes, which are named according to the bones of the skull under which they lie. These are the *frontal, parietal, temporal* and *occipital* lobes. An area of cortex buried within each hemisphere is sometimes described as a fifth lobe. This is the *insula* or *island of Reil*.

The cortex is responsible for three main activities — receiving and interpreting sensory impulses from all parts of the body; initiating and controlling voluntary movements; integrating functions such as consciousness and memory.

Some areas of the cortex are responsible for specialised functions, as shown in Figure 1.5.

The frontal lobe contains the *motor area*, which controls voluntary muscles, mainly on the opposite side of the body to the hemisphere. It also contains the *motor speech area* — Broca's area — which controls the muscles used in speech, and the *association area* (prefrontal cortex), which controls behaviour and higher mental functions such as judgement.

The parietal lobe contains the *sensory area*, which receives sensory impulses from the skin and deeper tissues. Like the motor area, each hemisphere is responsible for the opposite side of the body. The *vestibular area* is situated in the lower part of the parietal lobe and probably receives information for motor regulation and spatial orientation.

In both the motor and sensory areas, the body is represented in an inverted fashion in the cortex, i.e., face and head at the lowest part, followed by hand, arm, trunk and thigh, with the remainder of the leg and the peri-

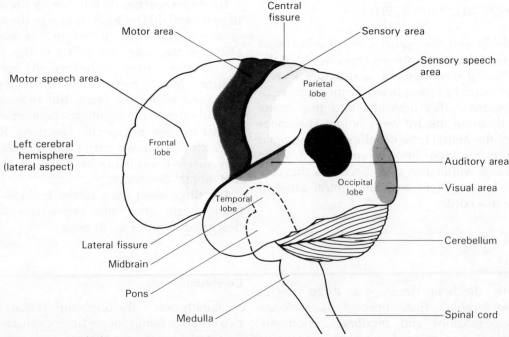

Fig. 1.5 The brain, showing areas of localisation of function.

neum on the medial surface of the hemisphere.

The temporal lobe contains the *auditory area*, with sound input mainly from the opposite ear to the hemisphere. However, there is substantial input from the ear of the same side. The *gustatory area* (taste) is often described as being located in the temporal lobe, with an extension into the insula. In fact, it is adjacent to the lower part of the sensory area in the parietal lobe, in the posterior wall of the lateral fissure. The *olfactory area* (which deals with the sense of smell) is classified as being in the temporal lobe, but is a rather more complex system.

The occipital lobe contains the *visual area*, mostly on the medial surface and extending over the occipital pole. This is the thinnest part of the cerebral cortex. About one-third of

the visual cortex deals with central vision, from the macula of the retina. Impulses from the temporal (outer) half of the retina pass to the hemisphere on the same side as the eye, whereas impulses from the nasal (inner) half of the retina pass to the opposite hemisphere (Fig. 1.6). This results in the left visual field being represented in the right hemisphere and vice versa.

The visual association cortex, surrounding the visual area in the occipital lobe, deals with complex visual roles. Its functions include relating past and present visual experiences, recognition and appreciation of what is seen. Nerve fibres from this area also connect with the midbrain, where the oculomotor, trochlear and abducens nerves originate. A reflex pathway exists for automatic scanning move-

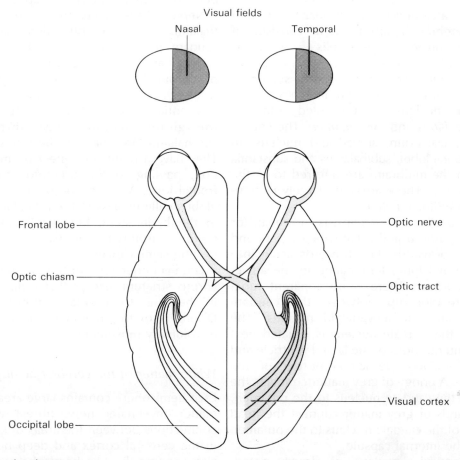

Fig. 1.6 Visual pathways.

ments and these nerve pathways also enable the focusing of near objects to take place.

The *association cortex* consists of areas of the cortex which are interconnected and responsible for complex functions such as integration of the senses, memory, learning, thought processes, behaviour and emotion.

Cerebral dominance refers to the hemisphere which deals with language. In the majority of people, it is the left cerebral hemisphere and, in about 65%, this hemisphere is larger than the right. The majority of people with a dominant left hemisphere are right-handed. The non-dominant hemisphere appears to be better in activities related to spatial activity such as drawing and constructing images.

Corpus striatum

This is an area of grey matter near the base of each cerebral hemisphere. It consists of groups of nuclei — nerve cells — known as the *caudate nucleus* and the *lenticular* (or *lentiform) nucleus*, which are partly separated by the internal capsule (white matter). The lenticular nucleus is subdivided into the *globus pallidus* and the *putamen*. The corpus striatum, claustrum, amygdaloid nucleus (in the temporal lobe), subthalamus and substantia nigra (in the midbrain) are referred to as the *basal ganglia*. These areas are largely responsible for motor functions.

The caudate nucleus consists of a head (or anterior portion) and a tail which tapers and extends backwards then forwards again into the temporal lobe, terminating in the amygdaloid nucleus. There is no apparent functional relationship between the caudate nucleus and the amygdaloid nucleus. The head of the caudate nucleus is situated next to the anterior horn of the lateral ventricle and the tail follows the lateral border of the ventricle. A bridge of grey matter connects the head of the caudate nucleus to the putamen, and strands of grey matter connect the head and tail of the caudate nucleus to the putamen across the internal capsule.

The lenticular nucleus, as already noted, consists of the putamen and the globus pallidus. The putamen is the larger, lateral portion and is bounded, laterally, by the external capsule of white matter. A thin, upward extension of grey matter — the claustrum — is connected to the putamen and lies between the external and extreme capsules. Lateral to the extreme capsule is the insula (island of Reil). Although it is connected to the putamen, the claustrum has no apparent functional relationship with the corpus striatum. It is probably derived from the insula and has connections with the frontal, parietal and temporal lobes of the cortex, but its role is not understood. The medial surface of the putamen is adjacent to the internal capsule.

The globus pallidus lies just beneath and medial to the putamen and consists of two, or possibly three divisions. It is so named because of its relatively pale appearance.

Nerve fibres from the cerebral cortex, thalamus and substantia nigra pass to the caudate nucleus and putamen through the internal and external capsules. Some fibres pass from the caudate nucleus and putamen to the globus pallidus and some return to the substantia nigra. Most of the neurones from the globus pallidus pass through the subthalamus and thalamus back to the cortex. They have a regulatory effect on motor function, passing to the premotor area in the frontal lobe. A few of the neurones from the globus pallidus pass to the reticular formation in the brain stem, but regulation of lower motor neurones by this pathway is probably of little significance.

Little is understood of the physiology of the corpus striatum, except that it has some role in helping to regulate motor function. Disorders of this region result in *dyskinesia* (involuntary movements).

White matter of the cerebral hemispheres

Each hemisphere contains large areas of white matter (myelinated nerve fibres) which form connections between the areas of grey matter in the cerebral cortex and deep nuclei; they also connect the two hemispheres with each

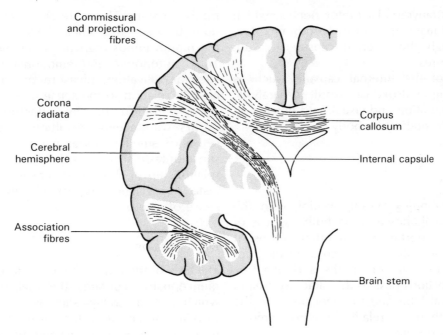

Fig. 1.7 White matter of the cerebrum.

other and with the spinal cord (Fig. 1.7). Generally there are two divisions of white matter — the *medullary centre* and the *internal capsule*.

The medullary centre consists of three types of nerve fibres, described according to the areas which they connect:

1. *Association fibres*, which connect areas of the cortex within the same hemisphere, and are the most numerous.
2. *Commissural fibres*, which connect the cortical regions of each hemisphere together. Most of these form the *corpus callosum*, a bridge between the two hemispheres; the remainder constitute part of the *anterior commissure*, which provides additional connections between the temporal lobes.

    Research has indicated that the commissural connections are responsible for bilateral memory traces, i.e., memory of the same order in each hemisphere.
3. *Projection fibres*, which radiate from the cortex to the corpus callosum and to the internal capsule — the latter being known

as the *corona radiata*. Some fibres form the external and extreme capsules, whose functions are not fully understood. Efferent motor fibres from the cerebral cortex pass through the internal capsule to the brain stem and spinal cord. Afferent fibres originating in the thalamus cross through the internal capsule and project to the cortex in various pathways. These fibres have sensory, motor, visual, auditory or association functions.

The internal capsule is a concentrated bundle of projection fibres from the corona radiata. It is described as having an anterior limb, a genu ('knee') and a posterior limb. The anterior limb lies between the caudate nucleus and the lenticular nucleus; the genu lies medial to the lenticular nucleus; the posterior limb lies between the lenticular nucleus and the thalamus. Motor nerves of the pyramidal system — i.e., those which pass to the cranial nerves in the brain stem and those which pass to the spinal cord — originate in the motor cortex of the frontal lobe and enter the posterior limb of the internal capsule. Extrapyramidal motor nerves, which originate in many areas of the cerebral cortex, pass through the internal capsule to subcortical centres.

Lesions of the internal capsule, such as those arising in stroke can result in paralysis, impaired sensation and visual field defects on the opposite side of the body.

Olfactory system

This is a complex system dealing with the sense of smell; however, in humans, it is of much less importance than other senses. It consists of the olfactory mucosa (in the roof of the nose), olfactory bulbs and olfactory tracts. Projections pass to the olfactory area in the temporal lobe and to other areas of the brain, and there are relationships to memory, emotions and taste.

The olfactory mucosa is capable of detecting a wide range of aromas, and there are probably different olfactory cells which are sensitive to different chemicals. (The mucosa is not described in detail here, being more appropriate to the structure and function of the nose.) Olfactory nerves pass from the olfactory mucosa, through the cribriform plate in the ethmoid bone, to the olfactory bulbs. The olfactory bulbs are the expanded terminal portions of the olfactory tracts which extend from the mucosa. There are neuronal connections between the two olfactory bulbs, through the anterior commisure. Neurones leaving the bulbs pass to the amygdaloid nucleus and temporal lobe (primary olfactory area), from where association fibres connect with other parts of the temporal lobe.

Some neurones supply the anterior perforated substance (intermediate olfactory area) which lies between the olfactory and optic tracts and is penetrated by many small blood vessels. Other neurones pass to the medial surface of the frontal lobe (medial olfactory area), which is probably concerned with some of the emotional aspects of the sense of smell. From this area, there are connections through the hypothalamus to the autonomic nuclei in the brain stem. There are also a few connections between the other olfactory areas and the hippocampus (part of the limbic system). Thus, autonomic and emotional responses, such as salivation, pleasure or nausea, can arise in relation to the sense of smell.

Degeneration of the olfactory mucosa occurs with ageing, resulting in a reduced sense of smell in older people. A reduced sense of taste also occurs because of the close relationship of these two senses — much of taste appreciation is actually through the sense of smell.

Diencephalon

The area of the brain which develops from the diencephalon contains the thalamic nuclei, which act as relay stations for impulses travelling to and from the cortex. It is divided into two halves by the narrow third ventricle and bounded laterally by the internal capsule. Each half consists of four regions — the thalamus, subthalamus, epithalamus and hypothalamus.

The thalamus is the largest area, containing several nuclei. It receives sensory impulses from the general areas of sensation, taste, vision and hearing, and transmits them to the relevant areas of the cerebral cortex. Also, it plays a part in emotions, associating sensations with pleasant or unpleasant feelings, and has a warning and protective function. The thalamus has an important role in the sleep-waking mechanism and in maintaining consciousness. It receives nerve fibres from the ascending reticular formation in the brain stem, and transmits impulses from this area throughout the cerebral cortex. Some motor fibres from the corpus striatum, substantia nigra and cerebellum also pass through the thalamus and transmit impulses to the internal capsule.

The subthalamus, which lies in front of thalamus, is a complex region containing a motor nucleus and sensory nerve fibres. The motor nucleus lies close to the internal capsule, with fibres crossing to and from the globus pallidus. Extensions of the reticular formation, red nucleus and substantia nigra — in the midbrain — enter the subthalamus.

The epithalamus is at the back and medial to the thalamus, lying next to the roof of the third ventricle. This area is concerned with autonomic responses of a more primitive nature in relation to the sense of smell and emotional drives. It also contains the pineal gland, which is an endocrine organ.

The hypothalamus, a relatively small but extremely important area, lies beneath the subthalamus. It is the main area for maintaining homeostasis, controlling the autonomic nervous system and integrating basic emotional drives with visceral responses. Connections with the frontal cortex, through the thalamus, affect moods, and it forms part of the *limbic system* of the brain. Its functions include the monitoring of osmotic pressure, temperature and hormone levels of the blood and responses to these. Direct links with the hypophysis (pituitary gland) exist — neurosecretory cells produce and transmit the hormones vasopressin and oxytocin to the neurohypophysis (posterior lobe of the pituitary gland) along nerve fibres. Releasing factors (peptides) travel via capillaries to the adenohypophysis (anterior lobe of the pituitary gland) to stimulate hormone production in that area.

Impulses originating in the hypothalamus travel to parasympathetic cells in the brain stem, where salivary, lacrimal and vagal functions are precipitated. Motor impulses to the trigeminal, facial and hypoglossal nerves have an important role in the functions of eating and drinking, with control of hunger and thirst in the hypothalamus. Regulation of body temperature is influenced by connections from the hypothalamus to motor neurones of the spinal cord, producing shivering when cold.

Nerve fibres concerned with the sense of taste and smell, and sensations from the erogenous zones of the body, are conveyed to the hypothalamus. Connections with the frontal cortex of the brain contribute to the subjective emotional experiences of these sensations. Visceral responses result from the connections between the hypothalamus and the autonomic nervous system.

Limbic system

Several references have been made in the preceding text to the limbic system. This system consists of a number of areas of grey matter in the cerebral hemispheres and the diencephalon, which have both anatomical and physiological connections. Included in the system are the *limbic lobe, hippocampus,* part of the *amygdaloid nucleus, hypothalamus* and part of the *thalamus*. Its functions are concerned with the emotions which are vital to survival, and visceral responses associated with these (through the autonomic nervous system), and also with memory.

The limbic lobe is a C-shaped portion of the cerebral cortex, on the medial surface of the hemisphere, and consists of the *cingulate* and *parahippocampal gyri*. These areas receive extensive communications from the cerebral cortex through association fibres. The parahippocampal gyrus is continuous with the hippocampus.

Developmentally, the hippocampus is an extension of the temporal lobe, and occupies the floor of the inferior horn of the lateral ventricle. Between the hippocampus and parahippocampal gyrus is the *dentate gyrus*. The hippocampus, in coronal section, is a C-shaped structure, and receives impulses from widespread areas of the cerebral cortex, through the parahippocampal gyrus. The dentate gyrus probably has a reinforcing or regulating effect on the hippocampus.

Efferent fibres from the hippocampus run parallel to afferent fibres in the cerebral cortex. In addition to these, there is also an efferent pathway in the *fornix*, which supplies the hypothalamus, thalamus and the medial olfactory areas. Reciprocal connections also exist between the hypothalamus and thalamus, and between the thalamus and cingulate gyrus. This results in an integrated system with provision of a feedback mechanism.

The amygdaloid nucleus, situated between the lenticular nucleus and the lateral ventricle, receives fibres from the olfactory bulb, thalamus, hypothalamus and cerebral cortex. Efferent fibres are distributed to the temporal and frontal lobes, thalamus, hypothalamus and reticular formation of the brain stem.

Studies indicate that the limbic system is responsible for emotions such as fear and anger and sexual behaviour — destruction or removal of the temporal lobe leads to docility, voracious appetite, increased (sometimes perverse) sexual behaviour, loss of recognition of people and memory defects. Electrical stimulation of the amygdaloid nucleus induces fear or anger. Visceral responses to these emotions are relayed mainly through the hypothalamus to the autonomic nervous system. The role of the limbic system in memory appears to be related to the retention of new information — people with lesions affecting the system have no short-term memory and are unable to commit new information to memory. However, memories of events prior to the loss of function are retained.

Brain stem

The brain stem (Fig. 1.8) consists of three parts — the midbrain, pons varolii and medulla oblongata. Each region has certain special features, but all have some common nerve tracts and contain the nuclei of the cranial nerves. The cerebral aqueduct (aqueduct of Sylvius), connecting the third and fourth ventricles, passes through the midbrain, and the fourth ventricle is situated partly in the pons and partly in the medulla.

Midbrain

This is continuous with the diencephalon and consists mainly of white matter, with some internal grey matter. It is described as having a roof, or tectum (notably on the posterior surface), and two cerebral peduncles which form the anterior and lateral surfaces. The third and fourth cranial nerves emerge from the midbrain and pass through the cavernous sinuses to the orbits.

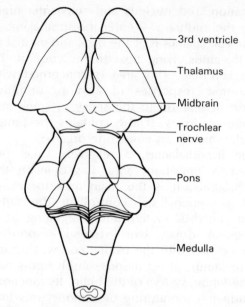

Fig. 1.8 Dorsal view of the brain stem.

The *tectum* contains nuclei of the auditory pathway, which transmit impulses to the thalamus and cerebral cortex. Some fibres pass to the cerebellum. There is also a reflex pathway connecting the auditory nuclei to nuclei which supply fibres to the extraocular muscles and motor neurones in the cervical region of the spinal cord. This enables the eyes and head to turn towards the source of sound. Cutaneous stimuli from the spinal pathway cause a similar reflex action — turning towards the stimulus. Another pathway between the occipital lobe and tectum accounts for reflex movements of the head and eye (scanning). Ocular responses for accommodation to near objects also occur through similar pathways. The role of the midbrain in other reflex actions includes closing of the eyes in response to a sudden visual stimulus (a protective function) and the pupillary response to light.

The *cerebral peduncles* can be divided into three regions:

1. *The tegmentum*, which contains nerve tracts, the red nuclei and grey matter surrounding the aqueduct of Sylvius. Sensory nerve fibres from lower regions pass through

the midbrain to the thalamus, in this region.

The red nucleus is a motor nucleus which receives nerve fibres from the cerebral cortex and the cerebellum. Efferent fibres are relayed to descending motor neurones, a few to the cerebellum, and there are reciprocal connections with the substantia nigra.

Pathways of the auditory, trigeminal, trochlear and oculomotor nerves are situated in the tegmentum.

2. *The substantia nigra* is a large motor nucleus which extends from the midbrain into the subthalamic region. Many of the cells contain melanin — a pigment which gives the nucleus its dark colour. The melanin is probably a by-product of chemical reactions involving the neurotransmitter dopamine. The cells bordering the substantia nigra do not contain melanin, but have iron within them. Fibres from the frontal, parietal and occipital lobes pass to the substantia nigra, and there are connections between it and the corpus striatum, red nucleus, reticular formation and thalamus. Although not all of the connections are fully understood, its significance as a motor centre is apparent. Degeneration of the melanin-containing cells in Parkinson's disease results in severe abnormalities of motor function.

3. *The basis pedunculi* (or crus serebri) consist of motor tracts, which relay impulses to the spinal cord and motor nuclei of the cranial nerves.

Pons varolii

This area is often referred to more simply as the pons. It is situated between the midbrain and the medulla, and appears, on anterior view, to connect the two cerebellar hemispheres. This appearance of a bridge between the cerebellar hemispheres resulted in its name. The pons consists of two distinct parts — the basal (frontal) and dorsal (posterior) sections. It has prominent cerebellar peduncles which connect the brain stem to the cerebellum. The basal region acts as a large relay station between the cerebral cortex and opposite cerebellar hemisphere, and contains motor nerve tracts. The dorsal region contains ascending and descending tracts and cranial nerve nuclei of the trigeminal, abducens, facial and auditory nerves. It also forms part of the floor of the fourth ventricle.

Medulla oblongata

This part of the brain stem is often referred to as the medulla. Its upper, wider portion lies just below the pons, and its lower junction with the spinal cord is at the level of the foramen magnum in the base of the skull. Part of the fourth ventricle is located within the medulla. The arrangement of grey and white matter within the medulla differs greatly from that in the spinal cord; the area of *decussation* (crossing over) of many motor fibres is in the medulla.

Grey matter in the lower part of the medulla consists of the *gracilis nuclei* and the *cuneatus nuclei*. The gracilis nuclei receive sensory fibres dealing with discriminatory sensations; the cuneatus nuclei receive some sensory fibres and proprioceptive fibres from the first four cervical nerves. The root of the spinal accessory nerve and motor cells of the olfactory nerve are situated near the lower border of the medulla.

On either side of the medulla is a prominent swelling — the *olive* — which is a nucleus of cells through which fibres pass to and from the cerebellum. It is an area which has a role in control of voluntary movements and equilibrium.

Numerous ascending and descending fibres pass through the medulla, and it is an area to which several cranial nerves are attached — the glossopharyngeal, vagus, spinal accessory and hypoglossal nerves.

Reticular formation

The reticular system is a network of neurones in the brain stem, which receives sensory information and transmits this to higher centres. It is also involved in relaying motor and autonomic impulses, and has an important role in the sleep-waking mechanism and in maintaining consciousness. Part of the reticular formation consists of nuclei which control the vital functions of the respiratory and cardiovascular systems. Other nuclei form the reflex centres for functions such as coughing and vomiting. Damage to the brain stem, particularly the medulla, may result in loss of sensory and motor function, loss of consciousness, and have serious — often fatal — consequences.

Cerebellum

The cerebellum lies beneath the posterior part of the cerebrum (Fig. 1.9), and is separated from it by a fold of dura mater — the *tentorium cerebelli*. It consists of two hemispheres, attached in the midline by a structure known as the *vermis*. Projections, or *peduncles*, connect the cerebellum to the brain stem. There are three regions in each hemisphere — the *anterior* and *posterior lobes*, which form the *corpus cerebelli* (main mass of the cerebellum), and the small *flocculonodular lobe*, which lies below the corpus.

The outer surface of the cerebellum — *cortex* — is composed of grey matter. It contains many transverse folds, providing a large surface area. There are several layers of different types of nerve cells.

The interior of the cerebellum is composed of a *medullary centre* of white matter and, embedded in this, four pairs of *central nuclei*. On a lateral view, the medullary centre appears to be a thin line of white matter, extending from front to back, in the centre of the hemisphere. The white matter branches in a tree-like pattern through the hemisphere. However, in cross-section, the white matter of the medullary centre extends quite widely through the hemisphere.

The central nuclei receive impulses from outside the cerebellum, which are then refined by impulses from the cerebellar cortex. The impulses are then transmitted out to the brain stem and thalamus, through the cerebellar peduncles. There are three pairs of peduncles — inferior, middle and superior, which connect with the medulla, pons and midbrain respectively.

Information from the cerebral cortex and most of the sensory systems of the body passes to the cerebellum. Its main function is to control equilibrium (balance), posture and skilled (fine) movements, and it operates at a subconscious level.

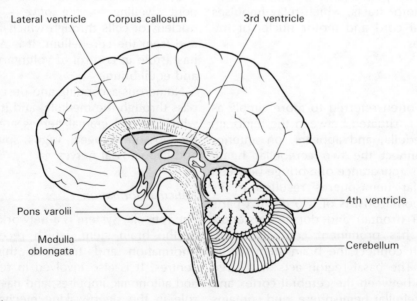

Lateral ventricle   Corpus callosum   3rd ventricle

Pons varolii

Medulla
oblongata

4th ventricle

Cerebellum

Fig. 1.9 Cerebellum

Ventricular system

The ventricular system consists of four fluid-filled spaces within the brain (Fig. 1.10). Continuous with these is the small central canal within the spinal cord. The ventricles also connect with the subarachnoid space, through small channels which leave the fourth ventricle.

Lateral ventricles

The two lateral ventricles — one in each cerebral hemisphere — each consist of a body and anterior, posterior and inferior horns. The body is situated in the temporal lobe and the horns extend into the frontal, occipital and temporal lobes, respectively. They are lined with ependymal cells and filled with cerebrospinal fluid. This fluid is produced by *choroid plexuses* (vascular connective tissue), which are situated along the floor of the body of the ventricle and the roof of the inferior horn.

Third ventricle

This is situated in the diencephalic region of the brain, dividing this area into two halves. It is connected to the lateral ventricles, above, by a small channel — the *foramen of Monro* — through which cerebrospinal fluid passes. Fluid is also produced in a small choroid plexus in the roof of the third ventricle.

Fourth ventricle

Situated partly in the medulla and partly in the pons, the fourth ventricle is connected to the third ventricle by the *cerebral aqueduct (aqueduct of Sylvius)*. A choroid plexus extends along the roof of the fourth ventricle and into its lateral recesses. The *foramen of Magendie* provides the main communication with the subarachnoid space, passing from the roof of the ventricle, along the undersurface of the cerebellum, to the cisterna magna near the occipital base of the skull. The *foramina of Luschka* are smaller openings which connect the lateral areas of the fourth ventricle to the subarachnoid space. These are situated at the cerebellopontine angles (junction of the medulla, pons and cerebellum).

Cerebrospinal fluid

The cerebrospinal fluid circulates within the ventricles and subarachnoid space (around the brain and spinal cord). It is produced

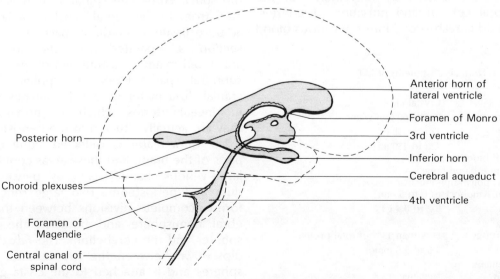

Fig. 1.10 Ventricular system.

mainly by the choroid plexuses in the ventricles. The choroid plexuses have a core of connective tissue containing many wide capillaries. They are covered by a layer of ependymal (cuboidal or columnar) cells in the ventricles, known as choroid epithelium. The surfaces of the choroid plexuses are folded, giving a greater surface area.

Cerebrospinal fluid is produced from the capillary blood in a complex way. Some components cross the capillary walls, which have permeable junctions between their cells, quite easily. Others are probably actively transported through the capillary walls and epithelial cells. The fluid is normally colourless and clear, and contains water, small amounts of protein, glucose, sodium, potassium, calcium, chloride, bicarbonate and urea. A few lymphocytes are also present. The pH is 7.3 and specific gravity 1005. Volume and pressure can vary slightly to accommodate for slight changes in intracranial pressure — the volume is approximately 120 to 150 millilitres, and the pressure is approximately 60 to 160 millimetres of water (see Table 1.1).

Cerebrospinal fluid flows from the lateral to the third and fourth ventricles and into the subarachnoid space, as previously described. A small amount passes into the central canal of the spinal cord. Movement of the fluid is slow; it is assisted by movements of the vertebral column and pulsation of arteries. The fluid is reabsorbed into the venous blood

Table 1.1 Normal constituents of CSF

Colour	Crystal clear
Pressure	80 to 160 mm water
Volume	120 to 150 ml
Cells	120 to 150 ml
a. red blood none	
b. white blood none	
(i) polymorphonuclear leucocytes	
(ii) lymphocytes 0 to 5 mm³	
Protein	0.2 to 0.4 g/l
Gamma globulin (IgG)	Less than 13% of total protein
Sugar	3.6 to 5.0 mmol
Wassermann reaction	Negative

through small projections (villi) in the arachnoid membrane. The arachnoid villi return the fluid to the venous sinuses which surround the brain.

Functions of the cerebrospinal fluid include:

- protection and cushioning of the brain and spinal cord
- provision of nourishment
- maintenance of intracranial pressure (in normal conditions)
- removal of waste products.

Meninges

The three membranes, or meninges, which surround the brain and spinal cord help to protect the central nervous system (Fig. 1.11). They are the external *dura mater*, the middle *arachnoid mater* and the internal *pia mater*. Between the arachnoid and pia is the subarachnoid space which contains the cerebrospinal fluid.

Dura mater

The dura mater is a tough, thick membrane which is attached to the periosteum below the skull. It is composed of collagenous connective tissue and extends as a tube to surround the spinal cord. The spinal section is separated from the vertebral canal by a layer of adipose tissue — epidural space. The cranial section is separated from the underlying arachnoid mater by a thin film of fluid in the subdural space. Blood is supplied to the cranial dura mater by small branches of the meningeal arteries, which are misnamed as they are actually situated in the periosteum.

The dura mater is reflected along certain parts of the brain, and these areas contain the large venous channels (sinuses) between the dura and periosteum. Two large reflections form incomplete divisions between the cerebral hemisphere and between the hemispheres and the cerebellum. The *falx cerebri* dips down between the two cerebral hemispheres and is attached to the crista galli of the ethmoid bone (at the front) and the occi-

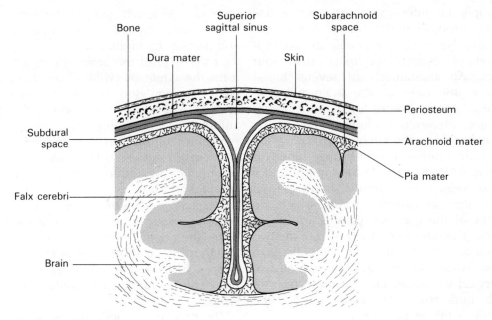

Fig. 1.11 Meninges of the brain.

pital protuberance (at the back). Between the occipital lobes of the cerebrum and the cerebellum is the *tentorium cerebelli*. This is attached to the falx cerebri along the midline, drawing it upwards and giving it a tent-like appearance. The outer edges of the tentorium are attached to the temporal bones.

A smaller reflection of the dura — the *falx cerebelli* — extends vertically between the cerebellar hemispheres.

The dura has its own nerve supply, mainly from the trigeminal nerve, which is responsible for sensation in the cranial dura. These nerve fibres result in the sensations associated with certain types of headache. Nerve fibres from the vagus nerve and upper cervical nerves supply the part of the dura which lines the posterior cranial fossa. The spinal dura is supplied by branches from the spinal nerves.

Arachnoid mater

The more delicate middle membrane is composed of collagenous and some elastic fibres, and is covered by squamous epithelium. Fine strands of connective tissue connect the arachnoid and pia, giving the webbed appearance which resulted in the archnoid mater's name (arachnoid = spider). There is no blood supply to the arachnoid mater.

Pia mater

The pia mater and arachnoid mater develop as a single layer of tissue, but become separated by the fluid filled subarachnoid space. The structure of the two membranes is thus the same, but the pia contains a network of small blood vessels and closely adheres to the surface of the brain and spinal cord.

Owing to their initial development from the same tissue, the pia and arachnoid are sometimes referred to as the *leptomeninges* (slender membranes).

Blood supply to the brain

Arterial supply

The brain requires a rich and constant supply of blood for the neurones to remain functional. Approximately 900 millilitres per minute circulates through the brain. Should the supply be interrupted for even a few seconds, irreparable damage to brain cells may result. Neurones are unable to survive if deprived of oxygen for more than four minutes. An anastamosis of several blood vessels at the base of the brain helps to provide alternative routes for blood if one of the major arteries is occluded. This anastamosis is known as the *circle of Willis.*

The main arteries which convey blood to the circle of Willis provide an anterior and a posterior supply. The anterior supply is from the two internal carotid arteries, which are branches of the common carotid arteries in the neck. The posterior supply is from the two vertebral arteries (branches of the subclavian arteries), which pass through the foramina of the cervical vertebrae. Both of these pairs of arteries thus arise from some of the first branches of the aortic arch.

The *internal carotid artery* passes through the base of the skull beside the sphenoid bone. It then bends forward in the cavernous venous sinus, turns upwards, pierces the dura and arachnoid to enter the subarachnoid space, turns back below the optic nerve and turns upward again at the side of the optic chiasm. This series of bends forms the *carotid siphon.* The internal carotid then joins the circle of Willis and branches into the anterior and middle cerebral arteries. Before dividing, the internal carotid gives off branches to pituitary gland and hypothalamus, the eyes and other frontal structures, the choroid plexus of the lateral ventricle and other areas of the brain, and forms the posterior communicating artery which joins up with the posterior cerebral artery.

The *vertebral arteries* pass through the foramen magnum and pierce the dura and arachnoid to enter the subarachnoid space. They pass slightly forward, beneath the medulla, and join together at the base of the pons to form the *basilar artery.* Branches of the vertebral arteries supply the upper cervical spinal cord and the cerebellum; very fine branches supply the medulla.

The *basilar artery* passes along the midline of the pons and divides into the two posterior cerebral arteries. It gives off branches to the cerebellum, labyrinth of the inner ear, pons and part of the midbrain.

At the base of the brain, the major arteries form the *circle of Willis* — the front of the circle is completed by the anterior cerebral arteries, which are connected together by the anterior communicating artery (Fig. 1.12). The remainder of the circle is formed by small segments of the internal carotids, the posterior communicating arteries and the posterior cerebral arteries.

The anterior cerebral arteries (one in each cerebral hemisphere)pass towards the midline over the optic nerves. They are joined together by the short anterior communicating artery. Each anterior cerebral artery then proceeds to supply the frontal and parietal lobes.

The middle cerebral arteries pass between the frontal and temporal lobes (one in each hemisphere) in the lateral fissure. They give off branches to the frontal, parietal, temporal and occipital lobes.

The posterior cerebral arteries curve around the midbrain (one on either side) and supply parts of the temporal lobe and the occipital lobe. Branches are given off to the choroid plexuses of the ventricles.

All the cerebral arteries pass across the surface of the cerebrum, forming a network of small vessels in the pia mater. Cortical branches supply the cerebral cortex and central branches supply the deeper parts of the hemispheres.

Venous drainage

Small veins drain from the brain stem and cerebellum into venous sinuses near the posterior cranial fossa. The cerebrum is drained by external cerebral veins — situated in the subarachnoid space — and internal cerebral veins beneath the corpus callosum, which drain the central parts of the cerebrum. Many of the small veins have no corresponding pattern with the cerebral arteries, unlike the situation in most other parts of the body, and empty directly into venous sinuses.

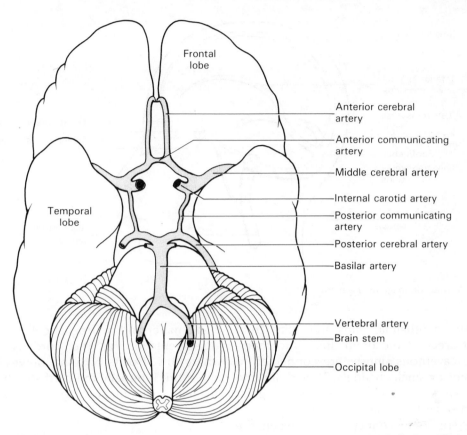

Frontal
lobe

Anterior cerebral
artery

Anterior communicating
artery

Middle cerebral artery

Internal carotid artery

Posterior communicating
artery

Posterior cerebral artery

Basilar artery

Temporal
lobe

Vertebral artery

Brain stem

Occipital lobe

Fig. 1.12 Blood supply to the brain, demonstrating the circle of Willis and main arteries at the base of the brain.

Some of the external and internal veins, which can more readily be identified, empty into one large vein — the *great cerebral vein* (or vein of *Galen*).

The *venous sinuses* — mentioned in the section on the dura mater — are large channels which collect the venous blood. The arachnoid villi also project into these sinuses and return cerebrospinal fluid to the venous circulation (Fig. 1.13).

Superior sagittal sinus — this is attached to the ethmoid bone at the front of the skull. It passes backwards toward the occipital region, along the border of the falx cerebri, and unites with other sinuses at the *confluence*.

Inferior sagittal sinus — this is smaller than the superior sagittal sinus and passes from front to back along the lower border of the falx cerebri, between the two cerebral hemi-

spheres. It joins the straight sinus where the falx cerebri and tentorium cerebelli are attached together.

Straight sinus — this receives blood from the inferior sagittal sinus and the great cerebral vein, and passes backward to the confluence.

Transverse sinuses — leaving either side of the confluence are the *right* and *left* transverse sinuses. These follow the border of the tentorium cerebelli which is attached to the occipital bones. At the petrous portion of the temporal bones the transverse sinuses turn downwards.

Sigmoid sinuses — these are continuous with the transverse sinuses, curving down to empty into the internal jugular veins.

Cavernous sinuses — the two cavernous sinuses lie one on either side of the sphenoid

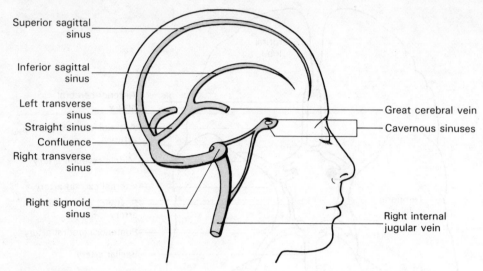

Fig. 1.13 Venous drainage of the brain.

bone. The ophthalmic veins and veins from adjacent areas of the brain drain into them. The two cavernous sinuses are connected to each other by small channels. They drain into the transverse sinuses and internal jugular veins, through two small channels.

There are some connections between the venous sinuses and veins outside the cranium. The connecting veins are known as *emissary veins*. Blood can flow in either direction through these, depending on the venous pressure within or outside the skull.

Spinal cord

The spinal cord (Fig. 1.14) is an oval-shaped cylinder, which lies within the spinal cavity of the vertebral column. It is approximately 45 centimetres in length, extending from the medulla oblongata to the level of the first or second lumbar vertebra. At the upper end, the cord passes through the foramen magnum in the base of the skull. Surrounding the spinal cord are the three meninges and cerebrospinal fluid, in the subarachnoid space. The epidural space is composed of adipose tissue, which contains a venous plexus.

The lower end of the spinal cord tapers slightly and is attached to the coccyx by a long filament — the *filum terminale*. This consists

of pia mater and neuroglial cells.

Segmentation of the cord is described where the 31 pairs of spinal nerves leave and enter, but internally the cord structure has no distinct segmentation to correspond with

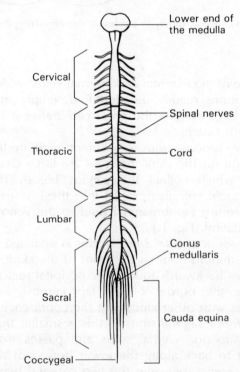

Fig. 1.14 Spinal cord.

these. The spinal nerves are named according to their distribution:

8 pairs of cervical nerves
12 pairs of thoracic nerves
5 pairs of lumbar nerves
5 pairs of sacral nerves
1 pair of coccygeal nerves.

The first 7 pairs of cervical nerves leave the spinal canal above the corresponding vertebrae, the 8th leaves between the 7th cervical vertebra and 1st thoracic vertebra. From there on, the spinal nerves pass through the foramina below the corresponding vertebrae, slightly above the intervertebral discs.

Because the spinal cord does not extend the full length of the vertebral column, the lumbar, sacral and coccygeal nerves pass downwards in the vertebral canal. These are progressively longer, the lower the nerves are, owing to the greater distances between the lower vertebrae. They form the *cauda equina* (horse's tail) in the subarachnoid space.

The spinal cord is enlarged in two regions: cervical and lumbar. The cervical enlargement, between C4–T1, contains the nerves supplying the upper limbs — most of them forming the brachial plexuses. The lumbar, or lumbosacral, region of enlargement extends between L2–S3, supplying the lower limbs.

Each spinal nerve is attached to the cord by two short roots — *anterior*, which contain motor fibres, and *posterior*, which contain sensory fibres. Although traditionally defined as motor and sensory roots, there is now speculation that the anterior roots may, in fact, carry some sensory pain fibres. The spinal nerve roots cross the subarachnoid space and pass through the arachnoid and dura mater. These two membranes become continuous with the epineurium of the spinal nerve. In the epidural space, between the intervertebral foramina, the posterior nerve roots have a ganglion (group of nerve cells). Immediately distal to the ganglion, the anterior and posterior nerve roots join together as the spinal nerve. Some of the spinal nerves also contain autonomic fibres.

In cross-section, the spinal cord has two deep grooves — the *anterior median fissure* (which is the deeper and wider of the two) and the *posterior median fissure* (Fig. 1.15).

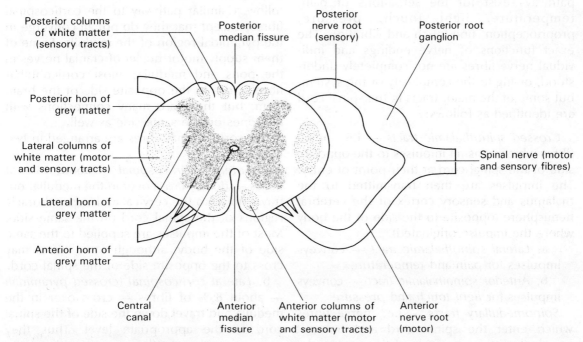

Posterior columns of white matter (sensory tracts)

Posterior median fissure

Posterior nerve root (sensory)

Posterior root ganglion

Posterior horn of grey matter

Lateral columns of white matter (motor and sensory tracts)

Lateral horn of grey matter

Anterior horn of grey matter

Spinal nerve (motor and sensory fibres)

Central canal

Anterior median fissure

Anterior columns of white matter (motor and sensory tracts)

Anterior nerve root (motor)

Fig. 1.15 Cross-section of the spinal cord.

The inner core is composed of grey matter and white matter. The grey matter is described as 'H-shaped' (appearing rather like a butterfly), with anterior, posterior and lateral horns. In the centre is the spinal canal, which contains cerebrospinal fluid. The neurones in the grey matter transmit sensory and motor impulses between various parts of the cord. White matter is arranged in columns (or tracts) along the length of the cord, and transmits impulses to and from the brain. The columns are arranged in the anterior, posterior and lateral areas of the spinal cord.

Although the arrangement of grey and white matter is generally the same throughout the length of the cord, there are some variations in different regions. There is more white matter higher up the cord; an increased amount of grey matter is found in the cervical and lumbosacral enlargements.

Sensory neurones

Stimuli of sensory nerve endings in the skin, muscles and tendons are transmitted to the posterior part of the spinal cord. Different pathways exist for the sensations of pain, temperature, light touch, pressure, proprioception, fine touch and vibration. The exact functions of nerve endings and individual nerve fibres are not completely understood, owing to the complexity of the system, but some of the major tracts in the spinal cord are identified as follows:

Crossed spinothalamic tracts — i.e., nerve fibres which transmit impulses to the opposite side of the spinal cord at their point of entry. The impulses are then transmitted to the thalamus and sensory cortex of the cerebral hemisphere (opposite to the side of the body where the impulse originated).

  a. *Lateral spinothalamic tract* — conveys impulses for *pain* and *temperature*.

  b. *Anterior spinothalamic tract* — conveys impulses for *light touch* and *pressure*.

Spinomedullary tracts — i.e., nerve fibres which enter the spinal cord and transmit impulses up the same side of the cord to the medulla. The impulses are transmitted in the *posterior columns* to the medulla, where they then cross over to the opposite side. Sensations of *proprioception, fine touch* and *vibration* are transmitted in this way to the sensory cortex.

Spinocerebellar tracts — these transmit impulses concerned with *unconscious detection of changes in position*. The impulses are thought to be conveyed to the cerebellum in the *lateral columns* on the same side of the body as their point of origin.

Motor neurones

Motor impulses to voluntary muscle originate in the motor cortex of the frontal lobe of the cerebral hemisphere. The impulses are transmitted to the cranial nerves or the spinal nerves, as appropriate. Major tracts are as follows:

Pyramidal tracts — these include the *corticospinal* fibres, which transmit impulses from the cerebrum to the medulla (pyramidal area of decussation — crossing over), and the *corticobulbar* fibres. The corticobulbar fibres follow a similar pathway to the corticospinal fibres, except that they do not all converge in the pyramidal region of the medulla. Some of them supply motor nuclei of cranial nerves in the pons and medulla; most corticobulbar fibres cross to the opposite side of the brain stem, but there are many connections with neurones on the same side as well.

The corticospinal fibres are arranged in two tracts:

  a. *Anterior corticospinal* — about 15% of fibres — do not cross over in the medulla, but travel down to the cervical and upper thoracic regions of the spinal cord on the same side. Most of the impulses are supplied to the same side of the body, although some fibres may cross to the opposite side of the spinal cord.

  b. *Lateral corticospinal (crossed pyramidal)* — about 85% of fibres — cross over in the medulla and travel down the side of the spinal cord to the appropriate level. Thus they convey impulses to the opposite side of the body from the hemisphere in which the impulses originated.

Extrapyramidal tracts — these are somewhat difficult to define in the light of present increased knowledge. Generally speaking, the extrapyramidal system consists of motor neurones within the central nervous system, exclusive of those in the pyramidal system. It includes neurones which have connections with areas such as the basal ganglia and cerebellum. Impulses are transmitted in various ways to cranial and spinal nerves. Some fibres are crossed, some direct, and fibres are conveyed in the lateral and anterior columns of the spinal cord.

Upper motor neurones is a term used to describe nerve cells and fibres within the brain and spinal cord, except those in the anterior horn cells (origin of the spinal or cranial motor nerves). Damage to these results in loss of voluntary muscle control, spasticity, exaggerated spinal reflexes, and possible weakness, paralysis or deformity. *Lower motor neurones* are the nerve cells and fibres of the anterior horn cells of the spinal cord and the peripheral motor nerves. Damage to these results in loss of muscle power, paralysis of the muscles supplied, flaccidity, muscle wasting, deformity, loss of spinal reflexes, and loss of sensation if the peripheral or spinal nerve is involved.

Spinal reflexes

Most of the input from stimuli is transmitted up the spinal cord in the *ascending sensory tracts*, as described previously. Motor responses are transmitted down the spinal cord in the *descending motor tracts*. However, a system exists whereby a more direct link between sensory and and motor neurones is established. These links, in the spinal cord, are the *spinal reflexes*, which basically serve as a protective mechanism. The 'reflex arc' may involve two or more neurones — sensory input to the posterior part of the spinal cord is relayed directly, through intermediate neurones of the grey matter, to the anterior part of the cord at the same level. Thus, a motor response is elicited without the information being relayed to and from the cortex.

Examples of these reflexes are the *stretch reflex*, such as the 'knee jerk', and the *flexor reflex*, such as withdrawal of the hand in response to a painful stimulus (Fig. 1.16). The latter type of reflex can be consciously overridden, e.g. picking up a hot plate containing food — it is desirable to hold the plate and the food, rather than drop it on the floor!

Blood supply to the spinal cord

The spinal cord is supplied along its length by three arteries — one *anterior spinal artery* and two *posterior spinal arteries*. The anterior spinal artery originates from the vertebral arteries, and runs down along the anterior median fissure of the spinal cord. It supplies the upper cervical sections of the cord, but, lower down, is supplemented by branches of the posterior intercostal arteries and radicular arteries. The radicular arteries are small branches of the spinal arteries which supply the vertebral column.

The posterior spinal arteries are branches of either the vertebral or cerebellar arteries, and form plexuses along the posterior part of the spinal cord, where the posterior nerve roots are situated. These are also supplemented by the branches described above. Because of its relatively poor blood supply, the spinal cord is very vulnerable to circulatory impairment.

Branches of the anterior spinal artery penetrate the spinal cord and supply the anterior grey horns, parts of the posterior grey horns and the anterior and lateral white columns. The posterior spinal arteries supply the remainder of the posterior grey horns and the posterior columns of white matter. A fine plexus of arteries also enters the pia mater on the anterior and lateral surfaces of the spinal cord.

The venous drainage of the spinal cord does not have a regular pattern, but there are essentially six main veins. The *anterior spinal veins* run along the anterior median fissure and the anterior nerve roots at either side of the cord. The *posterior spinal veins* run

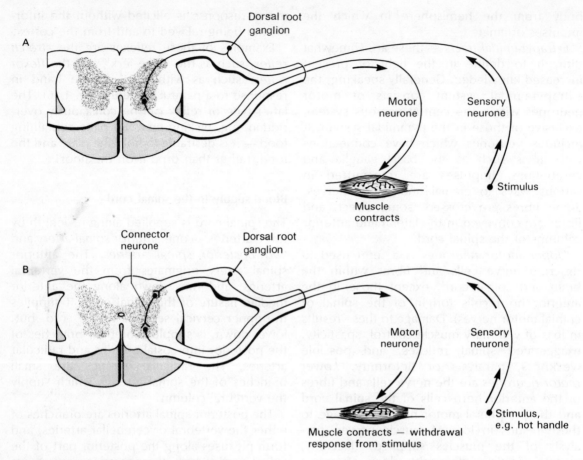

Fig. 1.16 (A) Stretch reflex (B) Flexor reflex.

along the posterior median fissure and one near the posterior nerve roots at either side of the cord. Drainage is into the anterior and posterior radicular veins, which empty into the epidural venous plexus. Venous blood then passes into an external vertebral plexus and into vertebral, intercostal and lumbar veins.

Spinal meninges

The three membranes which surround the brain — i.e., dura, arachnoid and pia mater — extend to cover the spinal cord in the vertebral canal. As previously noted, the spinal cord does not extend the full length of the vertebral column, but the dura and arachnoid continue to the lower lumbar region.

This is why access to cerebrospinal fluid is possible by lumbar puncture at about the level of the 3rd and 4th lumbar vertebrae.

Protection of the brain and spinal cord

The central nervous system is protected externally by the three meninges, cerebrospinal fluid, adipose tissue around the spinal cord, and the bony components of the skull and vertebral column. Internal protective mechanisms include the cerebrospinal fluid and cerebrovascular arrangement.

The cerebrospinal fluid thus acts externally and internally — externally, by helping to 'cushion' the brain and spinal cord, and internally, by helping to provide nourishment and remove waste products (as described in the previous section relating to the cerebrospinal fluid). The choroid plexuses also have an important role in the 'blood-brain barrier'.

As described in the section relating to the blood supply to the brain, the vascular anastomosis at the base of the brain (circle of Willis) ensures an adequate supply of blood.

Blood-brain barrier

This is an important protective component, which involves a selective transfer of substances passing between the cerebral arteries and nerve cells. It is a complex function, not fully understood, but appears to rely on the action of the capillaries of the choroid plexuses in the ventricles. Other capillaries in the brain probably act in a similar way. The capillaries are separated from underlying nerve tissue by a basement membrane; in the ventricles the ependymal tissue acts in the same way. Unlike capillaries elsewhere in the body, those in the brain have tight junctions between their endothelial cells. These two factors ensure that only selected substances can pass from the blood to the extracellular fluid and cerebrospinal fluid. Many potentially harmful substances are unable to cross.

The blood-brain barrier is not fully developed at birth, as demonstrated in icterus neonatorum. A severely jaundiced baby can develop encephalopathy because the harmful bile pigments can pass into the brain cells.

One drawback in medical treatment of patients, e.g., chemotherapy for cerebral tumours, is that many drugs are unable to pass through the blood-brain barrier.

PERIPHERAL NERVOUS SYSTEM

The peripheral nervous system consists of the spinal nerves and cranial nerves, plus components of the autonomic nervous system. The structure of peripheral nerves is described in the section on nervous system cells and nerve fibres. An account of the autonomic system is to be found later in the chapter. The peripheral nervous system serves to connect the central nervous system with other parts of the body. It does this by means of relaying sensory information from specialised receptor cells, e.g., in the skin and muscles, to the spinal cord and brain. Motor impulses are transmitted from the brain and spinal cord to muscles and various organs and glands.

Spinal nerves

Reference to the previous section on the spinal cord will give a description of the 31 pairs of spinal nerves. Each spinal nerve contains motor, sensory and autonomic fibres. Details of the distribution of spinal nerves are not included here, but they are of obvious clinical significance. For example, loss of function or sensation can be traced to peripheral or central origin, depending on the extent of the damage. Cutaneous sensation can be identified on a 'dermatomal map', which shows the distribution of sensation and relevent spinal nerve (although there is some overlap by adjacent nerves). In relation to clinical signs, it is also important to remember which nerve fibres cross over and where.

Cranial nerves

Some of the cranial nerves have been mentioned in the section relating to the brain stem, where many of them have their points of origin. A more detailed account is included in this part of the text. There are 12 pairs of cranial nerves, which pass through small openings in the skull from their site of origin (Table 1.2). Each pair of nerves is named according to its distribution or function, and is also numbered. Traditionally, Latin numerals have been used, but the trend is now towards the more familiar Arabic numbers — the latter are used in this text.

Some of the cranial nerves contain either sensory or motor neurones, and others contain both types (mixed nerves). A summary of the cranial nerves and their functions is included below:

The *olfactory nerve* contains sensory fibres and is concerned with the *sense of smell*. It

Table 1.2 Cranial nerves

No.	Name	Function
1	Olfactory	Sense of smell
2	Optic	Sense of vision
3	Oculomotor	Accommodation of the lens and constriction of the pupil; some eye movements
4	Trochlear	Eye movement, superior oblique muscle
5	Trigeminal	Sensory component: sensory nerve for head Motor component: mastication
6	Abducens	Eye movement, supplies the lateral rectus muscle
7	Facial	Sensory component: sense of taste Motor component: facial expressions
8	Vestibulo-cochlear	Vestibular branch: sense of balance Cochlear branch: sense of hearing
9	Glossopharyngeal	Sensory component: taste Motor component: swallowing
10	Vagus	Sensation and movement of the pharynx, larynx, thoracic and abdominal organs
11	Spinal accessory	Supplies muscles of the thoracic and abdominal organs, pharynx and larynx
12	Hypoglossal	Chewing, sucking and swallowing

originates from the sensory nerve endings in the olfactory mucosa (in the roof of the nose), and conveys impulses to the olfactory bulbs and temporal lobe. A more detailed description of the olfactory tract is included earlier in the text.

The *optic nerve* contains sensory fibres and is concerned with the *sense of vision*. It originates in the retina of the eye and conveys impulses to the midbrain, thalamus and occipital lobe.

The *oculomotor nerve* contains motor fibres and originates in the midbrain. It supplies the eye muscles (except for the superior oblique and lateral rectus muscles) and the ciliary

ganglia of the eye. The impulses to the ciliary ganglia are parasympathetic to the lens and iris. These result in accommodation of the lens and constriction of the pupil.

The *trochlear nerve* contains motor fibres and originates in the midbrain. It supplies the superior oblique muscles of the eye.

The *trigeminal nerve* is a mixed nerve which is the main sensory nerve for the head and the motor nerve for the muscles of mastication. It has three branches — ophthalmic, maxillary and mandibular.

a. Ophthalmic branch: originates as sensory nerve endings in the skin and mucosa of the front of the scalp, forehead, upper eyelid, conjunctiva and front of the nose. Impulses are transmitted to the trigeminal (or Gasserian) ganglion and the pons.

b. Maxillary branch: originates as sensory nerve endings in the skin and mucosa of the cheek and upper jaw and in the upper teeth and maxillary sinus. Impulses are relayed to the same areas as those from the ophthalmic branch.

c. Mandibular branch: originates in the skin and mucosa of the lower jaw and lower teeth (sensory fibres), from where impulses are transmitted in the same way as the other two branches. The motor fibres originate in the pons and supply the muscles concerned with mastication and a few other small muscles nearby.

The *abducens nerve* is a motor nerve which originates in the pons. It supplies the lateral rectus muscles of the eye. (It is worth noting that the *third, fourth* and *sixth* cranial nerves are all concerned with eye movements.)

The *facial nerve* is a mixed nerve. The motor fibres originate in the pons and supply the superficial muscles of the face and scalp — enabling various facial expressions to occur. Fibres also supply the submandibular and sublingual salivary glands and the lacrimal glands, carrying parasympathetic nerves.

The sensory fibres originate in the taste buds of the anterior two-thirds of the tongue, and are thus concerned with the *sense of taste*. These transmit impulses to the medulla and parietal lobe. A few sensory fibres also arise in the external ear, in the wall of the external auditory canal and external surface of the tympanic membrane.

The *vestibular cochlear nerve* contains sensory fibres and has two main branches — vestibular and cochlear.

a. vestibular branch: originates in the semicircular canals and vestibule of the inner ear. It transmits impulses to the medulla and pons, and is concerned with the sense of equilibrium (balance).

b. cochlear branch (or auditory branch): originates in the organ of Corti in the cochlea of the inner ear. It transmits impulses to the pons, medulla and temporal lobe, and is concerned with the sense of hearing.

The *glossopharyngeal nerve* is a mixed nerve. It contains sensory fibres from the pharynx and posterior third of the tongue (taste buds); other sensory fibres originate in the carotid sinus and carotid body and are concerned with reflex control of blood pressure and respiration. Sensory impulses are transmitted to the medulla.

The motor fibres originate in the medulla and supply the muscles of the pharynx to enable swallowing movements. Some motor fibres, which originate in the junction of the medulla and pons, are parasympathetic and supply the parotid salivary glands.

The *vagus nerve* is a mixed nerve with many functions. The motor fibres originate and the sensory fibres terminate in the medulla. It deals with sensation and movement of the pharynx, larynx, thoracic and abdominal organs. The vagus nerve also carries parasympathetic fibres to the heart, respiratory system and abdominal organs.

The *spinal accessory nerve* (sometimes referred to as the accessory nerve) is a motor nerve which originates in the medulla. It supplies motor fibres to the muscles of the thoracic and abdominal organs, pharynx and larynx. Movements of these areas and voice production are dependent on this supply. Some fibres originate in the anterior columns of the first five or six segments of the cervical cord and supply the trapezius and sternomastoid muscles of the shoulder and neck.

The *hypoglossal nerve* is a motor nerve which originates in the medulla. It supplies the tongue and has reflex actions connected with chewing, sucking and swallowing as well as enabling voluntary movement.

Although some of the cranial nerves are defined as having only a motor function, it is thought that they may have a sensory function in relation to proprioception.

AUTONOMIC NERVOUS SYSTEM

Autonomic nerves conduct impulses from the central nervous system to *cardiac muscle, smooth (involuntary) muscle* and *glandular tissue*. None of these tissues is under the control of the will and functions automatically. Essentially, the autonomic system contains motor nerves, but it can be influenced by sensory nerve input, acting on the reflex arc principle.

There are two divisions of the autonomic system — sympathetic and parasympathetic — which differ both anatomically and physiologically. Both types of autonomic neurones consist of preganglionic neurones, ganglia and postganglionic neurones. Preganglionic neurones transmit impulses from the central nervous system to the ganglia, which are groups of autonomic nerve cell bodies, and postganglionic neurones transmit impulses from the ganglia to the appropriate tissue.

Sympathetic nerves

The sympathetic ganglia lie at either side of the spinal column, connected to each other lengthways by short nerve fibres. This gives them a chain-like appearance, and they are often referred to as the *sympathetic chain of ganglia*. They are situated near the anterior aspect of the spinal column and extend from the level of the second cervical vertebra to the coccyx. The ganglia are connected to the spinal cord by short nerve fibres in the same pathway as the spinal nerves and motor nerve roots.

Sympathetic preganglionic neurones

These originate in the lateral horns of grey matter in the spinal cord — in the first three or four lumbar segments and the thoracic segments. They leave the cord with the anterior motor nerve roots and enter the spinal nerves. Soon after, a short branch — *white ramus* — leaves the spinal nerve to join one of the sympathetic ganglia. Some axons branch up or down the sympathetic chain to another level, and some of the preganglionic neurones leave the sympathetic chain to terminate in *collateral ganglia*.

Postganglionic neurones

These leave the sympathetic chain or collateral ganglia (there may be several from the same ganglion) and return to the spinal nerve as short nerve fibres — *grey rami* — or continue as separate sympathetic nerves. The neurones which supply blood vessels, sweat glands and the erector pili muscles (of the hairs) are carried initially with the spinal nerves. The separate autonomic nerves are more complex, forming *plexuses* — for example, the coeliac plexus, which supplies the abdominal organs, and the cardiac plexus, which supplies the heart. The coeliac plexus and sympathetic nerves to other abdominal structures are initially supplied by the *splanchnic nerves*, which are main branches of the thoracic sympathetic chain. Visceral effectors (i.e., tissues which are supplied by the sympathetic nerves) are widespread throughout the body; thus, sympathetic responses may affect many organs at the same time. (Figure 1.17 shows the sympathetic pathway in relation to the spinal cord.)

Parasympathetic nerves

Preganglionic neurones

The parasympathetic preganglionic neurones originate in the brain stem and in the sacral region of the spinal cord (in the lateral horns of grey matter). The neurones are carried in the *3rd, 7th, 9th, 10th* and *11th cranial nerves*

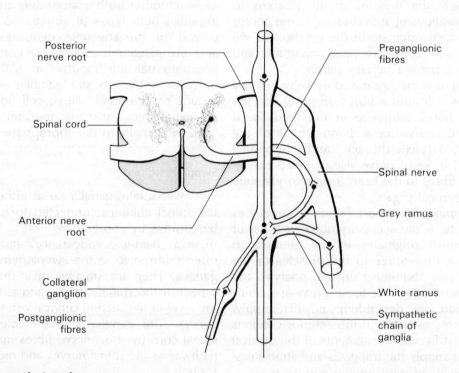

Posterior nerve root

Spinal cord

Anterior nerve root

Collateral ganglion

Postganglionic fibres

Preganglionic fibres

Spinal nerve

Grey ramus

White ramus

Sympathetic chain of ganglia

Fig. 1.17 Sympathetic pathway

and the *pelvic nerves*. They extend for some distance before forming synapses with the parasympathetic ganglia.

Postganglionic neurones

The parasympathetic postganglionic neurones have short axons which terminate in nearby structures. Stimulation is usually to one organ, unlike the more widespread effect of the sympathetic fibres.

All visceral effectors are supplied by sympathetic nerves, but only some have a parasympathetic supply. The sympathetic system increases its activity when the body is under stress. This is commonly known as the *'fight or flight'* mechanism, and enables the body to use maximum energy and physical resources. For example, the heart beats more strongly and faster, the bronchioles dilate, and blood sugar levels are increased.

The parasympathetic system is the main regulator of many organs and helps to restore homeostasis. Parasympathetic impulses can sometimes increase in stress — for example to the stomach (chronic stress may result in excess production of hydrochloric acid, leading to peptic ulceration).

As a whole, the function of the autonomic nervous system is to maintain or quickly restore homeostasis. The sympathetic and parasympathetic systems are antagonistic to each other, achieving a balance in those organs which are supplied by both types of neurones. Although the autonomic system was so called because it seemed to be an independent system, it is controlled by the central nervous system. The activity of the neurones is influenced by the cerebral cortex. In the opening paragraph of this section on the autonomic nervous system, it was stated that the system is responsible for the automatic functioning of various glands and tissues. It is now known, however, that responses can be influenced by voluntary action — this has been demonstrated in biofeedback techniques and the use of meditation (e.g., in helping to lower blood pressure).

CONCLUSION

The central, peripheral and autonomic nervous systems function as an integrated whole and are essential for the survival of the body. The human species also boasts highly developed mental functions, as well as physical ones, which are equally dependent on the nervous system. Many factors are of importance in the normal development of the nervous system. Similarly, many factors can cause a breakdown of this important communication and control system. An understanding of the normal structure, function and development of the nervous system forms an important basis for the nurse who is involved with people who have disorders related to this system.

It is not possible to explore all the known and speculative details of the nervous system in a chapter such as this. Should the reader wish to explore aspects of the nervous system in more detail, there are a number of textbooks written entirely on the subject. However, our knowledge of the nervous system is far from complete — the reader should also refer to current articles and research publications for up to date information. It is possible that some of the present beliefs about the nervous system may be changed in the future.

BIBLIOGRAPHY

Anthony C P, Thibodeau G A 1979 Textbook of anatomy and physiology, 10th edn. C V Mosby, St Louis
Barr M L 1979 The human nervous system, 3rd edn. Harper and Row, London
Hunt P, Sendell B 1983 The essentials of nursing — nursing the adult with a specific physiological disturbance. Macmillan, London

FURTHER READING

Campbell R, Heap M 1979 The divided self and the divided brain. New Scientist 82(1151):191
Cherfas J 1979 Singing in the brain. New Scientist 82(1156):649

2

Assessment of the nervous system

Neurological examination and assessment is a vital part of the management of a patient. It enables the medical practitioner to determine the most appropriate treatment for the individual. Similarly, the nurse has an important role in the assessment of each patient so that decisions about the relevant nursing care can be made.

A nursing assessment, or history, is performed when the patient is admitted to the unit. Initially it should provide information which will help the nurse to determine priorities of care. In many hospitals, a standardised questionnaire, or nursing history sheet, is used. An example is shown in Figure 2.1. Ideally, an experienced nurse should interview and assess the patient on admission, so that only pertinent questions are posed. Once rapport has been established and the patient is more settled into his new environment, further information can be obtained. Assessment should be viewed as an ongoing process. The patient is usually the primary source of information, but his next-of-kin, close family and friends, medical notes and other records are also valuable sources, particularly if the patient has problems with communication or is unconscious.

Neurological examination and assessment of the patient, in practice, form part of a total assessment. The patient must be seen as a whole person, because factors other than his particular illness play a part in his responses to that condition. Along with any specific tests or investigations, the initial assessment forms a basis for determining which specific problems or abnormalities exist. This leads to decisions about how best the individual can be helped.

When the doctor carries out his examination of the patient the nurse should be present if possible. Information can then be exchanged between the medical and nursing staff with maximum benefit to the patient. It is useful to remember that other members of the health care team — such as the social worker, physiotherapist and occupational therapist — assess each patient who is referred to them. Sharing information between all staff involved is useful.

This chapter aims to relate some specific details for both medical and nursing assessments. There is often some overlap, particulary when

recording basic details such as the patient's name, age, address and previous health history. Repetition of questions should be avoided. This will help the patient and his family to have confidence in the staff. If several people ask the same questions at different times, it may appear that there is a lack of co-ordination. Staff can consult with each other, as previously mentioned, and with written records which have already been completed (Fig. 2.1 A & B).

ASSESSING LEVEL OF CONSCIOUSNESS

A standardised method of measuring the patient's level of consciousness eliminates subjectivity and ambiguity. The Glasgow coma scale is widely used, and is the one described here. Other charts, or variations,

Date of admission ....

Full name ....

Preferred name/Form of address ....

Address ....

....

Telephone no. ....

Age .... Date of birth ....

Sex .... Marital status ....

Occupation ....

Religion .... Practising/Non-practising

Next of kin: Name ....

Relationship ....

Address ....

Telephone no. ....

Significant others:

Care/support at home:

Relevant social history:

Past medical history/surgery:

Allergies (if known):

Hospital no. ....

Brief history of present illness:

Patient's understanding of reason for admission:

Other current health problems:

Diagnosis:

Consultant: ....

Fig. 2.1A Nursing history — patient assessment.

Activities	Usual routines	Problems (Actual & Potential)
Maintaining a safe environment		
Communicating		
Breathing		
Eating and drinking		
Eliminating		
Personal cleansing and dressing		
Controlling body temperature		
Mobilising		
Working and playing		
Expressing sexuality		
Sleeping		
Worshipping		
Dying		
Promotion of health		

Fig. 2.1B Nursing history — assessment of activities of daily living (based on Roper et al, 1985).

exist — the importance is that the nurse is familiar with the chart in use and understands its interpretation.

The Glasgow coma scale is based on the assessment of eye opening, verbal response and motor response (Fig. 2.2). Changes in the patient's condition can be easily and quickly identified.

Eye opening
— Spontaneously (normal opening and closing of eyes)
— to speech (if the patient's eyes are closed, ask him to open them or call his name)
— to pain (apply painful stimulus, such as pressure on the nail bed)

— none (no response to any of the above, or lids are retracted due to flaccid eye muscles).

Peri-orbital swelling may prevent the patient from opening one or both eyes, and is recorded as C (=closed).

Verbal reponse
— Orientated (question the patient as to time, place and person; allowances are made for minor inconsistencies)
— confused conversation (able to converse but gives completely wrong answers)
— inappropriate words (minimal verbal response such as obscenities, or inter-changes 'yes'/'no')

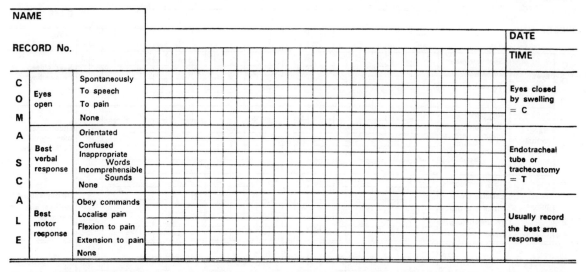

NAME				DATE	
RECORD No.				TIME	
C **O** **M**	Eyes open	Spontaneously			Eyes closed by swelling = C
		To speech			
		To pain			
		None			
A **S** **C**	Best verbal response	Orientated			Endotracheal tube or tracheostomy = T
		Confused			
		Inappropriate Words			
		Incomprehensible Sounds			
		None			
A **L** **E**	Best motor response	Obey commands			Usually record the best arm response
		Localise pain			
		Flexion to pain			
		Extension to pain			
		None			

Fig. 2.2 Glasgow coma scale. (Reproduced by kind permission of Nursing Times where this diagram first appeared on June 12, 1975, p. 917.)

— incomprehensible sounds (moans or grunts in response to verbal or painful stimulus)
— no verbal response (mute).

Certain factors may influence the patient's response, such as hearing difficulties, inability to understand the language, the presence of an endotracheal or tracheostomy tube (recorded on the chart as T), or speech difficulties.

Motor response
— Obeys commands (responds to being asked to lift his hand or perform other simple voluntary movements)
— localisation of pain (e.g., moves his hand to remove a source of irritation such as when pressure is applied to the supra-orbital ridge)
— flexion to pain (e.g., painful stimulus such as pressure applied to the nail-bed causes bending of the elbow and withdrawal of the hand, as a normal response to pain)
— extension to pain (painful stimulus to the the nail-bed results in extension of the elbow, an abnormal response to pain)
— no response (minimal or no observable response; leg movements may occur due to spinal reflexes).

The best arm response is recorded, if the right and left sides differ. Sometimes a 'decerebrate response' may be exhibited if there is damage to the upper brain stem or tentorial herniation. The patient lies completely still and has rigid muscles.

Other parameters are measured to provide further information on neurological status. These include:

Vital signs — respiration, pulse, blood pressure and temperature are recorded (Fig. 2.3). These are helpful in determining an increasing intracranial pressure or in indicating a disturbance of other body systems. For example:

— rising blood pressure (with a widening between systolic and diastolic pressures) and slowing pulse rate indicate a raised intracranial pressure
— falling blood pressure and rapid, weak pulse rate indicate haemorrhage and shock (signs of raised intracranial pressure usually override signs of shock)
— depressed respirations may indicate a raised intracranial pressure
— dyspnoea may indicate chest injuries
— pyrexia may indicate an infection

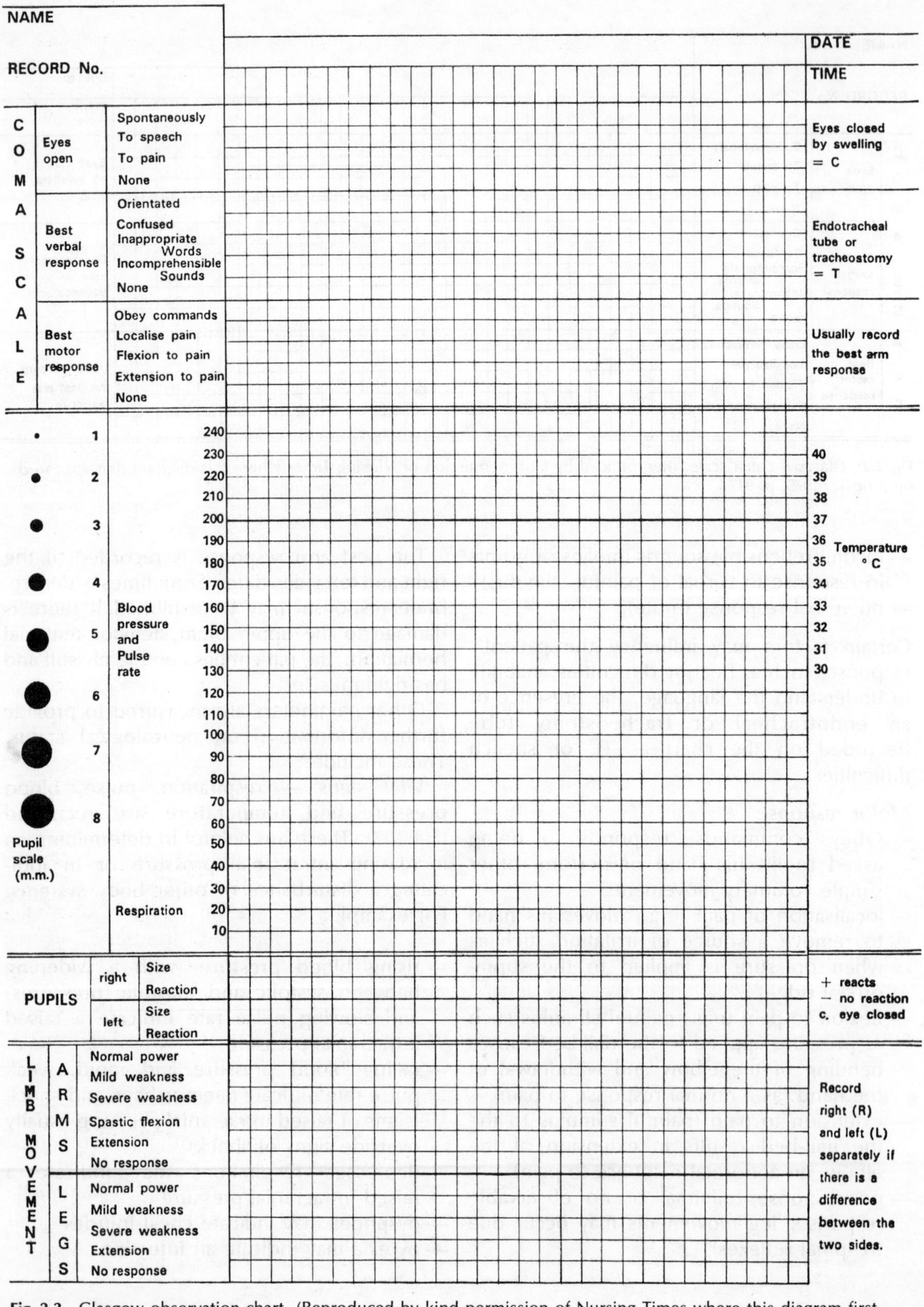

NAME				DATE
RECORD No.				TIME

COMA SCALE	Eyes open	Spontaneously		Eyes closed by swelling = C
		To speech		
		To pain		
		None		
	Best verbal response	Orientated		Endotracheal tube or tracheostomy = T
		Confused		
		Inappropriate Words		
		Incomprehensible Sounds		
		None		
	Best motor response	Obey commands		Usually record the best arm response
		Localise pain		
		Flexion to pain		
		Extension to pain		
		None		

Pupil scale (m.m.)
- 1
- 2
- 3
- 4
- 5
- 6
- 7
- 8

Blood pressure and Pulse rate

| 240 |
230	40
220	39
210	38
200	37
190	36	Temperature °C
180	35
170	34
160	33
150	32
140	31
130	30
120
110
100
90
80
70
60
50
40
30
Respiration	20
10

PUPILS	right	Size		+ reacts
		Reaction		− no reaction
	left	Size		c. eye closed
		Reaction		

LIMB MOVEMENT	ARMS	Normal power		Record right (R) and left (L) separately if there is a difference between the two sides.
		Mild weakness		
		Severe weakness		
		Spastic flexion		
		Extension		
		No response		
	LEGS	Normal power		
		Mild weakness		
		Severe weakness		
		Extension		
		No response		

Fig. 2.3 Glasgow observation chart. (Reproduced by kind permission of Nursing Times where this diagram first appeared on June 19, 1975, p. 972.)

— hyperpyrexia may indicate subarachnoid haemorrhage or damage to the hypothalamus

— subnormal temperature is evident in shock.

Any gross changes or changing pattern in vital signs should be reported.

Pupils

— The size of both pupils is compared; a millimetre scale is incorporated on a neuro-logical observation chart to help the nurse to estimate the pupillary size

— pupil reaction is observed, using a small–beamed bright light (e.g., a pencil torch), and is recorded on the chart as a positive (+) reaction or as no reaction, including fixed dilatation (−).

It is sometimes difficult to determine whether a pupil reacts briskly or slowly, and this infor-mation is not required on the chart. If the eyes are closed (e.g., peri-orbital oedema) this is recorded as C.

Limb movements — the arms and legs are examined for movement, and the right and left sides compared. If there is a discrepancy in the two sides, this can be recorded separ-ately — noting R (right) and L (left). The obser-vations are for

— normal power

— mild weakness

— severe weakness

— spastic flexion

— extension

— no response.

Response may be elicited by verbal commands (e.g., asking the patient to grip the nurse's hand or lift his arms) or by painful stimulus.

A paediatric version of the Glasgow coma scale has now been devised by neuro-surgeons in Adelaide, Australia.

It takes account of the child's age and appropriate neurological development and is suitable for use in the under 5 years' age group.

An overall picture of the patient's level of consciousness and physiological state can be seen by recording the observations as described above, and changes in his condition can be demonstrated. The nurse should also use general powers of observation as part of the assessment of the patient — looking at, listening to and touching the patient are important. One nurse observing the patient over a period is more likely to pick up changes in his condition.

The frequency of the observations and recordings will vary, according to the patient's condition, and is usually determined by the medical and/or experienced nursing staff.

MEDICAL EXAMINATION

When the doctor interviews the patient (and relatives or accompanying persons), and carries out the examination, it is useful for the nurse to be present. The nurse will then have a greater understanding of the patient's condition, which will help her make her own assessment and plan of care. The nurse can also assist the doctor and the patient during the examination procedure.

First, the environment in which the inter-view and examination are to take place should be considered. All patients and relatives have some degree of anxiety on admission to hospital — particularly so if they know or suspect that there is some disorder of the brain. The possibility of surgery to the brain can be extremely worrying. Therefore, the patient should be made to feel welcome and as relaxed as possible. Any accompanying persons should be treated likewise, and if they are not required to be present during the examination, the nurse should ensure that they have somewhere comfortable to wait if necessary. Refreshments such as a cup of tea or coffee should be offered.

The nurse should also ensure that any equipment the doctor requires for the exam-ination is at hand and ready for use. This usually includes the following items:

— sphygmomanometer and stethoscope

— ophthalmoscope

— a small, bright-beamed flashlight (e.g., pentorch)

— tendon hammer

— *sterile* needles and safety pins

— tuning forks

— auriscope
— tongue depressor
— small bottles containing various aromatic substances (e.g., oil of cloves, lavender water, asofoetida)
— small bottles containing salt and sugar solutions, quinine, and vinegar or lemon juice
— vials of hot and cold water (prepared as needed during the examination)
— orange sticks or cotton buds
— cotton wool
— tape measure
— paper and pen or pencil
— Snellen's eye chart and other visual testing charts if required
— syringes of various sizes
— common objects such as paper clips, coins and a key
— dividers
— blood specimen containers and laboratory request forms (if required)
— charts, as required, e.g., dermatome chart.

In some units, these items may be available for use on a tray or trolley, which can be checked and restocked after each use and prior to the next examination. After the equipment has been organised, and the patient's medical notes and any previous X-rays and other investigation results are made available, the doctor will take a history. This is very important in helping to identify the patient's diagnosis. Details such as the patient's name, age, address, occupation and previous medical history are checked, and noted. Any family history which may be of significance in familial or genetically related disorders is also elicited. The previous medical history may have some bearing on the patient's present problems — disturbed function in other organs or systems of the body may affect, or be affected by, the nervous system.

Personal details of the patient help to give a guide to level of intelligence; environmental factors which may have contributed to the illness can also be ascertained; the effect of the illness or any disability on the patient's future life can also be assessed.

A report of the present problems — e.g.,

nature, length of time these have been occurring, restrictions imposed by them — is sought. Any allergies or adverse reactions should be noted. If the patient is currently taking any medications — whether prescribed or self-administered — this should be recorded. When questions are asked and answers or information are given, it is important to make sure the words and terms used are understood.

It is helpful to clarify what the patient's own perception of his illness is, and what his expectations in seeking advice and treatment are. Close relatives or friends can be particularly useful in relating changes in the patient's behaviour and personality (especially if these are minor or have taken place gradually). They can help to give details which the patient himself may not be able to recall. An interpreter should be present if there are problems in interpreting communication due to a difference in native languages.

Specific, clear questions should be asked in order to elicit as much information as possible. The interview and examination should not be rushed so that the patient feels at ease and is able to recall relevant facts in what may well be a stressful situation. If the patient is a baby, young child, very frail or ill, or is elderly, some modifications will have to be made in the interview and examination procedure, as appropriate to the situation. The questions asked, and information given, can be related as the examination progresses. The areas of relevance to the examination, and some of the disorders which may arise, are detailed below.

Mental state

An assessment is made of any deterioration in, or loss of, memory, alteration in mood (depressed or euphoric), drowsiness, episodes of loss of consciousness, hallucinations, confusion or changes in intellectual function.

Assessment of mental function

General behaviour. Appearance, posture, dress and manner should be noted. Responses, body language and capacity for co-operation are also assessed. Allowances for ethnic/racial variations must be taken into account. Inability to co-operate may be due to temporary emotional instability, psychosis or impairment of special senses. Inappropriate crying or laughing is common in pseudobulbar palsy. Behavioural changes may be obvious in patients with head injuries or brain damage due to other causes. A note is made if the behavioural changes have occurred suddenly or progressively.

Memory. The patient is questioned on recent and past events (allowing for expected capacities in relation to age). A note is made on whether or not information is presented in a logical way. Simple exercises may be used, such as the following:

— asking what events have happened to the patient today
— asking what the patient was doing on the same day of the previous week
— giving the patient a name and address to remember and testing his recall of this about 5 minutes later
— asking the patient to repeat a series of seven numbers which have been stated.

Intellectual capacities. Orientation to time, person and place is assessed. The patient is questioned about common facts such as his name, age, address, day, date, year and name of the present monarch or Prime Minister. Mental arithmetic problems, such as the 'serial seven' test, can be posed. The patient is asked to subtract 7 from 100, and to continue subtracting 7 from the answer each time. (Most people can perform this task in less than 1 minute.) Simple addition and multiplication problems can also be given. Abstract reasoning can be assessed by asking the patient to explain the meaning of a well-known proverb, such as 'a stitch in time saves nine'.

In dementia, there is a loss of intellectual capacity and an inability to learn new information. The patient is asked to repeat a complicated sentence, such as 'The one thing a nation needs to be rich and great is a large,

secure supply of wood' (this is known as the Babcock sentence).

Powers of concentration and attention can be evaluated throughout the procedure. At this stage, quite a lot of information has been gained, some of which may require further exploration if there appear to be problems.

Speech and language problems

Language capacity is a process of reception, interpretation and response (verbal, written and body language). Any disorders of speech are assessed, including the following:

Aphasia. Literally means without speech, but is not necessarily the inability to speak due to interference with the muscles involved in voice production. The type of aphasia depends upon the area of the brain which is disrupted. Often, more than one type of language deficiency is seen in the same patient.

Dysphasia. This is a term more commonly used to describe a language disorder, which may be categorised as *motor* or *sensory*.

a. *Motor (expressive) dysphasia* is a difficulty in finding the correct word — i.e. when the patient is asked to name common objects, such as a pen or a watch, he may not be able to say the word 'pen'. A description of the object may be offered, such as 'something you write with', or he may demonstrate how to use the pen. The patient usually recognises the correct name of the object if it is offered to him.

b. *Sensory (receptive) dysphasia*, or 'word deafness', is an impairment in understanding the spoken word. It may be tested by asking the patient to carry out simple instructions, such as putting one hand on his head. As motor speech is directed by sensory information, expression is also disordered. The patient uses the wrong words, or puts them in the wrong order (jargon speech) and is unaware of his mistakes.

Sensory dysphasia is often associated with *dyslexia* — difficulty in understanding the written word — 'word blindness'. This can be tested by asking the patient to read some printed instructions and to explain what they mean.

Dysphonia. This is a reduction in the volume of speech, where the voice is very quiet or hoarse. It occurs when there is a disorder of the respiratory or laryngeal muscles, e.g., in Parkinson's disease.

Dysarthria. This is a difficulty in the pronunciation of words, owing to weakness or inco-ordination of the muscles involved in articulation (tongue, lips and cheeks), which is common in cerebellar disorders.

Preseveration. This is repetition of words or phrases and may occur along with other language disorders.

Dysgraphia. A disturbance in writing ability (in the absence of obvious physical handicap). This can be tested by asking the patient to write his name and to copy words in order to assess his ability (ensuring that he has previously learned writing skills). 'Mirror writing' is a phenomenon sometimes seen in stroke patients — perfectly spelled words are written, but the script is completely reversed.

Speech is a very complex function, involving different areas of the brain both anatomically and physiologically. The hearing and seeing of words are sensory impressions, while speaking and writing are dependent upon co-ordinated movements. Auditory memories and associations also influence speech. Similarly, patterns of speech movements are retained in the memory. Speech can be considered in two broad categories — *referential* (intellectual) and *emotive*.

Referential speech is associated with thinking and understanding, whereas emotive speech is an automatic expression of feelings (such as swearing). The latter may be encountered in patients who are unable to verbalise except when uttering an oath — emotive speech is the least severely affected in dysphasia.

In most right-handed persons, the main areas involved in speech are in the left cerebral hemisphere. Damage to these areas often results in some speech disorder. Owing to the importance placed on language development in humans, the hemisphere responsible for speech functions is referred to as the 'dominant hemisphere'.

The more language and its disorders are studied, the more complex they appear to be. The way in which speech disorders are classified is, perhaps, too simplistic, but provides a starting point to help to identify the patient's problems in communication and understanding.

Agnosia

This is an uncommon disorder in which the patient is unable to recognise objects or sounds, i.e., visual and auditory agnosia. It is tested by asking the patient to identify common objects shown to him, such as a key or paper clip. A differentiation between motor/sensory dysphasia and true agnosia should be made.

Astereogenesis

This is an inability to appreciate the size or shape of familiar objects by the sense of touch. The patient is asked to close his eyes and objects are placed in his hand. For size appreciation, two objects of the same shape but a different size — e.g., a complete and a broken matchstick — are placed in his hand consecutively. He is asked if the first or second is larger. For shape appreciation, familiar objects such as a pencil, key and coin are placed in his hand, and he is asked to identify them. The test is carried out in both of the patient's hands.

Apraxia

This may be present in the absence of paralysis, ataxia or sensory loss. The patient is unable to carry out normal movements such as combing his hair or putting on a cardigan.

Spatial orientation and distorted body image

If the patient has problems in visualising the relationship of different parts of an object, he will have difficulty when asked to draw or copy simple pictures, e.g., a house, clock face or geometrical figures. He may be confused about the left and right sides of his body, with failure to appreciate where his limbs are. This results in problems with self-care and safety.

Physical examination

The physical examination of the body should be carried out in an orderly manner so that relevant problems can be identified. A detailed examination of cranial nerve function and motor and sensory integrity is carried out when appropriate.

Examination of the head

The size and shape of the head are noted, along with an assessment of cranial symmetry; head circumference can be measured using a tape measure. Palpation of the suture lines, fontanelles (in infants) and the cranium (for any bony abnormalities) is carried out. In infants, the normal head circumference at birth is 35 centimetres. Any increase above 2.5 centimetres per month is abnormal. The anterior fontanelle should be closed by 18 months of age, the posterior fontanelle closes within a few months of birth. Any abnormally large or bulging fontanelles indicate an increased intracranial pressure (in infants).

Percussion of the skull is carried out, using the index and middle fingers. Auscultation is performed, using a stethoscope, to detect any bruits, which occur in arteriovenous malformations and vascular meningioma.

Meningeal irritation

An assessment of neck rigidity, Brudzinski's sign, and Kernig's sign is undertaken. Brudzinski's sign can be positive in two ways — the neck sign: when the patient is supine and his neck is flexed, he will flex his knees to reduce pain; the contralateral reflex: when the patient is supine and one leg is flexed, passively, a similar movement occurs in the other leg. Kernig's sign is positive when the patient

is in a supine position, his hip is flexed and he is unable to extend his knee without pain.

The neck

Apart from neck (nuchal) rigidity associated with meningeal irritation, there may be restricted movement in degenerative conditions of the cervical spine and in Parkinson's disease. Torticollis — repeated tonic or clonic movements of the neck to one side — is visually apparent. Auscultation for carotid bruits, using a stethoscope, may also be carried out.

The spine

The shape (curvature) of the spine is noted, looking for any deformities such as lordosis, kyphosis or scoliosis. Movement of the spine is checked — forward, backward and lateral motion, and any restrictions noted. If a ruptured lumbar disc is suspected, straight leg-raising is tested with the patient lying supine. The patient, in this case, would have a limited capacity for raising the extended leg on the side of the prolapse — Lasègue's sign. There may also be root pain on the side of the prolapse when the opposite leg is raised. Any tenderness of the spine can be detected by palpation.

Balance, co-ordination and gait

The patient's ability to maintain posture on sitting and standing is assessed. *Ataxia* (unsteadiness) due to cerebellar lesions is manifested by poor balance, inability to walk heel-to-toe in a straight line and a wide-based, reeling gait. The arms are extended, circular motions of the arms occur when walking and the patient has difficulty in turning when changing direction. If there is loss of *proprioception* (joint-position sense), due to damaged spinal or peripheral nerves, a positive Romberg's sign is elicited: when the patient is standing, with his eyes closed and his feet together, he will sway and fall (if not steadied); if his eyes are open, he can maintain balance by looking at a stable object. These patients have a wide-based, unsteady gait, look at their feet when walking, and stamp their feet down when walking. They have difficulty in walking and balancing in the dark.

In lower motor neurone diseases — foot drop — a stepping gait is seen. The knees are flexed and the feet lifted high off the ground and slapped down again, when walking — the patient appears to be walking 'up stairs'.

Upper motor neurone diseases — e.g., following a stroke — result in a stiff, outward swinging of the affected leg, with dragging of the toes.

In Parkinson's disease, the patient has a typical stooped appearance, with elbows flexed and arms held closely to his side. The arms do not swing, as normal, when walking, and steps are small and shuffling. There is a tendency to increase in speed and the patient has difficulty in stopping. Also, he will have difficulty in turning around and a tendency to fall.

Co-ordination of the arms and legs can be tested by asking the patient to carry out simple tasks, for example, to touch the tip of his nose and the tip of the doctor's finger alternately, with his index finger (Fig. 2.4); to close his eyes and touch the tip of his nose; to put his right heel on his left knee and run it along his shin.Wavering of the hand or foot occurs in cerebellar impairment. Loss of proprioception is demonstrated by wavering of the hand or foot only when the patient's eyes are closed.

The skin

Some neurological diseases are characterised by certain skin lesions. These include:

— cafe-au-lait spots and subcutaneous nodules in neurofibromatosis (Recklinghausen's disease)
— angiomas and naevi associated with neurological abnormalities
— rashes, allergies, herpes simplex and herpes zoster, which may be of significance
— melanoma (skin cancer) which can metastasize to the nervous system
— burns, scars or ulcers which may indicate sensory loss
— abnormal pigmentation or tufts of hair along the spinal region, associated with spina bifida occulta
— skin pallor (or a lemon tinge), in vitamin B_{12} deficiency (pernicious anaemia), which can result in neuropathy
— dry skin (inability to perspire) may result from disorders of the autonomic nervous system
— changes in normal skin colour (pallor, erythema or cyanosis) may arise in peripheral vascular disorders.

Other systems

A complete examination of other systems — e.g., cardiovascular, pulmonary, reproductive, endocrine — is undertaken, as primary conditions elsewhere can affect the

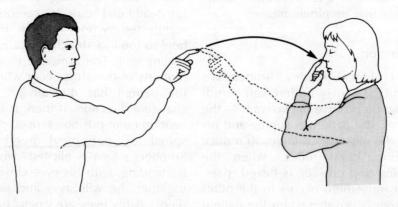

Fig. 2.4 Finger-nose test.

nervous system. Malignancies and infections can also spread to the central nervous system.

The cranial nerves

An assessment of the functions of the 12 pairs of cranial nerves is carried out, where appropriate (see Table 1.2):

1. **Olfactory nerve** — patency of the nasal passages should first be ensured. A selection of common aromatic substances is offered, in turn, to assess if the patient can detect and distinguish odours. He is asked to keep his eyes closed during the testing, and each nostril is tested separately.

2. **Optic nerve** — a. Visual acuity: distance vision is tested in each eye, using Snellen's chart (which should be 6 metres away from the patient); near sight is tested by asking the patient to read printed paragraphs from a newspaper or magazine held in his hand. Printed paragraphs of different sized print, e.g., the Jaeger chart, can be used. If the patient normally wears spectacles or contact lenses, he is requested to perform these tests with and without these. Patients with severely reduced vision are asked to count fingers held up by the doctor, to observe movements or to detect light. If there is no visual perception, i.e., the patient is blind, this is recorded as such. Also, it must be borne 'in mind that some people are unable to read.

b. Visual fields: each eye is tested separately, with the other eye being covered. The doctor sits in front of the patient and moves one of his fingers from the periphery of each visual quadrant towards the centre of the

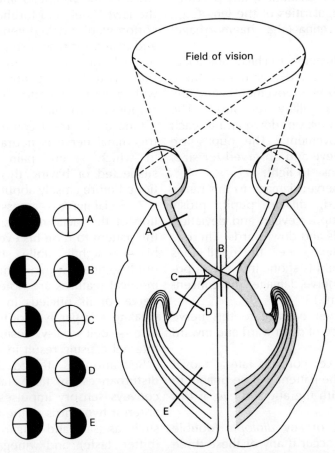

Fig. 2.5 Visual field defects. Shaded area in circles indicates loss of vision according to site of lesion.

patient's gaze (the patient should be looking at a fixed point, such as the doctor's nose). The temporal (outer), nasal (inner), upper and lower quadrants are checked in turn, by asking the patient to indicate when he first sees the moving finger. Visual loss in any of the quadrants is termed *hemianopia*; a complete or partial loss of vision in the nasal quadrant of one eye and the temporal quadrant of the opposite eye is termed *homonymous hemianopia* (see Fig. 2.5).

c. Fundi: the interior of each eye is examined, using an ophthalmoscope. Papilloedema (swelling of the optic disc) may indicate raised intracranial pressure; pallor or atrophy of the retina may be an early sign of multiple sclerosis. If the pupils are small, and it is difficult to view the retina, dilating drops should only be used under expert supervision.

When the eyes are examined, any previous eye surgery or irregularities of the lens (e.g., opacity), pupil or retina (e.g., haemorrhage) are noted.

3, 4, and 6. **Oculomotor, trochlear and abducens** nerves can be tested together — these are concerned with eye movements (and the oculomotor with pupillary response). The patient is asked to look up, down and to each side to check movements. The pupils are compared in each eye and observed for size, equality and response to light.

a. Oculomotor nerve: damage to this nerve results in a fixed, dilated pupil, ptosis (drooping) of the upper eyelid and deviation of the eye outwards and downwards. There is no consensual reflex — i.e., the pupil does not react when a light is shone into the opposite eye. (In optic nerve damage, the consensual reflex is present.)

b. Trochlear nerve: damage to this nerve results in an absence of downward and inward eye movement.

c. Abducens nerve: controls lateral movement of the eye. The patient will be unable to look to the side with the affected eye, if this nerve is damaged.

A note is made of any *diplopia* (double vision), which can occur if any of these three cranial nerves are damaged. (Diplopia also occurs if there is damage to the pons or midbrain.) Any unusual ocular movements are observed, such as *nystagmus* (flickering movements of the eye) — these may be horizontal, vertical or rotary movements. The patient is asked if he is aware of these himself.

5. **Trigeminal nerve** — motor function is tested by asking the patient to clench his teeth together, then to open his jaw and withstand pressure from the doctor's hand to close it. Any distortion in movement or asymmetry is noted. The maxillary reflex is tested by tapping the centre of the chin with a tendon hammer, while the patient's mouth is open — the normal response is rapid closure of the mouth.

Sensory function is tested in each of the three branches of the trigeminal nerve — ophthalmic, mandibular and maxillary. Both sides of the forehead and face are checked: the jaw, cheek and forehead are stroked with cotton wool, pricked gently with a sterile pin, and tested for response to hot and cold water (in vials held against the skin). The corneal reflex is tested by gently touching the cornea with a wisp of cotton wool — the normal response is to blink.

One of the most common disorders of the trigeminal nerve is neuralgia (tic douloureux), in which severe pain occurs. A patient suspected of having this condition is questioned more closely about relevent symptoms.

7. **Facial nerve** — assessment of motor function of the facial muscles is made by asking the patient to raise his eyebrows, frown, close his eyes tightly, smile, show his teeth, blow out his cheeks with air and whistle. Any asymmetrical features are noted. Disorders of the nerve, or its nucleus in the pons, result in weakness or paralysis of the whole side of the face — Bell's palsy. Lesions of the cortex or internal capsule result in a lower facial palsy.

Sensation is tested by observing any disturbances in taste (as the facial nerve conveys sensory impulses for taste from the anterior two-thirds of the tongue). Substances such as salt and sugar solutions, quinine (bitter taste) and vinegar (acid taste) are placed onto the patient's tongue. Each side of the tongue is tested separately, and a small amount of water should be drunk between each substance to remove the previous taste. If taste is diminished or absent, there may be a disorder of the sensory part of the facial nerve, or of its nucleus in the medulla.

The patient can also be questioned about salivation and lacrimation, as the facial nerve supplies the submaxillary and submandibular salivary glands and the lacrimal glands.

8. **Acoustic nerve** — a. Auditory portion: this is tested by assessing the patient's hearing ability. A distinction between conductive deafness (disease of the middle ear) and sensori-neural deafness (disorder of the inner ear or auditory nerve) must be made. An auriscope is used to examine the external ear canal and tympanic membrane, to exclude problems such as wax in the ear or otitis media, which can cause deafness.

Bone and air conduction of sound are tested by using a vibrating tuning fork — Rinne's test. The foot of the tuning fork is placed on the mastoid process, until the patient indicates that he can no longer hear the ringing sound. The open end of the tuning fork is then held, vibrating, near the ear canal and, normally, the ringing sound can still be heard.

Lateral hearing discrimination can be evaluated by using Weber's test (Fig. 2.6) — the foot of the vibrating tuning fork is placed either in the centre of the patient's forehead or in the centre of the top of the head. Normally, the ringing sound can be heard equally in both ears, or is perceived in the midline. More detailed hearing tests can be undertaken using audiometry.

b. Vestibular portion: this is assessed by caloric testing, if the patient has a history of dizziness, imbalance or tinnitus. Each ear is irrigated in turn with warm water, followed by cold water, which normally produces nystagmus, and sometimes a feeling of nausea. Damage to the brain stem results in a lack of these responses. (The caloric test is performed using ice-cold water in comatosed patients — there is no resulting nystagmus if the brain stem is damaged.)

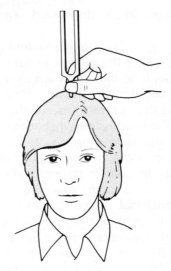

Fig. 2.6 Weber's test.

9. **Glossopharyngeal nerve** — sensation of the posterior part of the tongue and pharynx is tested by touching the sides of the pharynx with an orange-stick or tongue-depressor. The 'gag reflex' is normally present, which is manifested by a choking sensation and spluttering.

10. **Vagus nerve** — motor function of the pharynx, larynx and soft palate is tested. If the nerve is intact, normal swallowing and speech are present. Damage to the nerve or its nucleus in the medulla results in dysphagia, hoarseness, a tendency to regurgitate fluids through the nose when drinking, and asymmetrical movement of the palate when the patient says 'ah'. The autonomic functions of the vagus nerve are usually assessed separately.

11. **Accessory nerve** — the patient is observed for movement of the head, neck and shoulders. Any wasting of the trapezius or sternomastoid muscles is noted. The head falls forward if there is severe weakness of the trapezius muscle, and falls backward if there is severe weakness of the sternomastoid muscle. To test the strength of the trapezius muscle, the patient is asked to shrug his shoulders against resistance from the doctor's hands. When one side is affected, the shoulder on that side droops, and the scapula

is displaced in a downward and lateral direction.

The strength of the sternomastoid muscle is tested by asking the patient to turn his head to one side, then the other, against the resistance of the doctor's hand. Normally, the muscle on the opposite side to the direction in which the head is turned should stand out. If both sternomastoid muscles are affected (as in muscular dystrophy and poliomyelitis), the patient has difficulty in raising his head when sitting up from a supine position.

12. **Hypoglossal nerve** — the extended tongue is inspected for any signs of weakness, wasting or involuntary movements (fasciculation — flickering of muscle fibres — may occur in some disorders). Lateral deviation of the tongue occurs if there is weakness on that side. The patient is asked to move his tongue from side to side, against the resistance of a tongue-depressor, to assess the strength of movements.

Motor function

Muscles are assessed for size, tone, power, movement and co-ordination; reflexes are also tested. Any obvious abnormalities are noted — such as flexion, tremors or gross wasting.

Muscle size. The girth of limbs is measured, using a tape measure, and both sides are compared. Any missing muscles or abnormal contours are noted. Signs of malnutrition should be taken into account, as this affects growth and bulk of muscles. Muscle wasting (atrophy) due to lower motor neurone disease is commonly accompanied by fasciculations (tremors of individual muscle fibres). Enlargement of muscles (hypertrophy) can occur in some types of muscular dystrophy.

Muscle tone. This is the degree of tension in a muscle at rest, which is difficult to assess under normal circumstances. Abnormal responses to passive movement can be assessed, but it is important to have the patient as comfortable and as relaxed as possible.

a. Flaccid movement occurs when there is

decreased muscle tone — *hypotonia*. This is seen as less resistance to movement, limpness, possible increase in the range of joint movement and difficulty in maintaining the limb in a given position.

b. Spastic movement occurs when muscle tone is increased — *hypertonia*. Three forms of increased tone are recognisable:

- resistance to passive movement which is more pronounced in one group of muscles than its antagonist group, but the resistance suddenly gives way — known as 'clasp-knife spasticity'; the extensor muscles of the lower limb and the flexor muscles of the upper limb tend to form contractures of the knee and elbow
- an equal amount of resistance in both agonist and antagonist muscles of the same group, with constant resistance to passive movement (muscles may remain rigid at rest and there is immobility of the limbs) — known as 'lead-pipe rigidity'
- rapid, alternating contractions of agonist and antagonist muscles during passive movement — known as 'cogwheel rigidity'.

Myotonia is a condition where muscle contraction continues into the period of relaxation. It can be assessed by asking the patient to close his eyes tightly and then to open them again. Opening of the eyelids is delayed. True myotonia can be temporarily relieved by injecting adrenocorticotrophic hormone (ACTH).

Muscle power and movement — This is assessed by asking the patient to put his joints through a range of movements, both with and without resistance (Fig. 2.7). Opposite sides of the body are compared for strength. Any obvious deformity or injury is taken into account. Fine movements, e.g., of the fingers, are assessed by asking the patient to wriggle his fingers, or to place the tip of each finger of one hand on the tip of his thumb of the other hand in turn. Children can be given toys which require manipulation with the hands and fingers.

Involuntary movements are observed during the assessment — e.g., is the involuntary

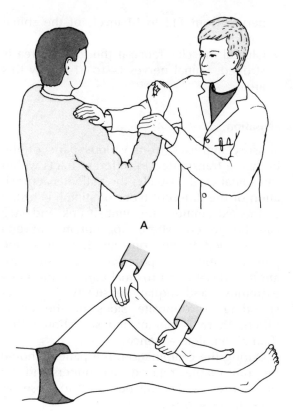

Fig. 2.7 Test of muscle power and movement.

movement constant or intermittent, does it occur at rest or is it related to voluntary movement? Epilepsy, chorea, dystonia or tics are some of the causes of involuntary movements; sometimes there may be a habit spasm with no organic cause.

Tremors may be evident, which may be described as fine or coarse. There are many causes for tremors, e.g., Parkinson's disease, multiple sclerosis, anxiety. Fasciculations, which have been previously mentioned, are irregular contractions of muscles at rest, which increase after voluntary activity. Fibrillations are very fine movements which are not visible to the eye, but can be detected on electromyography.

Muscle co-ordination. This has been discussed earlier in the text, in the section relating to balance, co-ordination and gait (under general examination of the patient).

Both sides of the body are assessed, noting speed and accuracy of movement.

Reflexes

1. **Primary reflexes** in the newborn and young infant include the following:

- Moro reflex (startle reflex) — the baby is lifted a few centimetres off the bed by its hands, and is suddenly allowed to fall back; the normal response is extension of the head, arms and fingers, which is present up to about 6 months of age.
- Grasp reflex — the baby closes its fingers around the examiner's finger when placed in the palm of its hand; this develops over the first few months of the infant's life into a true grasp reflex.
- Automatic walking — stepping movements — which occur when the infant is held upright with its feet in contact with a firm surface; scissoring of the legs may occur, normally, up to about four months of age.
- Rooting and sucking reflexes — these are responses to tactile stimuli around the baby's mouth, and are essential for feeding.

More details on these and other primary reflexes can be found in textbooks on neonatal and paediatric care.

2. **Deep (tendon) reflexes** are evoked by tapping muscle tendons with a tendon hammer. Reflex contraction can be observed in some muscles, if the patient is relaxed.

- Muscles of the upper limbs — the biceps, triceps and supinator muscles (supplied by spinal nerves C5 to C8).
- Muscles of the lower limbs — the quadriceps muscle contracts when the patella is tapped — knee-jerk — and the calf muscles contract when the Achilles tendon is tapped — ankle jerk. These are supplied by spinal nerves L2 to L4 and L5 to S2, respectively.
- Contraction of the abdominal muscles can also be elicited by tapping the abdomen.

Repeated contraction and relaxation of a muscle is termed *clonus*. This may result when a muscle is stretched. An example of this can be seen when the calf muscle is stretched by forcibly dorsiflexing the ankle. Clonus occurs when the muscle is hypertonic, or in someone who is very tense.

3. **Superficial reflexes** are elicited by stroking the skin, using adequate, but not too much, pressure. Some examples of superficial reflexes are:

- Plantar reflex — the lateral, lower surface of the foot is stroked from heel to toes, using an orange-stick or spatula. Normally, after about 18 months of age, the toes should flex downwards. An extensor reflex — spreading of the toes and extension of the great toe — is abnormal, except in young infants. The extensor reflex is known as *Babinski's sign* and indicates a lesion of the pyramidal tracts in S1/S2 segments of the spinal cord (Fig. 2.8).
- Abdominal reflex is seen as contraction of the abdominal muscles, with retraction of the umbilicus to the stimulated side, when the abdomen is stroked. This reflex is absent in upper motor neurone lesions affecting T7 to T12 segments of the spinal cord.
- Cremasteric reflex can be elicited in males by lightly scratching the inner surface of the upper thigh. The testicle on the same side should elevate. This area is supplied by

nerves from T12 to L1 levels of the spinal cord.
- Gluteal muscles tense if the gluteal area is stroked. Spinal nerves L4 to S1 supply this area.

Sensation

Sensory impulses from various parts of the body are transmitted in different tracts within the spinal cord. Usually, the patient's appreciation of the different types of stimuli is tested at the extremities; the limbs, trunk and face can be tested where appropriate. Several points need to be considered, such as the patient's ability to perceive sensation, variation in distal and proximal parts of the same extremity, and equal sensitivity in corresponding or opposite sides of the body. Often, there is diminished sensation rather than a complete absence.

During the examination, the patient should be comfortable, relaxed, and understand the procedures, as he will be asked to close his eyes (if conscious).

1. **Primary sensation** includes perception of superficial stimuli to the skin, vibration sense, deep pressure and proprioception. These can be tested in the following ways:

- Light touch — touching the skin lightly with a piece of cotton wool
- Superficial pain — carefully pricking the skin with a sterile needle or pin
- Temperature discrimination — tubes containing hot and cold water are held against the skin (taking care with the hot water, to avoid scalding)
- Pressure — pressing on the skin
- Deep pressure pain — squeezing the Achilles tendon, calf and forearm
- Vibration sense — placing a vibrating tuning fork on bony prominences, such as the wrist — the patient should be able to feel the vibration in the extremity of the limb
- Proprioception — by passive movement of one of the patient's fingers or toes, which should be held lightly on its lateral aspects

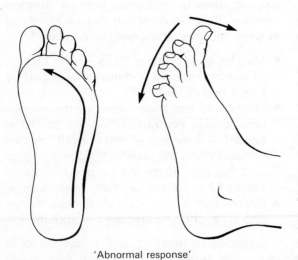

'Abnormal response'

Fig. 2.8 Babinski reflex.

— the patient is asked to indicate if the digit is moved up or down.

2. **Discrimination** may be tested if a lesion of the sensory area of the parietal lobe is suspected. Two-point discrimination is checked to see if the patient has the ability to distinguish sensation in two close areas. Metal dividers are used for this, so that two parts of the body can be touched simultaneously.

Discrimination of texture is assessed by placing different materials into the patient's hand, e.g., cotton, velvet and glasspaper. The patient should be able to distinguish the different textures, under normal circumstances.

Steregnosis — recognition of shapes — is tested by placing familiar objects such as a key, pen or coin into the patient's hand, and asking him to identify the object.

Graphaesthesia is tested by tracing figures and letters on the patient's skin, using an orange stick, and asking him to identify the tracings.

Extinction is tested by touching two opposite sides of the body simultaneously — the patient should feel the touch on both sides at the same time.

Brain death

It is sometimes necessary for the medical staff to decide whether or not the patient is clinically dead, although sustained on life support equipment.

A full explanation of how this is performed can be found in the chapter on the care of the unconscious patient.

CONCLUSION

This chapter on neurological examination has included information on both nursing and medical aspects. The two are often interdependent and the nurse must appreciate what steps have been taken by the doctor in arriving at a diagnosis. With most patients, a provisional diagnosis is made from the presentation of signs and symptoms and the history given. It is not usually necessary to carry out all the procedures mentioned here, only those which are relevant to the individual patient. Further assessment may be required, involving special tests and investigations. These are dealt with in a separate chapter.

The nurse's own assessment of the patient, enhanced with information from other sources, such as the medical examination, is an important step. Without this assessment, the patient's problems in relation to his activities of daily living cannot be identified and dealt with in a logical manner.

BIBLIOGRAPHY

Allan D 1984 Glasgow coma scale. Nursing Mirror 158(23):32

Collins S, Parker E 1983 The essentials of nursing — An introduction to nursing. Macmillan, London

Coltheart M 1979 Mysteries of reading in brain defects. New Scientist 82:1140

Conway-Rutkowski B L 1982 In: Carini & Owens Neurological and neurosurgical nursing, 8th edn. C V Mosby, St Louis

Henderson V, Nite G 1978 Principles and practice of nursing, 6th edn. Macmillan, New York

Pemberton L 1979 Nursing an unconscious patient. Nursing Mirror, 149(11):41

Purchese G, Allan D 1984 Neuromedical and neurosurgical nursing, 2nd edn. Baillière Tindall, London

Roberts A 1982 Systems of life. Nursing Times, supplement 78(18):89, 78(22):90, 78(27):91, 78(31):92

Roper N, Logan W, Tierney A 1985 The elements of nursing, 2nd edn. Churchill Livingstone, Edinburgh.

Simpson D, Reilly P 1982 Paediatric coma scale. Lancet 2:450

3

Neurological investigations

The investigative period in any disorder is of a variable length of time and the extent and number of tests to which the patient may be subjected, will depend on the provisional diagnosis. Neurological investigations have changed dramatically over the last decade, with the advent of sophisticated, largely non-invasive techniques replacing previously hazardous methods. This has led to, in some instances, a reduction in physical pre- and post-investigative nursing intervention but does not preclude the value of psychological preparation.

Most of the tests performed in neurology are considered as 'special' in that, to perform them, the patient needs to be transferred to another department, e.g. radiology, theatre.

A study by Wilson-Barnett & Carrigay (1978) demonstrated significantly more anxiety on 'special test' days than on any others and that 78% of all patients' comments about 'special tests' were negative. These reflected anxiety over what would happen and how much discomfort would be experienced. Furthermore, the degree of reported anxiety was often not related to the amount of discomfort or the seriousness of the test.

Many studies (Elms & Leonard, 1966; Moran, 1963; Franklin, 1974) have indicated that the amount of information given to patients by staff was inadequate.

PATIENT PREPARATION: GENERAL CONSIDERATIONS

The nurse has an important part to play in teaching and support of the patient during the pre-test phase. A properly prepared patient will co-operate and be more relaxed, necessitating only one performance of the test and producing the best results.

No assumptions should be made of the patient's understanding of the test and a clear concise explanation of what will happen should be provided. An explanation must be provided based on the patient's level of knowledge and desire to know about the test. If the co-operation of the patient is needed special manoeuvres must be explained, e.g. lying still, holding breath etc.

When providing explanations the nurse should note the patient's ability to comprehend what is being said. Patients with a disorder of the central nervous system may be suffering from poor concentration, loss of memory, knowledge deficits and sensory problems. A diminished conscious level may mask all of these signs, in which case it may be necessary to obtain the patient's family's consent for the procedure.

Faulkner (1985) reminds us how easy it is for the nurse to become familiar with common tests and subsequently fail to appreciate the patient's anxiety and apprehension.

It is necessary to let the patient know where and when the test will take place. He should be informed of any delay and provided with an explanation. It might be reassuring for the patient to know that a familiar nurse from the ward may accompany him to the X-ray department. Where this is not the usual practice, a nurse from recovery/X-ray department may visit the patient, prior to the test in order to introduce herself.

When talking to the patient about the diagnostic procedure, it is worthwhile to remember that the patient may be aware of the provisional diagnosis. This will be stress-provoking if the diagnosis is potentially life-threatening, e.g. tumour.

PLAIN RADIOGRAPHY

Skull

Skull films are usually obtained in lateral and anterior-posterior (AP) views. Other, more specialised views are less often used. Interpretation of skull films centres around:

— **Presence of a fracture.** This may be described as linear, depressed or comminuted. Found most often in tumour patients.
— **Displacement of structures**, e.g. the pineal gland may, in the presence of a lesion, be displaced from its usual midline position.
— **Unusual calcification**. A patient with a metastatic tumour may have some bone thinning as a result of bone erosion. Bone thickening may be seen in Paget's disease.
— **Sutures** may be widened in hydrocephalus or prematurely fused.
— **Intracranial air** may be seen in the patient with a basal skull fracture.

Spine

Views may be obtained in an anterior-posterior, lateral or oblique projection. Interpretation of spinal films will centre around:

— presence of any congenital defects, e.g. spina bifida
— bony erosion caused by a tumour
— widening of the foramina
— narrowing of the vertebral canal
— fractures or dislocations
— degenerative changes of the bone
— spondylosis.

COMPUTERISED AXIAL TOMOGRAPHY (CT OR CAT SCAN)

This safe, non-invasive (for most patients) procedure has changed the face of neurological investigations, since its introduction in 1972. The earlier scans were sometimes marred by artefact caused by patient movement but with the considerable reduction in scan-

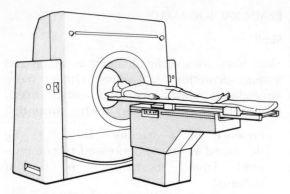

Fig. 3.1 Computerised tomography machine.

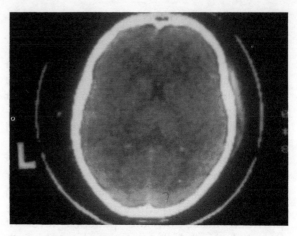

Fig. 3.2 Normal CT scan.

ning time with the present generation of CT scanners, this is now a rare occurrence. CT scans have now become a common investigation for many patients. It is particularly suited to outpatient use.

An image is produced based on the tissue density of the structure being scanned. The patient lies on a motor driven couch and his head is placed in a hole in the scanner. For whole body scans, the entire body passes through. A series of X-rays are beamed through the head, in a trans-axial slice of varying sizes (2.0–15.0 mm) and, depending upon the density of the tissue, are either transmitted or absorbed. The transmitted X-rays are detected by a battery of sensitive crystals and this information is then fed into a computer for analysis and creation of an image on a screen or on film. Once one set of data is collected, the machine moves round 1° and the whole process is repeated until the arc (180°) is complete.

On the image, bone appears white, CSF is black and the brain appears as various shades of grey. Review of a CT scan may reveal alterations in tissue density, displacement of structures and abnormalities. CT scanning has a widespread use in neurological investigations, being utilised in virtually every patient with suspected intracranial pathology.

Contrast enhancement may be used. An intravenous dye is injected and the patient scanned shortly afterwards. Contrast may enhance the diagnosis of certain abnormal structures. Serial scans may be required to

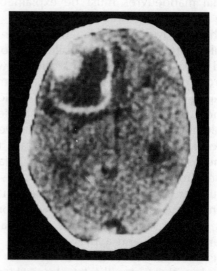

Fig. 3.3 Glioblastoma multiforme of the frontal lobe. (Reproduced with permission from Burrows & Leeds 1981.)

follow the progress of a disorder and its treatment and this is easily done. The patient does not necessarily need to be conscious to be scanned; many unconscious patients are successfully scanned provided body movement is kept to a minimum.

Pre-test care

Adequate explanation of the procedure, including mention of what is expected of the patient, where and when the test is being performed, that it is painless and a description of the noises which the machine will make. The patient should not wear any metal jewellery on or around his head and neck. The need for the patient to lie still should be emphasised. If the patient is very confused or agitated, administration of a general anaesthetic may be considered, therefore appropriate preparation for this will be necessary. Some light sedation may be all that is necessary.

Post-test care

None specific. The patient who has received contrast should be observed for a possible delayed reaction. This reaction may manifest itself as a skin rash or at its very worst, anaphylactic shock, which is very rare. The patient who has had a general anaesthetic will need adequate nursing for a safe recovery.

MAGNETIC RESONANCE IMAGING

Magnetic resonance imaging (MRI) produces high definition images of the nervous system using a system of varying radio pulse waves and a magnetic field instead of the traditional radiation associated with CT scanning. The procedure is non-invasive and painless and presently takes longer to perform than a CT scan.

The patient lies on a couch and is then completely enclosed in a 'tunnel' within the scanner. A strong magnetic field is applied and the nuclei within the tissues, which were previously spinning in a random manner, line up in a north-south magnetic field orientation. At this stage a radio pulse wave is introduced at a right angle to the magnetic field and the nuclei are tipped out of alignment causing uniform resonance. The pulse waves are stopped and the resonating nuclei will return to their previous state. Minute radiofrequency signals are given off as the nuclei enter this relaxed state and these are monitored by the scanner. By pre-programming the computer to simulate a non-uniform magnetic field, the protons (positively charged particles) in different parts of the magnetic field will resonate at different speeds. Varying the radio pulse waves will result in differences in the emission of radio frequency data. The computer assimilates this data and constructs a tissue image. The introduction of different radio pulse wave patterns will result in different types of images being produced. T_1 is based on the hydrogen tissue density and its relative solidity. The T_1 parameter is based on the amount of time that it takes for the hydrogen protons to relax to their prior magnetic state. The T_1 time leads to markedly improved differentiation between grey and white matter, thus the plaques of multiple sclerosis are easily located.

The T_2 parameter is based on the relationship of the hydrogen atoms to each other. Some protons are accelerating on their spinning axis while others are decelerating; this creates differences within different tissues resulting in the T_2 relaxation pattern. This again provides valuable data for the computer to analyse in terms of early biochemical changes in a disease pattern prior to structural changes. MRI has a particular application in detecting cerebral and spinal oedema and cerebral and spinal blood flow related disorders such as infarction, haemorrhage and arteriovenous malformation. Tumours are also easily located particularly in the prevously difficult to scan area of the posterior fossa. Early changes in degenerative disorders such as multiple sclerosis and dementia may well lead to more effective detection and treatment in the future.

Pre-test care

An adequate explanation of the procedure and what is expected of the patient is provided. The patient should be reassured that he will be given a call button which he can press whilst in the scanner should he wish to come out.

It should be ascertained that the patient is not wearing metallic jewellery, a cardiac pacemaker or any metal prostheses including aneurysm clips. These objects will all be displaced by the effects of the magnetic field. General anaesthesia or sedation may be required to ensure that the patient lies still for up to 30 minutes.

Post-test care

None specific.

POSITRON EMISSION TOMOGRAPHY (PET)

This technique is still being developed. The patient inhales or is injected with a compound, deoxyglucose with radioactive fluorine. Positrons are emitted and collide with electrons to produce photons that are detected and analysed by a computer. Essentially, this produces a colour map of the levels of glucose metabolism within the brain.

Uses for this type of scanning may be producing a better understanding of diseases such as epilepsy and dementia, and of cerebral blood flow. Presently, access to PET is very limited due to its expense.

LUMBAR PUNCTURE

This is the commonest test used in relation to investigation of the nervous system. It involves the insertion of a trocar and cannula into the spinal canal and the withdrawal of a sample of cerebrospinal fluid (CSF) for analysis. Other methods include cisternal puncture or direct puncture of a lateral ventricle.

The needle is inserted between lumbar vertebrae 3 and 4 or 4 and 5 (Fig. 3.4). This avoids accidental penetration of the spinal cord which terminates at lumbar vertebra 1 level. Lumbar puncture may be performed for diagnostic or therapeutic reasons.

Diagnostic

The appearance of CSF may be checked by taking samples of fluid. Table 3.1 outlines the

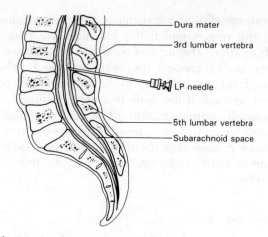

Fig. 3.4 Lumbar puncture needle in situ.

Table 3.1 Values of cerebrospinal fluid

Colour	Crystal clear
Pressure	80 to 160 mm water
Volume	120 to 150 ml
Cells	120 to 150 ml
a. red blood none	
b. white blood none	
(i) polymorphonuclear leucocytes	
(ii) lymphocytes 0 to 5 mm^3	
Protein	0.2 to 0.4 g/l
Gamma globulin (IgG)	Less than 13% of total protein
Sugar	3.6 to 5.0 mmol
Wassermann reaction	Negative

normal constituents of CSF. Samples are usually taken for laboratory analysis including biochemistry, bacteriology and viral studies depending on the tentative diagnosis and history.

Pressure measurement. Isolated measurements of lumbar spinal pressure may be of use in diagnosis. Pathology which may result in an increase in pressure will include space occupying lesions. It should be noted however, that the performance of lumbar puncture in the presence of raised ICP is extremely dangerous. The release of pressure at the lumbar spine will exacerbate any herniation or coning which may take place. This will produce a marked deterioration in the patient's condition, resulting in some cases in death.

Injection of material such as contrast or radioisotope's to outline the spinal canal or ventricular system.

Therapeutic

The administration of drugs into the theca is facilitated with lumbar puncture. It may be desirable, for example, to give intrathecal antibiotics in the treatment of meningitis. Special precautions need to be observed while administering drugs this way. They should be specially formulated without preservatives for this purpose. A meticulous checking system should be implemented prior to injection.

Reduction in pressure may be desired following surgery in a patient with a persistent CSF leak. This would necessitate repeated lumbar punctures, once daily for several days.

Contraindications to lumbar puncture

Raised ICP. As already mentioned, all reasonable precautions should be adopted to ascertain that the patient does not have markedly raised ICP. If some doubt exists as to whether intracranial hypertension is present, a decision will be made as to whether the benefit outweighs the risks to the patient. Where possible, CT scanning will confirm the existance of raised ICP.

Infection or deformity of the lumbar vertebrae. This would preclude lumbar puncture. Infection may be spread into the CSF or a deformity can hinder safe insertion of the needle. If it is essential to obtain a sample of CSF this may be achieved with cisternal puncture or direct cannulation of the lateral ventricle.

THE PROCEDURE

A thorough explanation is given to the patient prior to the procedure. He should be reassured that his back will be anaesthetised and that it is not a painful procedure. The patient should be informed of the after care and what is expected of him. An oppor-

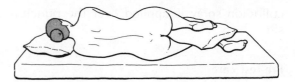

Fig. 3.5   Patient position for lumbar puncture.

tunity is given to the patient to empty his bladder. The patient is placed in the right or left lateral position with his spine parallel to the edge of the bed. The patient is instructed to flex his knees and place his head forward, this has the effect of opening the spaces between the vertebrae facilitating easier and safer insertion of the needle. Once the appropriate area has been anaesthetised the needle and stylet of the correct size is inserted until the resistance of the dura is overcome. Once in the subarachnoid space the stylet is removed and CSF should drip out of the needle. If the pressure is to be measured, the manometer is attached and a reading is taken prior to removal of CSF. The normal range is 80–160 mm water. Fluctuations of the pulse and respiration can be seen.

Queckenstedt's test may be performed to determine if the CSF pathways are patent. Pressure is applied to the jugular veins for a brief period of time. This will dam back the blood flow from the head producing a rise in ICP. If the pathways are patent a rise in the pressure recorded on the manometer is noted. A blockage of the pathway, for example, by a tumour would prevent this rise in the reading. The patient should be forewarned prior to this procedure as placing the hands on the patient's throat may be misinterpreted. The test should not be performed in the presence of raised ICP or cerebral haemorrhage because brain stem herniation or rebleeding may occur.

Once this is complete, samples of CSF are then obtained and placed in the appropriate collection containers. The amount of CSF taken and the number of containers required is determined by the laboratory tests performed. The needle is removed from the patient's back and an adhesive covering or collodion spray is applied over the puncture site.

Pre-test care

Adequate explanation must be provided for the patient by the physician and this may be reinforced or clarified by the nurse. This explanation will assist in reassuring and relaxing the patient thereby ensuring a more comfortable procedure.

The patient should be reassured and observed throughout the procedure, including pulse and respirations and any report by the patient of discomfort. The correct position will optimise the successful performance of the procedure.

Post-test care

Opinions vary as to the length of time which the patient should remain on bed rest following lumbar puncture. Traditionally 24 hours was deemed appropriate however the tendency has been to shorten this to as little as 6 hours. Generally speaking, within limitations, the patient should remain on bedrest while any headache persists. Analgesia should be provided. Fluids are encouraged to stimulate replacement of the removed CSF volume.

Neurological observations are maintainad to monitor conscious level and limb movements in particular. Any deterioration should be reported immediately because of the dangers of coning. The puncture site should be checked frequently for, possible leakage. Other minor manifestations which may occur include back pain, problems with urination and a slight pyrexia. These are all of a temporary nature and should be managed conservatively.

COMPLICATIONS OF LUMBAR PUNCTURE

— **Coning**. Brain stem herniation is encouraged when lumbar puncture is performed in the presence of raised ICP. This can be fatal.

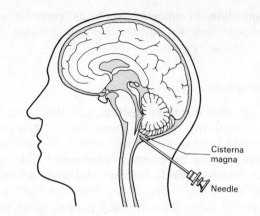

Fig. 3.6 Cisternal puncture.

— **Infection**. A poor aseptic technique may lead to the introduction of infection into the subarachnoid space leading to meningitis.
— **Traumatic tap**. During the procedure the needle may pierce a small blood vessel. This might give the wrong impression that a bloody CSF had been obtained. A traumatic tap is not uniformly bloodstained.
— **Injury to the nerve root**. This is very rare and is due to the tip of the needle touching a nerve root.
— **Leaking puncture site**. A slow leak from the puncture site will exacerbate any headache which the patient may already have.

CISTERNAL PUNCTURE

When a specimen of CSF cannot be obtained by lumbar puncture, cisternal puncture may be considered. This involves inserting a needle into the cisterna magnum from a posterior approach (Fig. 3.6). This is a potentially dangerous procedure due to the close proximity of the medulla, puncture of which would be disastrous. In order that the doctor knows precisely to what depth the needle has been inserted, a special graduated needle is used.

The nape of the patient's neck is shaved up to the occipital protuberance and the procedure is performed with the patient sitting with his head tilted slightly forward. The administration of a sedative prior to the performance of the procedure is often advocated.

Post-test care

This is as for a lumbar puncture, with particular emphasis on respiratory assessment and observation of neurological status. Indications for performance of cisternal puncture may also include injection of contrast medium to demonstrate lesions of the upper cord, cervical vertebral abnormalities and blockage of the subarachnoid space.

A further extension of this procedure is the cisternogram. A radioisotope is injected into the subarachnoid space and is taken up by the CSF. Periodic scans are then performed which demonstrate the length of time it takes for the radioisotope to be cleared from the CSF. Cisternogram may be indicated in the diagnosis of hydrocephalus or to establish the presence of otorrhoea or rhinorrhoea.

ANGIOGRAPHY

Angiography involves outlining the intracranial and extracranial blood vessels with the injection of contrast medium. The following abnormalities may be demonstrated:

- aneurysm or arteriovenous malformation (AVM)
- displacement of blood vessels by a space occupying lesion
- narrowing, thrombosis or occlusion of the blood vessels.

The contrast medium can be administered directly into the carotid or vertebral arteries or indirectly via the femoral artery. Using the indirect route precludes the need for general anaesthesia. Serial rapid radiographic films are then taken as the contrast medium progresses through the cerebral circulation.

Another technique used is termed *digital subtraction angiography*. This produces a clearer image by abolishing surrounding anatomical structures. This is done by obtaining images before and following injection of the contrast medium and then subtracting the first image from the second.

Pre-test care

Although the patient may not be scheduled for general anaesthesia he is prepared as though he were. An adequate explanation is provided following which written consent is obtained by a member of the medical staff. The patient is fasted and prepared as for

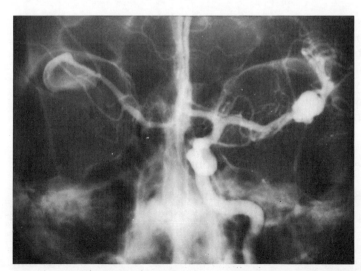 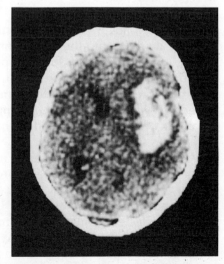

Fig. 3.7 Bilateral middle cerebral artery aneurysms. (Reproduced with permission from Burrows & Leeds 1981.)

general anaesthesia. Baseline pre-angio-graphic neurological observations and vital signs are noted.

Post-test care

On completion of the test the patient is continued on bed rest. The nurse should be aware which puncture site has been used and if any difficulties were encountered with cannulation. If the femoral artery was used, a close check should be maintained on the pulses in that leg. Frequent neurological observations and vital signs are noted. Any excessive swelling around the puncture site may be treated with a local cold application. If the carotid artery was cannulated the de-velopment of a haematoma could endanger respiratory function. Rare complications which the nurse should be aware of include:

— development of a stroke; there may be hemiparesis and/or dysphasia
— seizure activity
— an allergic reaction to the contrast medium; the patient should be questioned prior to the procedure with regard to any allergies; if any doubt arises, a test dose is given.

Any changes in the patient's condition should be reported immediately.

MYELOGRAM

Myelography involves the injection of a contrast medium into the subarachnoid space via a lumbar puncture for the purpose of outlining the spinal cord and vertebral column. The contrast medium may be oil based or water soluble; it is important to establish which has been used as the post-test care varies for each one.

Myelography may be performed at a particular level although it is more usual to visualise the entire spinal canal. Following lumbar puncture a quantity of CSF is removed and the selected contrast medium injected. Films are then taken, serially. A significant finding would be indicated by a partial or complete obstruction to the flow of the

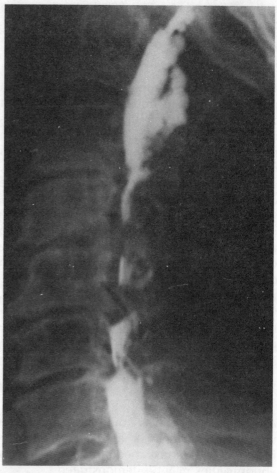

Fig. 3.8 Myelogram demonstrating cervical spondylosis. (Reproduced with permission from Burrows & Leeds 1981.)

contrast. A myelogram will be performed in those patients suspected of having a prolapsed disc or spinal tumour. Alternatively, it may be ordered to exclude other causes in a patient who may have, for example, multiple sclerosis.

Pre-test care

Written consent is obtained by the doctor following explanation of what is involved. On the morning of the investigation the patient is prepared. Policy varies — in some places the patient is fasted although general anaesthesia is not used. This is advocated in case the patient must proceed to surgery following myelography. An open-backed gown is put on to preserve the patient's modesty. As many of these patients are suffering from back pain, adequate pre-myelogram analgesia should be provided as they may have to lie in a position that is very painful. The patient should empty his bladder immediately prior to the investigation.

Post-test care

As already stated this will vary according to which type of contrast medium is used. Care relevant to whichever type of contrast includes the following:

— continuing neurological and vital signs recordings; particular note is taken of lower limb movements
— observation for signs of reaction to the contrast
— provision of adequate analgesia
— ensure adequate fluid intake
— note any difficulty in voiding
— observe puncture site for leakage.

If an oil-based contrast medium is used the patient is nursed flat; sitting the patient upright produces headache. If a non-ionic water soluble contrast medium is used the patient is nursed in the sitting position for at least 7 hours.

With the advent of newer and more sophisticated imaging techniques some tests are used less frequently or have become completely obsolete. These include:

Brain scan. In this procedure an intravenous radioisotope is given following the administration of a blocking dose of potassium perchlorate. This reduces selective absorption of the isotope by the choroid plexus. Shortly after, depending on which isotope is used, images are obtained with the use of a gamma camera. This technique is unable to distinguish what the lesion is but will confirm its presence by an increased uptake of the isotope, the so-called 'hot spot'.

While isotope scans have reduced in number other techniques have been developed. These include:

Dynamic scan. This assists in determining the efficiency of cerebral blood flow. This data is useful for diagnosing changes in flow during certain disease processes and for predicting outcome. The procedure involves using inhalational xenon which can then be traced to the cerebral cranial probes. Values for blood flow can then be estimated.

Pledget test. This is used to confirm the presence of a CSF rhinorrhoea and otorrhoea. An isotope is administered via lumbar puncture into the CSF. Plugs are placed in either the patient's nose or ears, for up to 1 hour. If radioactivity is detected, the patient has a CSF leak. Local regulations with regard to the administration of isotopes should be observed.

Lumbar air encephalogram (Pneumo-encephalogram). This procedure carried a number of risks and is seldom performed now. It has been largely superseded by the much safer CT scan.

The procedure involves the injection of air into the subarachnoid space, following removal of a quantity of CSF. The patient is strapped to a chair which is then slowly moved through 360° to outline the ventricular system. The air acts as a contrast medium. Radiographic films are obtained and abnormalities in the outline of the ventricular system are noted. Again, this only provided an indication of the presence of a lesion without actually identifying what it was.

Possible complications include severe headache, nausea and vomiting. The patient often took up to 1 week to recover from the test. Other complications included shock, haemorrhage, air embolism and seizures aside from the other complications of lumbar puncture.

Echoencephalography. This is another investigation made obsolete by CT scanning. The principal relies upon sonic waves being reflected from a structure, in this case inside the head, back to the receiver and from these data calculating if that structure was abnormally displaced. It still finds some application in neonatal units, but rarely in neurosurgical units.

Ventriculogram. Again the advent of CT precludes performance of this technique. The patient had a small catheter placed in the lateral ventricle and contrast medium was then injected into it. This outlined the ventricular system. This investigation took on the status of minor surgery, with its attendant potential complications.

ORBITAL VENOGRAPHY

A small volume of contrast medium is injected into one of the frontal veins. A specialised technique involving the placement of elastic bands around the patient's head, permits the insertion of a small intravenous cannula and the injection of contrast. This flows through the ophthalmic veins and radiographic films are obtained. This test may be indicated in patients with pituitary gland lesions, aneurysms and tumours. No specific pre- or post-test care is needed.

DOPPLER IMAGING

An ultrasonic probe is placed on the skin over the carotid artery and then moved slowly from here to the bifurcation between the internal and external carotid artery. The probe emits high frequency sound waves which are reflected against the red blood cells back to the probe, providing an indication of the velocity of the blood flow. This technique is used to assess occlusive disorders of the carotid arteries. It is safe, non-invasive and no specific pre- or post-test care is needed.

ELECTROENCEPHALOGRAPHY (EEG)

An electroencephalogram is a graphic record of the electrical activity of the brain. Small electrodes are placed on the scalp in a standard pattern and a recording is obtained on paper. A number of different types of rhythms have been identified in the 'normal' adult and variation from these may be noted (Fig. 3.9).

An EEG is useful for classifying different types of seizure disorders, for monitoring threatened cerebral ischaemia during trial occlusion of the cerebral arteries, location of focal supratentorial lesions and in some countries is included as part of their brain death criteria.

The patient either sits in a chair or lies on

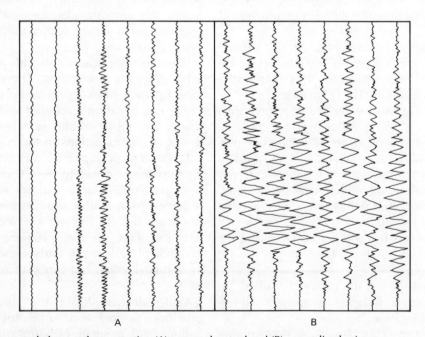

Fig. 3.9 Electroencephalogram demonstrating (A) a normal record and (B) generalised seizure.

a bed while the recording is being made. It is useful to have the patient's co-operation but not essential. If the resting EEG is normal, certain manoeuvres may be used to increase the instability of the electrical activity. These may include the use of hyperventilation or photic stimulation. In this technique, a flickering light is shone on the patient with his eyes closed. It may be possible to demonstrate an abnormal waveform which was previously not shown. Sometimes for similar reasons, a sleeping EEG may be performed. Some patients are at their most susceptible as they are falling asleep or upon waking and an EEG performed at this time may be beneficial. An attempt is made to allow the patient to fall asleep naturally and failing this, a sedative may need to be given.

A sphenoidal EEG may be indicated in the classification of temporal lobe epilepsy. As the abnormal discharge is deep-seated this may not be detected by ordinary surface electrodes. Wire electrodes are placed close to the undersurface of the skull through needles inserted into the cheeks.

Some patients may have a 24 hour ambulatory EEG performed. This may be indicated in patients in whom a one-off recording is not of value or where there may be the possibility of an hysterical component. Patients suffering from absence attacks may be suitable candidates for this type of monitoring. Small electrodes are glued to the patient's scalp and the wires are connected to a portable recorder which can be attached to the patient's waistband. The patient can then go about his normal business throughout the day. A device is included which permits the patient to 'mark' the tape when he feels a seizure starting.

The cassette tape is then analysed and possible patterns of seizures or seizures related to certain activities or times of the day may be seen.

Pre-test care

It should be emphasised to the patient that this is an entirely painless procedure. An explanation of what will happen is useful.

Prior to attending for EEG the patient's hair is washed and any hair oil removed. Hairgrips should also be removed. It may be that the doctor will order witholding certain types of medication. Certain drugs such as tranquilizers can affect the result.

Consent is needed for a sleeping EEG in which a sedative is to be given. Once sedated the patient should not be left alone.

Post-test care

There is no specific post-test care.

ELECTROMYOGRAPHY (EMG)

Like the EEG, electromyography also records electrical activity but this time of the muscles. It is the electrical activity within the muscles which results in contraction and in some disorders the normal 'pattern' of activity is distorted and this may be apparent on the EMG.

Small needle electrodes are placed in the muscle to be examined. These are connected to sensitive machinery which is capable of detecting the electrical activity within a muscle, both at rest and during activity. These signals are amplified and then displayed on a screen or as hard copy, for interpretation. It is a useful diagnostic tool in disease of muscle or of its nerve supply.

There is no specific pre- or post-test care apart from explanation.

EVOKED POTENTIAL MEASUREMENTS

An evoked potential is a minute electrical change that occurs in response to a sensory stimulus. This is not to be confused with an EEG in which the recorded electrical activity is at random. A sophisticated computing process facilitates the interpretation of collected data and will produce an average curve. This can then be compared with abnormal responses which may be obtained from some patients in the presence of disease of the peripheral and central nervous system.

Small electrodes are applied to the patient's scalp and recordings made. It is painless and non-invasive.

Three sensory systems can be tested as follows:

Visual evoked responses

The stimuli are usually patterned boards or flashing lights. In this procedure the integrity of the pathway between the retina and the occipital cortex is tested. Delayed potentials may be seen in the patient with multiple sclerosis or an optic tumour.

Evoked potential audiometry (auditory evoked responses)

Headphones are placed over the patient's ears and an auditory stimulus consisting of clicks is introduced. As before, the patient's response is detected with the use of appropriately placed scalp electrodes and analysed. This type of testing will provide information regarding the integrity of the cochlear and auditory nerve pathways.

Somatosensory evoked potentials

This version tests the integrity of the ascending pathway and provides information regarding its efficiency. Scalp electrodes are placed over the sensory cortex and commencing at the median nerve and progressing upwards, small electrical charges are introduced at each of these sites in turn. The patient's responses are noted. There is little or no nursing intervention in these procedures.

VISUAL FIELD TESTING

The direct confrontation method of examination of the visual field may be indicated in those patients who are suspected of having a central nervous system lesion interfering with the visual pathway. Such lesions would

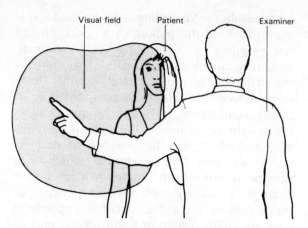

Fig. 3.10 Direct confrontational technique.

produce a deficit within the patient's visual field. The examiner sits in front of the patient and asks the patient to close one eye and to concentrate on the examiner's nose with the other. The examiner presents a moving finger from the peripheral area and the patient is asked to indicate when he becomes aware of it. This would indicate if the patient has a visual field defect.

More sophisticated means of detecting visual field defects are available. The Bjerrum's screen is a large black screen with a white fixation point in the middle. A moving spot (fixed on the end of a long black wand) is moved across the screen in different direc-

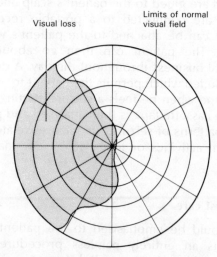

Fig. 3.11 Visual field deficit.

tions. Again, the patient is asked to close one eye and indicate when the moving spot comes into vision. Using this method allows a more accurate graphic representation to be made of the patient's visual field.

BIBLIOGRAPHY

Ambrose J 1973 Computerised transverse axial tomography. 2, Clinical application. British Journal of Radiology 46:1023

Bradshaw J R 1985 Brain CT: an introduction. Wright, Bristol

Burrows E H, Leeds N E 1981 Neuroradiology, volume 1. Churchill Livingstone, New York

Bydder G M 1983 Brain imaging by NMR. The Practitioner 277(1377):497

Byers V, Gendell H 1982 Using metrizamide for lumbar myelography: adverse reactions and nursing implications. Journal of Neurosurgical Nursing 14(6):315

Elms R R, Leonard R C 1966 Effects of nursing approaches during admission. Nursing Research 15:39

Faulkner A 1985 Nursing: a creative approach. Baillière Tindall, London

Franklin B L 1974 Patient anxiety on admission to hospital. RCN, London

Hall J W, Spielman G, Gennarelli T A 1982 Auditory evoked responses in acute severe head injury. Journal of Neurosurgical Nursing 14(5):225

Hickey J 1986 The clinical practice of neurologial and neurosurgical nursing. J B Lippincott, Philadelphia

Houndsfield G N 1973 Computerised transverse axial tomography, 1, Description of the system. British Journal of Radiology 46:1016

Lyons M, Wilson D 1981 Regional cerebral blood flow — a newer non-invasive diagnostic test. Journal of Neurosurgical Nursing 13(6):286

Maida M 1982 Regional cerebral blood flow: Patient correlation. Journal of Neurosurgical Nursing 14(5):309

McManus J C, Hausman K A 1982 Cerebrospinal fluid analysis. Nursing 82 12(8):43

Moran P 1963 (quoted by Janis I 1971 Stress and frustration, Harcourt Brace, New York) Unpublished thesis, Yale University

Peterson H O, Keiffer S A 1975 Introduction to neuroradiology. Harper and Row, London

Wilson-Barnett J, Carrigay A 1978 Factors affecting patients' responses to hospitalisation. Journal of Advanced Nursing 3(3):221

Wilson-Barnett J 1979 Stress in hospital. Churchill Livingstone, Edinburgh

Young J A 1981 Head injuries. 2. Advances in diagnostic equipment. Nursing Times 77(19):819.

4

The unconscious patient — the nursing perspective

MECHANISM OF COMA

The complex mechanism which maintains consciousness in the human body relies upon a close interrelationship between the cerebral cortex and the reticular activating system (RAS), located in the dorsal aspect of the upper brain stem.

Two parts of the RAS have been identified: the mesencephalic part, consisting of areas of grey matter within the pons and midbrain and responsible for general wakefulness, and the thalamic part, comprising grey matter within the thalamus, which is responsible for arousal.

The state of wakefulness, which we term consciousness, is the direct result of complicated feedback systems. Once an individual is aroused, following stimulation of the thalamic part of the RAS, consciousness is maintained by sustained activation of both the cerebral cortex and the RAS, via several feedback circuits. One of these circuits connects with the spinal cord which permits impulses from the stimulated RAS to be transmitted to skeletal muscles where activation causes proprioceptors to return impulses that stimulate the RAS. The RAS in turn constantly stimulates the cerebral cortex resulting in consciousness, until fatigue supervenes and sleep is induced. Under normal circumstances, the level of consciousness is dependent upon the number of feedback circuits in operation at a given time. Loss of consciousness, however, can be due to abnormal circumstances, and these can be divided into these categories:

1. Damage to the RAS

The proper functioning of the RAS may be interrupted by one or more of the following:

a. compressive lesions of the brain stem, e.g. by a cerebellar haematoma
b. infarction of or haemorrhage into the brain stem
c. disruptive lesions of the ascending connections between the RAS and cerebral cortex
d. depression of the RAS due to toxic substances such as drugs.

Interruption of the function of the RAS will lead to coma, in varying degrees depending upon prevailing circumstances.

2. Lesions of the cerebral cortex

Diffuse and extensive lesions such as those caused by an anoxic episode, will result in coma.

The medical management of the unconscious patient will vary according to the original cause, but fundamental to any care is the contribution and constant vigilance provided by the nursing staff. The totally dependent unconscious patient demands meticulous nursing care to ensure that vital functions are supported until a successful outcome from coma is achieved.

NURSING MANAGEMENT

An individualised approach to the nursing of the unconscious patient will greatly assist and enhance the care given. To illustrate the concepts involved in this approach the Roper, Logan & Tierney model for nursing, based on the activities of living, will be adapted to show how effective and worthwhile care can be implemented.

Maintaining a safe environment

The unconscious patient's ability to process sensory information is absent and this leads to a loss of normally functioning protective mechanisms. The two mechanisms principally affected which have implications for nursing practice are those protecting the eyes and the skin.

The corneal reflex is often absent in the unconscious patient which leaves the cornea exposed to damage by dryness and debris. Instillation of artificial teardrops and regular cleansing of the eyes with sterile normal saline, followed by taping down of the eyelids or application of an eyeshield is indicated. The condition of the patient's eyes will determine how often such care has to be given. The presence of infection, crusting or peri-orbital oedema will require more frequent attention. Some centres advocate the use of prophylactic ophthalmic antibiotic drops or ointment and these are instilled after the eyes are cleaned.

The lack of sensory input will also mean that the patient will be unaware of imminent danger from the external environment. The patient will not feel pressure on the side of his body as he lies immobile, and therefore will not be able to move and relieve potentially dangerous pressure. Likewise the use of heating devices such as hot water bottles are contra-indicated for similar reasons. In contrast, the restless patient who may be indiscriminately thrashing about the bed will require padded cot sides to prevent injury and may require constant supervision. The use of 'boxing glove' restraints on both hands may be required in order to prevent the patient from interfering with intravenous infusions, urinary catheters and head bandages.

Communicating

Communicating with the unconscious patient is a one-way process and the lack of response from the patient often results in the carer quickly giving up this activity. It is important that this is not allowed to happen. Conversing with the patient about everyday activities and topics such as the weather, his family and the current news is worthwhile. The patient's relatives will seek guidance on this and if they see the nurse talking to the patient quite normally this will encourage them to do likewise. A degree of controlled stimulation, e.g. music, for the patient is useful and so it is worthwhile asking the family about the patient's musical tastes, if any. Conversing with the patient in a normal speaking voice is essential; unconscious patients do not need to be shouted at or spoken to in baby talk to make them understand what is being said.

After recovering consciousness, many patients are able to recall with acute accuracy certain words or phrases which were spoken by staff caring for them. This reinforces the usefulness of conversations and a planned sensory input for the unconscious patient, and also serves to remind us that we should be guarded in our conversation lest the patient hears something which we do not intend him to.

The importance of touch should not be underestimated. The patient will receive a considerable amount of tactile stimulation in the course of his nursing care and relatives should be encouraged to do likewise when they visit. The importance of gentle handling while working with the patient, e.g. when turning, should be remembered. The patient is unable to express his feelings and reactions and it is important that we do not harm the patient while administering care. Some patients will indicate their discomfort with the use of non-verbal cues, and the nurse will quickly become adept at detecting these signals. Rest-lessness or an increase in heart rate and/or respirations may be indicative of pain.

Breathing

Maintenance of a patent airway in the unconscious patient must receive the utmost priority if adequate gaseous exchange within the lungs is to be facilitated. Positioning of the patient is crucial. The patient should be semi-prone, with a slight head up tilt (10–30°) to ensure that the patient's tongue does not fall back and obstruct his airway and to permit secretions to dribble out of the corner of the patient's mouth. If these measures are insufficient to maintain the airway, the use of artificial aids needs to be considered. This will be especially important in the patient with a depressed cough reflex. The simplest of these aids is the oropharyngeal or Guedel airway. These disposable plastic devices can be easily inserted and changed by a nurse. However, it should not be assumed that a patient's airway is patent, because they have an artificial airway in situ. The lumen of the airway can, if the secretions are particularly tenacious, be blocked thereby leading to obstruction. If the oropharyngeal airway proves to be inadequate, endotracheal intubation may be considered. The decision to intubate a patient lies with the doctor, although the nurse's observations will be taken into account. Endotracheal intubation is best performed as an elective procedure, in a department equipped for this task and with adequately trained staff.

Once it has been decided to perform intubation the procedure is explained to the

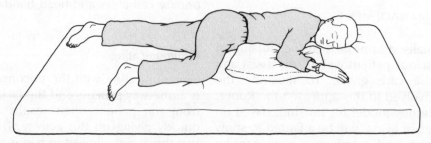

Fig. 4.1 Ideal position of patient to maintain patent airway.

patient, and reassurance must be given that he will be unable to speak while the tube is in place but that speech will return upon removal of the tube. The patient is placed in the supine position with his neck flexed. This is the only time that an unconscious patient is placed in this position, and during this time he is kept under close observation and never left unattended. The equipment for intubation should be prepared and checked; a non-functioning piece of equipment can lead to the difference between success or failure of the procedure or indeed could cost the patient his life.

If endotracheal intubation has to be prolonged beyond what is considered to be a safe period, tracheostomy may be indicated. This is a surgical opening in the anterior wall of the trachea, through the 2nd and 3rd or 3rd and 4th tracheal rings, to facilitate ventilation. The presence of a tracheostomy can itself lead to problems and further complications.

A respiratory assessment schedule should be instituted in the unconscious patient. The nurse should note the depth, rate, frequency and pattern of the patient's respirations, along with colour. Noisy breathing is obstructed breathing but obstructed breathing is not always noisy.

The nurse needs to be alert to the dangers that can be posed by the following factors:

Blood: bleeding into the oropharynx from, e.g. a chest injury could cause respiratory obstruction.

Vomitus: the patient with a full stomach and/or a depressed cough reflex is at particular risk of vomiting and possibly aspirating gastric contents into the lungs resulting in a deterioration in the patient's respiratory status. The insertion of a nasogastric tube and emptying of the patient's stomach in the early stages of the patient's coma, will help to avoid this.

Mucus: patients with a pre-existing chest disorder or history of heavy smoking may produce excess amounts of secretions which are often thick and tenacious. This may lead to respiratory obstruction. In order to remove

secretions, suctioning using an aseptic technique will be performed as often as required to maintain a patent airway. Routine 2 hourly or more frequent turning of the patient will assist with pulmonary drainage and toileting. Some centres advocate hyperinflating the patient's lungs with an Ambu bag on a regular basis, prior to suctioning and/or increasing the oxygen intake for 5 minutes prior to and following suctioning.

Dentures: if present, these should be removed in the initial stages in order to eliminate a possible cause of obstruction. However, in the long-term, a comatose patient's dentures can safely be inserted in order to improve the patient's general appearance.

Oxygen therapy is often prescribed for the unconscious patient and the nurse should administer it as directed. Determination of the amount of oxygen to be administered will depend upon the patient's arterial blood gases and respiratry status. Blood gases are drawn either by the doctor or in some departments by nursing staff. A sample of arterial blood is processed to determine the pH, the partial pressure of oxygen and carbon dioxide. Normal results are as follows:

pH   7.42
pCO_2 33–43 mmHg
pO_2 91–100 mmHg

Deviations from these parameters can be corrected in some circumstances by increasing or decreasing the amount of oxygen therapy that the patient receives. In most practical situations, however, a multifaceted approach to the patient's respiratory status is often adopted to correct deficiencies. It is important that the patient receives the correct amount of oxygen as indicated on his prescription sheet. This may involve using different oxygen delivery systems depending upon the patient's condition. Humidification of the patient's respiratory tract will prevent drying up of the secretions and facilitate easier removal by suctioning.

Prevention of infection of the respiratory tract falls within the remit of the nurse. Use of an aseptic technique during suctioning procedures is very important. One such protocol is as follows:

The nurse will first don a mask and a sterile glove. Sterile water is poured into a bowl to irrigate the dirty catheter afterwards.

A sterile catheter is selected and connected to the suction source. Using the ungloved hand, the nurse removes the patient's oxygen mask or cap over the swivel connector on the endotracheal or tracheostomy tube. The catheter is inserted as far as it will easily advance, no force should be applied. Suction is applied only while withdrawing the catheter which should be gently rotated between the thumb and forefinger. The catheter should be used once only and then discarded. The procedure is repeated until all the secretions are removed. The patient's mouth and nose are suctioned at the end of the procedure.

Cross infection is further reduced between patients if the nurse uses a meticulous handwashing technique between procedures.

The patient with a tracheostomy presents further potential infection problems, because the stoma requires to be treated as an open wound. This involves dressing it as often as is necessary, using an aseptic technique and the application of a sterile absorbent, non-adherent dressing following cleansing of the stoma with an antiseptic solution, according to local policy. Some centres advocate changing the disposable tracheostomy tube every few days in order to prevent infection.

Detection of any respiratory tract infections forms part of the assessment procedure. An increase in and/or change in the character of the secretions, an increased respiratory rate and pyrexia are all indicative of an infective process. A specimen of sputum is obtained for bacteriological examination. Treatment consists of the prescription and administration of antibiotics and active pulmonary toileting. The advice and practical assistance of the physiotherapist should be sought at each stage of the patient's respiratory care. Sometimes, despite these measures a number of patients will require ventilatory support in order to facilitate adequate gaseous exchange. This is achieved by artificially ventilating the patient via a sealed endotracheal or tracheostomy tube and a mechanical ventilator. Whenever this is necessary, the patient should be cared for in a department suitably equipped and staffed for this purpose.

Hypoxia is the most common cause of neurological deterioration and this serves to underline the importance of maintaining the patient in an optimum respiratory condition.

Eating and drinking

The maintenance of an adequate dietary and fluid intake in the unconscious patient is essential in order to preserve homeostasis and combat infections.

It was once thought that the calorie requirements of a severely injured patient needed to be increased during the recovery stage, but this is not so. The average male adult would probably require an intake of approximately 2500 calories/24 hours, although this would be adjusted according to circumstances. The patient with raised intracranial pressure may need to have his fluid intake restricted in order to underhydrate him. This would necessitate prescribing a feeding regime which permitted a sufficient intake of calories within a restricted fluid volume. It is important that the dietitian is involved in the patient's dietary care from an early stage.

A nutritional status profile should be coordinated by the nurse, so that an estimation of the patient's requirements and subsequent progress can be made. There are four parts to the profile, and these are as follows:

1. An estimation of the patient's weight loss. Knowledge of the patient's normal weight is required and either an estimation of his current weight or, if practical, the patient is weighed using sophisticated bed scales. From this information any weight loss can be determined.

2. An estimation of the patient's muscle mass and available fat stores is obtained by two measurements:

a. triceps skinfold measurement, achieved with the use of skin forceps
b. mid upper arm circumference, obtained by measuring the girth of the upper arm at the mid point.

If parenteral nutrition is being considered, the following additional information is needed:

3. Estimation of serum urea and electrolytes, glucose, liver function tests, albumin, calcium, phosphate, magnesium, pre-albumin, osmolality, creatinine and red cell folate level.

4. Routine ward urinalysis, and, in particular, glucose and acetone detection. Specimens of urine are also collected for osmolality and creatinine levels along with a 24-hour collection for urea and electrolytes.

Information for parts 1,2 and 4 of the profile are collected by the nurse and blood samples for part 3 are obtained by the doctor. Once the information is available, it is collated, preferably on a single chart designated for this purpose in order that an appropriate regime can be designed for a particular patient's needs. There are many different enteral feeding regimes in existence and there are now various pre-prepared proprietary feeds available. Regimes will vary according to local policy and the nurse caring for the unconscious patient should be aware of the content of the patient's feed. In order to minimise weight loss in the unconscious patient it is imperative that a feeding protocol is started as quickly as possible, and certainly within 48 hours from the onset of coma. Every unconscious patient should have his fluid balance carefully monitored and recorded on a fluid balance chart.

Methods of feeding

Two basic methods of feeding the unconscious patient are available. The simpler and more natural of the two methods is enteral feeding facilitating the use of a nasogastric tube. Oral fluids are completely contraindicated in the unconscious patient, owing to impairment or absence of the cough and/or swallow reflex. Nasogastric feeding is often advocated as the method of choice for several reasons:

— utilises the gastrointestinal tract in its normal function
— can be instituted and performed by the nurse
— does not require direct medical supervision
— has fewer potential complications than parenteral nutrition
— less expensive than parenteral nutrition.

A nasogastric tube will probably already be in place, having been inserted for the purpose of emptying the patient's stomach, in order to prevent vomiting, in the early stages of coma. An alternative to the conventional nasogastric tube is the fine bore feeding tube which is now available. Such tubes are purported to be more comfortable for the patient, although they can be considerably more difficult to pass. If the patient has a history of head injury, it is necessary to check that he does not have a basal skull fracture. Passage of a nasogastric tube via the nasal route is contraindicated in these patients for fear of penetrating the fracture site and, whenever doubt exists as to the presence of such a fracture, the oral route must be used.

Once the nasogastric tube has been passed, its placement in the stomach should be confirmed by the usual methods, and always prior to each feed. The tube must be anchored to the patient's face in order to prevent slippage and if an adhesive fastener or tape is used, this needs to be changed routinely to prevent excoriation of the skin. Rotation of the tube will discourage the formation of crusts and/or pressure necrosis at the point where it leaves the patient's nose or mouth. The gastric contents are aspirated prior to each feed in order to determine whether the previous fluid has been tolerated. Most centres will have a local policy on this issue; some will advocate that if the aspirate exceeds a certain amount, no further feed should be given and as the aspirate is a valuable source of electrolytes, it should be returned to the patient. Others may advocate discarding the aspirate and feeding the patient with a fresh solution. The nurse is advised to check her own unit's policy. In order to minimise the risk of vomiting, the patient is fed in either the semi-prone or head up position.

Enteral feeds can be given either as a bolus, in which the quantity of the feed is given at timed intervals, e.g. a 24-hour intake of 2400 ml could be given as 8 bolus feeds of 300 ml, or the feed may be administered using a slow continuous drip method. A quantity of feed, say, 1000 ml is made up and hung in an appropriate infusion container and allowed to drip with the aid of gravity at a predetermined rate. Alternatively the use of a feeding pump may be considered, in which case a quantity of feed is made up and the rate of flow pre-set by the pump. The continuous feeding method is often used in conjunction with a fine bore tube, although this precludes the ability to test or quantify gastric aspirate.

An alternative to the nasogastric tube is the gastrostomy tube, although this is rarely used. A surgical incision is made in the abdominal wall through which a large bore tube is passed directly into the stomach. Feeding a patient via a gastrostomy tube is similar in many respects to any other method and the usual precautions are adopted prior to feeding.

The second and more complex method of providing nutrition for the unconscious patient is by the use of hyperalimentation. This would be indicated in those patients for whom feeding via the nasogastric route had consistently failed. It requires the placement of a central line, as the constituent fluids are irritant to the sensitive lining of the peripheral veins. The feeding will be determined by the medical staff. Most fluids contain hypertonic dextrose as a calorie source, amino acids as a source of nitrogen and electrolytes, multi-vitamins and trace elements. Several brands of appropriate parenteral fluids are available and these are selected according to the doctor's preference. The patient needs to have regular blood chemistry performed while the regime is in progress, in order to establish the feeding status. Problems pertaining to parenteral nutrition centre around those of infec-

tion and metabolic reaction to the infused solution. Parenteral nutrition is the most complicated method of feeding and should only be performed in those departments equipped to deal with it and with staff who are familiar with techniques and possible complications.

Intravenous fluids

Peripheral intravenous fluids may be indicated in some patients for electrolyte and fluid imbalances. It is important that the nurse monitors the patient's vital signs during infusion and is alert to signs of overinfusion. The cannula site is inspected at frequent intervals for inflammation and the nurse must ensure that the correct fluids are hung and infused at the proper rate. An accurate record of fluid balance is required.

Eliminating

Bladder

Despite the acknowledged dangers of urinary bladder catheterisation, performance of this procedure should be undertaken in the early stages of coma, and certainly within 18–24 hours of onset. It permits an accurate record of urinary output to be maintained, which may be especially important in the patient receiving osmotic diuretic therapy and avoids local irritation and possibly serious breakdown of the skin. The danger of urinary tract infection cannot, of course, be underestimated, and the nurse must endeavour to minimise this risk as far as possible. A urinary catheter management protocol could consist of:

— strict aseptic technique for the insertion of the catheter. Selection of the correct size is important in order to avoid bypassing of urine.
— scrupulous catheter care should be performed every 4 hours, according to unit policy.
— system should remain closed, with breaches only permitted for absolutely essential purposes.

— use a urine bag with a valve to permit drainage of urine without disconnection. Each patient should have his own container for this purpose and it should be sterilised between emptyings. The instillation of an antiseptic solution into the emptied bag is recommended. The catheter should be taped to the thigh to prevent urethral traction. Collections of urine within dependent loops of tubing is discouraged by attaching the tubing to the bed.

— drainage bag is situated below the level of the bladder to provide for an efficient, free flow of urine. The bag should not be placed on the bed, for example, when the patient is being transported to another department.

— carry out regular bacteriological monitoring of urine.

— educate all members of the caring team about the importance of preventing infection in the catheterised patient, and in particular, the role of good handwashing techniques.

If coma is prolonged consideration must be given to removing the urinary catheter at the earliest opportunity and replacing it, in the case of a male patient, with an external penile collection device such as a Uro-dome. Unfortunately an equivalent device does not exist for female patients. If it is possible that the patient can be bladder trained, this should be encouraged. Urinals or bedpans should not be left in place for prolonged periods of time but rather should be offered to the patient on a regular, frequent basis. Mishaps will occur often at the start of such a regime, but perseverance usually pays dividends and the patient can be 'trained' to urinate at specific times of the day. An accurate record of urinary output should be kept for all unconscious patients.

Bowels

The maintenance of regular bowel movements can be a difficult problem to overcome in the unconscious patient. The lack of roughage in the diet and inactivity lead readily to constipation and impaction. The use of laxatives in an aggressive bowel management protocol is virtually essential in every case. In order to avoid major problems this needs to be considered at an early stage. The use of an enema is contra-indicated in the patient who is suspected of having raised intracranial pressure, as its use will initiate Valsalva's manoeuvre, resulting in a further rise in intracranial pressure. A record of the patient's bowel motions should be maintained.

Personal cleansing and dressing

A daily bed bath is essential for the unconscious patient and this may need to be performed more often if the patient is incontinent or prone to excessive perspiration. The opportunity is taken at this time to inspect the patient's skin, particularly over bony prominences, to ensure that it is intact. Any breakdown in the integrity of the skin will lead to pressure sore formation which will impede the patient's recovery and delay rehabilitation. The identification of patients 'at risk' through the use of a scoring system, such as the Douglas scale, will assist in alerting the nurse to the patient's vulnerability to skin breakdown. Two hourly positional changes will ensure that the vital skin microcirculation is unimpeded by pressure. Any reddening area which does not 'recover' its usual colour once pressure is relieved must be left pressure free until such time as it does. It is important that the reddening stage does not pass unobserved; the unrecovered reddened area is the first stage in the process toward skin breakdown and pressure sore formation. Dryness of the skin may occur, and the application of a lubricant cream will help to alleviate this. Male patients should be shaved each day.

Finger and toe nails should be kept short and clean; this is particularly pertinent in those patients who clench their fists tightly. Hair should be washed and combed as required.

Oral hygiene is performed 2–4 hourly

depending upon the condition of the patient's mouth. Many unconscious patients breathe through their mouth or may be receiving oxygen therapy, both of which have the effect of drying the mucous membranes, increasing the patient's susceptibility to oral infections and ulceration. Attention should be directed toward the teeth which are brushed twice daily with toothpaste. In the early critical stages of coma dentures are removed as they may constitute a danger to the airway. In the long-term comatosed patient, dentures can be inserted in order to improve the patient's general appearance.

Controlling body temperature

Many unconscious patients experience a rise in body temperature either due to infection as a result of lowered resistance or damage to the temperature regulating centre in the hypothalamus following head injury. The implications of this are serious; for each degree of risen temperature a proportionate increase in oxygen demand is also made. In the patient whose oxygen supply is crucial this can have devastating effects, bearing in mind that the most common cause of neurological deterioration is hypoxia.

It therefore becomes essential to reduce the patient's body temperature to within normal levels as soon as possible. Various techniques are available and will be used according to the preference of the medical staff. The following are some measures that may be adopted:

— tepid sponging with or without the addition of a small amount of alcohol solution in the bath water
— administration of aspirin suppositories
— nursing the patient naked and with as few bedclothes as possible but ensure that the patient's dignity is maintained
— use of cooling rooms which blow cold air into the atmosphere around the patient or less effectively, a cold air fan (this must not be pointed at the patient's eyes).

Control of body temperature reduction methods must be exercised; if the patient begins to shiver in response to cooling measures this will produce a further rise in body temperature creating more danger for the patient. While the temperature remains elevated, the patient is at increased risk of dehydration and therefore an increase in the fluid intake may be ordered by the doctor.

Hypothermia can occur in some circumstances. Following surgery some patients will demonstrate a subnormal temperature and they will have to be warmed gradually until normal body temperature is achieved.

Mobilising

Careful positioning of the unconscious patient is essential in order to aid rehabilitation. Maintaining the body in straight alignment with paralysed or weakened limbs supported will help to prevent contractures, loss of muscle tone, foot and wrist drop and joint injury. Proper positioning encourages good chest expansion. Difficulty will be experienced with restless patients, who will move from the optimum position as quickly as they are placed in it.

In this instance returning the patient to his original position is all that can be done. Passive range of movement exercises are performed on the patient with each of the joints being put through its full range of movement, two or three times each day. The physiotherapist will be involved in this aspect of patient care and the nurse will supplement the exercise programme.

Working and playing

It is important, for the reasons already outlined, that the patient is assisted in his recovery from unconsciousness in order that he may return to his occupation and resume previous hobbies with as little inconvenience as possible. Long absences from work may create financial and social hardships for the patient's family and the help of the medical social worker may be required.

Expressing sexuality

The unconscious patient is unable to express feelings and desires. The menstruating female patient will require special attention and intimate parts of the body will have to be touched at this time. The nurse should remember this and maintain the patient's dignity at all times.

Sleeping

An important part of the process of returning the patient to consciousness is assessment of conscious level. This can be easily performed using a standardised system such as the Glasgow coma scale. It logically evaluates three modes of behaviour, i.e. eye opening, verbal response and motor response, and provides an indication of overall brain dysfunction. Results are recorded on a convenient bedside chart, which also includes a section to record other parameters including vital signs, observation of pupil size and reaction, and limb movements. This produces an indication of local abnormalities. Elaboration of this system can be found in Chapter 2. The frequency of the observations are determined by the nurse in charge according to the patient's condition but observations are usually made 2–4 hourly.

Dying

While the unconscious patient's feelings regarding death and dying cannot be elicited, the nurse must consider and support the role played by the relatives and significant others. A dying unconscious patient will present practical and psychological problems for the relatives; an awareness of these by the nurse will allow her to deal effectively with them as they arise.

Many relatives experience feelings of helplessness and are often understandably unsure how to behave in these circumstances. Occasionally relatives will request to perform an act of nursing care in order to reduce this feeling of helplessness and this should, within reason, be encouraged and facilitated. The relatives should be told that their visits are worthwhile and they should be permitted access to the patient as frequently as possible.

Once the reality of the situation becomes apparent many questions will arise and the nurse should answer these honestly and sympathetically within the bounds of her responsibility. Relatives will require repeated reassurances and explanations and need to feel free to express fears and doubts without reproach from the nurse.

The need to prepare relatives for the death of their loved one is essential, especially in the case of the patient who is declared brain dead. These relatives will require sympathetic handling and the news given to them at the appropriate moment and under proper circumstances. Often a nurse will accompany the doctor when this is being done. Painful decisions require to be made prior to the switching off of life support machinery and an understanding of these decisions will help in supporting not only the relatives but also one's colleagues caring for the patient.

DIFFERENTIAL DIAGNOSIS

Occasionally, some patients will appear to be in coma but are in fact in a state of markedly reduced responsiveness. Several syndromes have been identified, including:

The locked-in syndrome: in which the motor pathways in the ventral pons are interrupted by, for example, infarction. The patient is tetraplegic and mute but continues to be responsive. Communication is only possible by developing a limited code consisting of eye blinking.

Vegetative state: this may occur as a result of diffuse cerebral hypoxia or ischaemia or extensive damage to the white matter connecting the cortex to the arousal centres of the brain stem. This results in a spontaneously breathing patient who lies with his eyes open and demonstrates day and night sleep rhythms. The patient does not speak and may show primitive grasp reflexes when stimulated. The vegetative state can persist for a considerable period of time, with the patient making no further progress from this stage.

Brain death

The new procedures and complex machinery in today's highly technological intensive care units have been responsible for saving many patient's lives. However, we have now produced an unfortunate and unique group of patients who later prove to be brain dead. The confirmation of brain death is a vitally

important and profound concept. Continuing heroic treatment and resuscitation measures beyond a reasonable point prevents death with dignity and needlessly prolongs the distress of the patient's family. It is also judged to be an inappropriate use of staff and facilities.

The criteria for determining brain death in the UK is that laid down by the Medical Royal Colleges and their faculties. Consideration of brain death cannot take place until at least 6 hours have elapsed since the onset of coma and should not be made if the cause is unknown. The criteria consists of two principal parts; the second part, the test for action

---

Diagnosis to be made by two doctors, one a Consultant and the other a Consultant or Senior Registrar.

Diagnosis should not be considered until at least 6 hours after the onset of coma; 12–24 hours will be more usual.

Name ....   Unit No ....

Pre-conditions   Time of event leading to
Nature of irremediable brain damage   Coma
Dr A ....
Dr B ....
Do you consider that apnoeic coma is due   *Dr A*   *Dr B*
to:
    Depressant drugs
    Neuromuscular blocking (relaxant) drugs
    Hypothermia
    Metabolic or endocrine disturbances

Tests for absence of brain stem function
Is there evidence of: *Dr A*   *Dr B*
    Pupil reaction to light
    Corneal reflex
    Eye movements with cold caloric test
    Cranial nerve motor response
    Gag reflex
    Respiratory movements on
    disconnection from ventilator to allow
    adequate rise in $PaCO_2$

Date and time of First Testing ....
Date and time of Second Testing ....

Dr A   *Dr B*
Signature ....   Signature ....
Status ....   Status ....

Fig. 4.2 Criteria for diagnosis of brain death

of brain stem function, cannot be performed until the stated pre-conditions are fulfilled.

The pre-conditions include ascertaining beyond all reasonable doubt the nature of the irremediable brain damage and the time of the event leading to coma. The doctor must satisfy himself that temporary depression of the brain stem reflexes has not occurred as the result of the ingestion of a large quantity of depressant drugs in an overdose, the use of neuromuscular blocking agents to facilitate mechanical ventilation, hypothermia or the presence of a severe metabolic or endocrinological disturbance, such as uncontrollable diabetes.

The second part of the criteria consists of testing for the presence of brain stem reflexes. The pupillary reaction to light is tested; a non-reactive pupil indicates loss of the reflex. Before accepting this result, it must be established that paralytic eye drops have not been instilled to aid examination of the fundi. Loss of the light reflex could be due to a third nerve palsy or optic nerve damage. The corneal reflex is tested, as is also the cranial nerve motor response and gag reflex. Absence of function indicates depression of the reflex. Cranial stimuli such as pressure over the supra-orbital ridge must be included, because a cervical cord injury may co-exist with head injury and impair the response to stimuli below the neck.

The oculovestibular reflex is tested by injecting 20 ml of ice cold water into each ear in turn, following confirmatory visualisation of the tympanic membrane. If the brain stem is still functioning a deviation of the eyes to the stimulated side occurs.

The presence of apnoea is determined by several tests. The patient is disconnected from the ventilator to allow the $PaCO_2$ to rise to a threshold level1 (50 mmHg); this provides maximum stimulus to breathe. While the patient is disconnected, he is oxygenated via a tracheal catheter at 6L/minute to maintain tissue perfusion and avoid hypoxia. The chest wall is observed closely for any movement indicative of respiratory effort.

If the patient fulfils the criteria, he is not considered dead, until examined by a second doctor who repeats the process. Both doctors sign, time and date the necessary forms.

BIBLIOGRAPHY

Allan D 1984 Patients with an ET or tracheostomy tube. Nursing Times 80(13):36
Allan D 1982 Nursing aspects of artificial ventilation. Nursing Times 78(24):1006
Allan D 1984 Brain death. Nursing 2(23):671
Allan D 1984 Glasgow coma scale. Nursing Mirror 158(23):32
Allan D 1984 Patient care in hyperalimentation. Nursing Times 80(18):28
Borsig A, Steinacker I 1982 Communication with the patient in the intensive care unit. Nursing Times 78(12):2 (supplement)
Diagnosis of brain death. Statement issued by the secretary of the Conference of Medical Royal Colleges and their Faculties in the UK on 11 October 1976. British Medical Journal 2:1187
Faulkner A 1985 Nursing — a creative approach. Baillière Tindall, London
Hickey J 1986 The clinical practice of neurological and neurosurgical nursing. J B Lippincott, Philadelphia
Jenner E A et al 1983 Catheterisation and urinary tract infection. Nursing (supplement) 2:13
Jennett B 1981 Brain death. British Journal of Anaesthesia 53 (11):1111
Jennett B, Teasdale G 1981 Management of head injuries. F A Davis, Philadelphia
Maus-Clum N 1982 Bringing the unconscious patient back safely. Nursing 12(8):34
Miller M 1981 Emergency management of the unconscious patient. Nursing Clinics of North America 16(1):59
Myco F, McGilloway F A 1980 Care of the unconscious patient: a complementary perspective. Journal of Advanced Nursing 5:273
Nikas D 1982 The critically ill neurosurgical patient. Churchill Livingstone, New York
Pritchard V 1986 Calculating the risk (Douglas Scale). Nursing Times 82(8):59
Purchese G, Allan D 1984 Neuromedical and neurosurgical nursing. Baillière Tindall, London
Roper N, Logan W, Tierney A 1985 The elements of nursing, 2nd edn. Churchill Livingstone, Edinburgh
Tortora G J, Anagnostakos N P 1981 Principles of anatomy and physiology. Harper and Row, London

5

Raised intracranial pressure

Intracranial pressure (ICP) is the measurable pressure exerted by the brain tissue, blood and cerebrospinal fluid (CSF) within the rigid bony skull. For the majority of individuals it is automatically maintained within a set of normal limits rising in response to such activities as coughing or stooping and returning to its normal level thereafter. However, this simple statement belies the complex inter-relationship between the main structural components and other external factors and influences which exist within and outwith the human body, to maintain and in some instances, adversely affect, intracranial pressure.

The normal range of intracranial pressure is considered to be between 0–10 mmHg; levels over 15 mmHg are deemed to be abnormal. It is convenient to consider measurements of intracranial pressure in mmHg as this permits critical correlation with arterial pressure.

PHYSIOLOGY OF INTRACRANIAL PRESSURE

An alteration of, or addition to, the volume of one of the non-compressible components, i.e. brain tissue, blood or cerebrospinal fluid, due to disease or trauma, within the confined space of the rigid adult skull, will result in displacement of the other two, leading to a rise in intracranial pressure. This in essence is an appropriate interpretation of the modified Monro-Kellie hypothesis and assists in understanding the pathophysiology of intracranial pressure.

The three main intracranial components involved are the brain, the largest constituent accounting for 80–85% of the volume, the circulating cerebrospinal fluid constituting 10–15% and blood 5–7%. Knowledge of these components at this stage is useful as it will help to identify and explain the causes of raised intracranial pressure, discussed later in this chapter.

Volume pressure relationship

As intracranial pressure begins to rise, compensatory mechanisms will be utilised initially to accommodate a degree of compression within the skull. However, at a critical moment the intracranial pressure will start to rise dramatically with only minor increases in intracranial volume; this is as a result of a rise in intracranial elastance. Intracranial elastance plays a crucial role in intracranial pressure. It is the element that determines cerebrospinal fluid volume and pressure at which the production and subsequent absorption of cerebrospinal fluid is maintained in a state of equilibrium. The walls of the cerebrospinal fluid compartments and pathways possess a degree of elasticity which accommodates changes in order to maintain homeostasis. If the degree of elasticity is reduced, and the compartmental walls become more rigid, this will result in an increase in intracranial pressure, as the ability of the system to adapt to change is overcome. This is sometimes referred to as the 'tight brain' syndrome.

The significance of elastance will now become apparent if the volume/pressure graph is reviewed again. There are small increases in intracranial pressure as a result of an increase in volume as indicated in the compensated (flattened) part of the curve, However, when the same increase in volume is created at a later point, the increase in intracranial pressure is more dramatic. There are progressive increases in elastance as a space occupying lesion expands; thus creating the volume/pressure response. Several factors can influence intracranial elastance, e.g. hypercapnia ($PaCO_2 > 40$ mmHg), hypoxia ($PaO_2 < 50$ mmHg) and REM sleep will lead to increased elastance (and therefore increased intracranial pressure); hypothermia and the use of barbiturates will result in decreased elastance. This is important for the nurse caring for the patient with an abnormal intracranial pressure.

Of the three components involved, it is believed that cerebrospinal fluid is the one that is most frequently and easily displaced as intracranial pressure begins to rise in response to the presence of an expanding intracranial space occupying lesion. The displaced cerebrospinal fluid is accommodated in the distensible spinal dural sac in the initial period. This displacement of cerebrospinal fluid is only one of several factors which constitute part of the compensatory mechanisms involved in the early stages of raised intracranial pressure. Four stages have been identified:

Stage 1 The compensation phase: there is no rise in intracranial pressure, and conscious level remains unaltered.

Stage 2 The early phase of reversible decompensation: a slight increase in brain mass will produce an elevated intracranial pressure. Early signs of de-

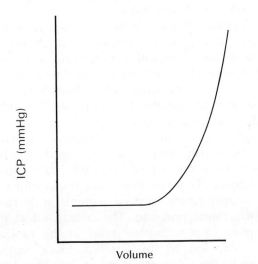

Fig. 5.1 Relationship between intracranial pressure and volume of space occupying lesion.

terioration in conscious level noted.

Stage 3 The late phase of reversible decompensation: intracranial pressure now very high and conscious level deteriorating rapidly. Detrimental changes occur in the respiratory rate and pattern. Intracranial pressure will soon equal mean arterial pressure with, ultimately, cessation of cerebral blood flow.

Stage 4 The irreversible decompensation phase: in which further deterioration leading to death will occur if intervention is not initiated.

Cerebral blood flow (CBF)

A critical relationship exists between cerebral blood flow and intracranial pressure. The cerebral blood flow is essential for the supply of oxygen and other nutrients to the cerebral tissues in order to maintain function. This is an accurately controlled system, the mechanics of which are still not fully understood. It has however been clearly demonstrated that cerebral blood flow is disadvantaged in the presence of raised intracranial pressure. Cerebral perfusion pressure (CPP) is the pressure required to maintain an adequate cerebral blood flow, ensuring proper perfusion of the brain cells and therefore their continued function. It is dependent upon the opposing difference between the incoming systemic arterial pressure and the intracranial pressure. This implies that if we are aware of the patient's blood pressure and intracranial pressure we can calculate the cerebral perfusion pressure with the following equation:

Mean arterial pressure — Intracranial pressure = Cerebral perfusion pressure

Therefore if the mean arterial pressure is 90 mmHg and the intracranial pressure 10 mmHg, the cerebral perfusion pressure would be 80 mmHg. These are normal parameters for a healthy adult. However, if we look at the example of a hypotensive multiple head injured patient the results are considerably different. Assuming a mean arterial pressure

of 63 mmHg (obtained by adding the diastolic pressure to one-third of the pulse pressure, in a blood pressure of 90/50) and an abnormally high intracranial pressure of 50 mmHg, cerebral perfusion pressure is now 13 mmHg; any pressures below 30 mmHg cause cessation of cerebral blood flow and death of vital brain cells.

Autoregulation, the automatic adjustment of blood vessel diameter, is an important factor involved in maintaining a constant cerebral blood flow during changes in cerebral perfusion pressure. A hypertensive episode within the systemic arterial system would cause the cerebral blood vessels to decrease their diameter which causes a proportionate increase in pressure within the vessel. The vasoconstriction acts as a protective mechanism, as the rise in pressure has been reduced from what it would be if the full impact of the raised systemic arterial pressure was brought directly to bear on cerebral tissue. Conversely hypotension produces vasodilation which increases the size of the blood vessel diameter. Alterations in systemic arterial pressure have little or no effect on cerebral venous pressure. Unfortunately, the controlling mechanism of autoregulation only operates within certain limits and, once a critical stage is reached, it may cease to function effectively. It can be impaired by ischaemia, hypoxia or hypercapnia.

Carbon dioxide, which is a potent vasodilator, can produce untoward effects on cerebral blood flow and subsequently, intracranial pressure. The process of cell metabolism is constantly producing carbon dioxide which is passed into the blood for disposal. The carbon dioxide level in blood may be raised even higher as a result of hypercapnia. This could conceivably occur as retained tracheal secretions impair respiratory efficiency, causing hypoxia. This has important implications for the respiratory care of patients with raised intracranial pressure. The overall effect of a raised carbon dioxide level in the blood is vasodilation of the cerebral blood vessels, producing an increase in cerebral blood flow and exacerbation of intracranial hypertension.

Cerebral oedema

The final consideration in the physiological aspects of intracranial pressure is the effect of cerebral oedema. Cerebral oedema can precipitate a rise in intracranial pressure or exacerbate pre-existing intracranial hypertension. It occurs as a direct result of trauma to the brain tissue following head injury or surgery or in response to pathophysiological changes, as found in the presence of a cerebral tumour or infarction. Areas of oedematous tissues are usually localised to the region of trauma or change.

Two different types of oedema are thought to occur; the first, and most common, is vasogenic oedema. An abnormality in the cerebral blood vessel walls is thought to permit an increased outflow of fluid which accumulates in the precious extracellular spaces. The larger protein molecules are forced out between the cells of the blood brain barrier along with electrolytes, the process being accelerated in the presence of increased arterial pressure. This breach occurs across the normally, closely regulated and highly organised blood-brain barrier where even the smallest molecules are rarely permitted to cross over, under normal circumstances. Vasogenic oedema predominates in the white matter. Cytotoxic oedema, wich is not so common, tends to be confined to the grey matter. The mechanism involved is not entirely understood.

The implications for the patient with an already compromised intracranial pressure are serious. The increase in the overall bulk of the cerebral tissue leads to further rises in intracranial pressure, which may lead to further complications such as transtentorial herniation. The danger period for the patient is 2–4 days following the onset of oedema, the degree of oedema being directly proportionate to the severity of the trauma or extent of the disease.

CAUSES OF RAISED INTRACRANIAL PRESSURE

The principal causes of intracranial hypertension can be conveniently subdivided according to the three components, i.e. the brain, blood and cerebrospinal fluid.

Brain

An increase in the brain tissue volume such as that caused by an expanding intracranial lesion and/or cerebral oedema will produce raised intracranial pressure as a result.

Cerebrospinal fluid

Increased production, decreased absorption or blockage of a cerebrospinal fluid pathway will lead to hydrocephalus resulting in a raised intracranial pressure.

Blood

Cerebral blood flow may be increased as a result of hypoxia and/or hypercapnia leading to congestion within the cerebral circulation culminating in a raised intracranial pressure. This would occur as a result of inadequate care of the patient's airway.

HERNIATION OF BRAIN TISSUE

When two compartments of adjoining areas of pressure differences occur, there is a strong likelihood that the tissue contained within the area of high pressure will become compressed and herniate through any opening that may be present into the area of low pressure. Just such a situation can occur in the presence of an expanding space occupying lesion which will exert pressure on cerebral tissue as a result of brain shift and produce further deterioration in the patient's conscious level due to compression and herniation of vital structures.

In order to categorise the different types of herniation the cranial cavity can be divided into the supratentorial and infratentorial compartments. The supratentorial compartment, as the name implies, comprises the region above the tentorium, and the opening which facilitates, under appropriate circumstances, supratentorial herniation is termed the tentorial notch. The infratentorial compartment is that part below the tentorium where the cerebellum is located. The opening which permits herniation is the foramen magnum. Each of the herniation syndromes produces characteristic clinical signs depending upon the site of the lesion.

Supratentorial herniation

There are two classifications of supratentorial herniation: central tentorial and lateral transtentorial herniation.

Central tentorial herniation

The downward displacement of the cerebral hemispheres, diencephalon and midbrain in symmetrical herniation through the tentorium can be produced by a supratentorial midline lesion, simultaneously compressing bilateral lesions or generalised swelling. The displaced tissue is relocated in the posterior fossa. The nerves and posterior cerebral arteries are stretched, as they are fixed from above. Compression of the occulomotor nerve produces clinical signs involving eye movements and occlusion of the artery may result in haemorrhagic infarction of the affected area. The subsequent increase in pressure within the posterior fossa may produce a further downward displacement of the cerebellar tonsils, creating an uncal herniation.

The signs and symptoms of central tentorial herniation are fairly characteristic and occur in a progressive fashion; the effects of pressure on the diencephalon are noted first, followed by those on the midbrain, pons and lastly the medulla. Therefore, in the early stages, the patient will display drowsiness or agitation, pupils will be small and reactive and he may have a contralateral hemiparesis. As the herniation progresses, the patient will have difficulty with upward gaze, conscious level will have deteriorated further and there may be impairment of respiration. In the final sequence pupils will dilate and become fixed, the extra-ocular signs will remain, deep coma will supervene, Cheyne-Stokes respiration will be evident (eventually resulting in apnoea), limbs will become unresponsive to painful stimulus, temperature is elevated, pulse will increase and then gradually decrease with an associated fall in blood pressure. Death eventually results if herniation is allowed to proceed unchecked.

Lateral transtentorial herniation

An expanding lesion located in or very close to the temporal lobe located in the middle fossa will produce lateral and downward displacement. The uncus and hippocampus, which is the medial part of the temporal lobe, are forced down into the cisterna ambiens, causing compression and displacement of the diencephalon and midbrain. While the endpoint is the same as for central tentorial herniation the preceding signs and symptoms are different.

In the early stages, conscious level remains unchanged, but the patient may become restless and agitated. The most significant and characteristic sign is an ipsilateral dilated pupil which reacts sluggishly to light and possibly ptosis. This occurs as a result of entrapment of the nerve and posterior cerebral artery, between the swollen uncus and the tentorium falx cerebelli. This occurs on the same side as the expanding lesion. As the herniation continues there is a dramatic deterioration in conscious level, the ipsilateral dilated pupil becomes non-reactive and the ptosis more pronounced. Eventually both pupils become fixed and dilated. The patient will develop a contralateral hemiparesis which progresses to a hemiplegia. It is interesting to note that a false localising sign may occur. This results from compression of the cerebral peduncle against the tentorium on the opposite side to the herniating uncus, producing a hemiparesis on the same side as the lesion. This is termed Kernohan's notch.

The end stages of herniation will also cause Cheyne-Stokes respirations which will eventually lead to apnoea, bradycardia and elevated systolic blood pressure and a hyperpyrexia.

Infratentorial herniation

This less frequently occurring type of herniation most often results from a lesion in the posterior fossa which in turn bears down on the cerebellum, forcing the cerebellar tonsils into the foramen magnum, where compression of the medulla ensues. It is in the medulla that vital centres are located for respiratory and cardiac function and damage to these areas because of oedema, ischaemia or infarction can result in respiratory and cardiac arrest. Infratentorial lesions are known to encroach upon part of the ventricular system causing hydrocephalus.

HYDROCEPHALUS

Hydrocephalus is characterised by an increase in the volume of cerebrospinal fluid within the ventricular system, which may or may not be under increased pressure (see Ch. 1 for normal CSF production process). This section will deal with hydrocephalus in adults, and the reader is referred to Chapter 15 for elaboration of this condition in children. In adults, abnormalities can occur at three different stages in the cerebral CSF circulation.

1. CSF may be overproduced
2. An abnormality in, or encroaching on, the pathways results in a blockage
3. Decreased absorption.

Different methods are used to classify hydrocephalus, but essentially there are two important ones which are often used together. Hydrocephalus may be described as communicating or non-communicating (obstructive).

In communicating hydrocephalus all the ventricular spaces freely communicate with each other and so the cause is usually due to overproduction of CSF or faulty re-absorption. Overproduction may be caused by a tumour within the choroid plexus (papilloma), although this is rare. Decreased absorption is more likely and may be caused as a result of subarachnoid haemorrhage, when blood blocks the arachnoid villi, thereby preventing effective absorption.

Non-communicating hydrocephalus implies that free communication is not possible and an obstructive lesion, e.g. a tumour, may

Table 5.1 Classification of hydrocephalus

Acquired	Intracranial haemorrhage	Broken down blood products block absorption by the arachnoid villi
	Infection	Purulent exudate blocks absorption by the arachnoid villi
	Trauma (traumatic subarachnoid haemorrhage)	Broken down blood products block absorption by the arachnoid villi
	Neoplasm	Tumour will obstruct the narrow ventricular pathways
Congenital	Neoplasm	As above
	Malformations Arnold-Chiari	A downward displacement of the fourth ventricle and medulla resulting in obliteration of the cisterna magna
	Aqueduct stenosis	Narrowing of the aqueduct of the midbrain which impedes CSF flow
	Cysts	Cysts will obstruct the narrow CSF pathways

block one of the pathways causing a damming effect, resulting in dilated ventricles and a rise in ICP. This obstruction occurs between the point of production of the CSF (choroid plexus) and the foramina of Luschka and Magendie. Hydrocephalus in adults, therefore, should be viewed as a clinical syndrome rather than as a disease entity. The second classification is based upon whether the hydrocephalus is acquired or congenital. Obviously most of the congenital causes will be seen in childhood, although some of them do not manifest themselves until early adulthood. Table 5.1 summarises how each of these conditions can arise.

Diagnosis of hydrocephalus is usually by CT scanning, when enlarged ventricles will be noted. Prior to this, signs and symptoms of raised ICP and the presence of characteristic features on skull X-ray will arouse the clinician's suspicion. Signs and symptoms will include those of raised ICP (usually associated with non-communicating hydrocephalus). In communicating hydrocephalus, a more protracted pattern is seen, comprising dementia, disturbances of gait and balance and incontinence of urine.

Treatment will include the insertion of a shunt to bypass the system and/or removal of the cause of the hydrocephalus. Shunts divert the flow of CSF from the ventricles to either the peritoneum or atrium (for more detailed information on shunts see Ch. 15). Stenosis of the aqueduct of the midbrain is treated by diverting the CSF into the cisterna magna (Torkildsen's procedure). Initially, a temporary external drainage system may be used until the primary problem is dealt with. Elaboration of the treatment and the nursing care are discussed later in this chapter.

Normal pressure hydrocephalus, a particular type of hydrocephalus, usually presents in the elderly with signs of raised ICP, dementia, incontinence and disturbance of gait but when CSF pressure is measured it is found to be within normal limits (80–180 mm of water). CT scanning will demonstrate enlarged ventricles with periventricular lutency but the sulci are not separated. Normal pressure hydrocephalus is usually of the communicating type and may follow head injury, subarachnoid haemorrhage, craniotomy or meningitis and in some patients no preceding cause can be identified. In addition to CT scanning, lumbar CSF infusion studies may be performed. These involve introducing artificial CSF via a lumbar puncture, at twice the normal production rate. Under normal circumstances the patient can cope by adapting to the increase in volume of CSF but the patient with normal pressure hydrocephalus is unable to. ICP monitoring may reveal A or B waveforms.

Dementia with an associated ataxia could be due to other causes, e.g. degenerative cerebral atrophy (for which there is no treatment), and it is imperative to ascertain the correct diagnosis, as normal pressure hydrocephalus may respond to shunting and therefore is potentially treatable.

Benign intracranial hypertension is thought to be due to impaired absorption and usually presents in young, usually obese females. Causes may include a history of minor trauma, endocrine disorders and toxic side-effects of certain antibiotics. CT scanning will reveal normal sized ventricles and the patient usually presents with signs and symptoms of raised ICP. Progressive optic nerve damage can occur and treatment is aimed at preventing this. Treatment of the primary disorder includes a weight reduction diet, symptomatic treatment of the effects of raised ICP and the insertion of a lumbo-peritoneal shunt. Drug therapy may include acetazolamide, a carbonic anhydrase inhibitor and steroids.

SIGNS AND SYMPTOMS OF RAISED INTRACRANIAL PRESSURE

The nurse should have a working knowledge of the signs and symptoms of raised intracranial pressure in order that she recognises them properly when they occur. An understanding of why certain signs and symptoms present themselves helps to explain the processes involved and the reason they happen. Many patients' lives have been saved by the alertness and prompt action of the nursing staff. The most reliable method of determining the presence of raised intracranial pressure is to 'tap' the brain itself with a sensor which would directly detect the presence of raised pressure. This is quite possible through the use of continuous intracranial pressure monitoring, but for various reasons it may not always be possible to use the tap in every situation. Whether or not the technique of pressure monitoring is employed, reliability is placed on accurate and frequent observation of the patient. As the nursing staff are with the patient on a continuous basis they are best suited to perform this task. This would include observing the level of consciousness and any loss of motor or sensory function, changes in pupillary responses, alterations in vital signs and any complaints of headache and nausea or vomiting. Papilloedema may also feature, but detection of this does not fall within the remit of the nurse in the UK.

Traditionally, the clinical correlates of headache, vomiting and papilloedema formed the so-called Cushing triad. It has now been discovered that these signs and symptoms are not always present or may occur so late in the process that it is too late to help the patient. When they do occur they indicate a need for urgent intervention.

Most clinicians agree that a number of more reliable indicators have now been identified, in order to alert us to the presence of raised intracranial pressure.

The signs and symptoms of raised intracranial pressure are summarised in Table 5.2.

DIRECT MEASUREMENT OF INTRACRANIAL PRESSURE

In some patients direct measurement of intracranial pressure to determine the extent of hypertension is indicated. The monitoring system will consist of a sensory device which should be placed in the area of abnormal pressure and then connected up to a recording device to provide data.

Indications and reasons for monitoring

Direct intracranial pressure monitoring is most commonly used following head injuries although its use may be indicated in patients with an intracerebral haemorrhage, brain tumour, hydrocephalus and benign intracranial hypertension.

The benefits to the patient of monitoring the progress of intracranial hypertension are as follows:

— Diagnosis and/or detection of early rises in intracranial pressure
— Evaluation of the effectiveness of treatment particularly in the postoperative period following craniotomy and to provide an indication for intervention
— To act as a prognostic guide to outcome.

The methods involved in measuring intracranial pressure all rely on direct invasive techniques incorporating the use of a catheter, transducer and a chart recorder or oscilloscope.

The first method measures the ventricular fluid pressure with the use of a small catheter placed in the lateral ventricle in the non-dominant hemisphere. The catheter is connected to capillary tubing which has previously been purged with sterile normal saline and then connected to a pressure transducer. The transducer converts pressure in the capillary tubing to an electrical signal which is then displayed on a chart or oscilloscope for interpretation. Unfortunately with this method there is a small risk of ventriculitis and this underlines the importance of the nurse using a strict aseptic technique when working with the system. Blood or debris may block the ventricular catheter resulting in a loss of the waveform.

The advantages of the system, however, include ready access to the lateral ventricle for sampling cerebrospinal fluid, instilling drugs and injecting contrast media.

The second method involves the use of a subarachnoid screw or bolt. A small hole is made in the skull through which a special hollow metal bolt is inserted until the tip

Table 5.2 Signs and symptoms of raised intracranial pressure

Clinical parameter	Signs/symptoms	Reasons
Conscious level	Deterioration in conscious level	Raised intracranial pressure will reduce the amount of oxygen received by the oxygen sensitive cells of the cerebral cortex.
Respiration	Deterioration in respiratory pattern	A particular respiratory pattern will be seen in relation to the non-functioning area in the medulla and pons. *Breathing pattern* — *Non-functioning area* Cheyne-Stokes — affects various areas Apneustic — Pons varolii Ataxic — Medulla Central neurogenic hyperventilation — Lower mid-brain–upper pons Cluster breathing — Medulla
Pupils	a. Alteration in pupil size b. Reaction to light c. Blurring of vision/diplopia d. Ocular muscle paresis/paralysis	All the pupillary and eye movement responses to raised intracranial pressure are as a result of compression of the 3rd cranial nerve (occulomotor). The ipsilateral pupil is usually affected first followed by the other one.
Blood pressure	a. An increase in systolic blood pressure followed by b. a fall	The increase in blood pressure occurs as a result of ischaemia, due to raised intracranial pressure, of the vasomotor centre. Implicated in this is a widening pulse pressure. If this is not corrected, the intracranial pressure continues to rise, and the blood pressure then begins to fall dramatically until it is unrecordable
Pulse	Initially bradycardia (< 60 bpm) develops with a full and bounding pulse. In the later stages the pulse becomes weak and thready.	This is brought about as a result of increased workload on the heart which is attempting to overcome cerebral blood vessel resistance by pushing more blood into the cerebral circulation.
Motor function	Contralateral hemiparesis/hemiplegia	The raised intracranial pressure affects pyramidal tract function and continued deterioration will ensue until the limbs are unresponsive to deep painful stimuli.
'Cushing's triad'	Headache usually in the early morning	Headache due to raised intracranial pressure is thought to be the result of displacement of the cerebrospinal fluid cushion producing dilation of cerebral blood vessels, stretching of arteries at the base of the brain and traction of bridging veins. Intracranial pressure will be adversely affected following REM sleep and by the retention of carbon dioxide during sleep resulting in exacerbation of intracranial pressure in early morning.
	Vomiting: may occur with early morning headache.	The mechanism involved is not well understood.
	Papilloedema	Occurs as a result of raised intracranial pressure being transmitted down the optic nerve to produce a swollen nerve head. This may be seen on direct fundoscopy. An unreliable sign, which is not constantly seen in all patients with raised intracranial pressure.

No order is implied within the above set of signs and symptoms. Any combination in varying degrees can occur in each patient. Individually, each of the signs and symptoms can be caused by other pathology, including extracranially.

indents the subarachnoid space. The bolt is attached to fluid-filled pressure tubing which in turn is connected to a transducer and recorder. The risk of infection is the same as for the intraventricular method and the bolt can become blocked with blood resulting in loss of data.

The newest method of monitoring intracranial pressure relies on the use of an extradural (or epidural) sensor, which is positioned between the skull and the dura. The pressure transducer is located at the tip of the catheter, with the sensing membrane facing against the dura. The system is connected directly to a chart recorder, completely eliminating the need for fluid-filled tubing. This implies that there is no access to the ventricles for sampling or withdrawal of cerebrospinal fluid.

Interpretation of the data

Once the monitoring system is operational the data can be interpreted. The following should be noted and reported:

— Any rise in intracranial pressure, or the presence of waveforms
— Loss of the pulsatile waveforms.

Detection of elevated pressure is the most significant; readings over 15 mmHg are above normal, over 20 mmHg moderately elevated and readings over 40 mmHg severely elevated. These elevated readings may be continuous or transient.

Three main types of transient wave elevations have been identified:

A Waves. Starting from an elevated base line, intracranial pressure will rise suddenly to over 50 mmHg for a period of 5–20 minutes before falling again below the original level. Sometimes referred to as plateau waves because of their shape on the graph paper, A waves are of significant clinical importance.

B Waves. These are sharp rhythmic waves occurring every 0.5–2 minutes and peaking between 10 and 15 mmHg often seen in conjunction with a fluctuating respiratory pattern such as Cheyne-Stokes breathing.

C Waves. These are of little significance,

occur at 4–8 per minute and may raise intracranial pressure by up to 20 mmHg. They can be related to changes in the cardiovascular system.

FACTORS AFFECTING INTRACRANIAL PRESSURE

A number of factors have been identified as causing a rise in intracranial pressure; in patients with intracranial hypertension the presence of these factors could be detrimental to their outcome. Some of these factors are associated with body functions, e.g. the level of carbon dioxide in the blood, over which we have some external control, and other factors, such as isometric muscle contraction, which we can avoid by good nursing care.

The principal factors exerting an influence are:

Hypoxia and/or hypercapnia. These are probably the most significant factors involved. Hypoxia is a cellular oxygen deficiency resulting in a decrease in the level of arterial oxygen levels. P_aO_2 of less than 50 mmHg is the usual standard. This implies that there is less oxygen available for the sensitive cells of the cerebral cortex, which in turn will lead to an increase in cerebral blood flow culminating in raised intracranial pressure. Hypoxia can arise as a result of mismanagement of respiratory care, e.g. inadequate ventilation during surgery, or by the patient refusing to wear his oxygen mask.

Hypercapnia is caused by an increase in the level of carbon dioxide in the blood; levels over 40 mmHg are abnormal. The build up of carbon dioxide arises as a result of underventilation. Carbon dioxide acts as a potent vasodilator on the cerebral blood vessels, increasing the congestion within the cranial cavity and resulting in a rise in intracranial pressure. Causes of hypercapnia include sleep and coma.

Body position. The head should be placed in a neutral position avoiding any flexion or extension movements of the neck, especially while turning the patient. Obstruction of the blood vessels of the neck will result in a decrease in venous outflow from the head, producing a rise in intracranial pressure.

Isometric muscle contractions. An isometric exercise is one which involves contraction of the muscle without lengthening. Such a situation will result if a patient pushes down on his hands or feet to move up the bed, and therefore should be avoided. Isometric exercising will cause a rise in intracranial pressure as a sequel to a rise in blood pressure.

Valsalva's manoeuvre. An increase in intrathoracic pressure will result, following Valsalva's manoeuvre, which will impede venous outflow encouraging intracranial pressure to rise. It occurs when the patient exhales against a closed epiglottis and this may happen while straining at stool or turning in bed.

Coughing, sneezing, REM sleep and emotional upset will all cause rises in intracranial pressure. Prevention of these is almost impossible therefore it is essential to restrict other activities during the course of their duration.

Vasodilation. Certain drugs are known to produce vasodilation of the cerebral blood vessels, and probably the best known culprit is halothane, an anaesthetic agent, the use of which should be avoided. Other drugs to be used cautiously include cyclandelate (Cyclospasmol) and histamine.

MEDICAL MANAGEMENT OF THE PATIENT WITH RAISED INTRACRANIAL PRESSURE

The general medical management of the patient with raised intracranial pressure is dealt with here, although recognition of the important contribution made by skilled nursing care should be acknowledged. Broad principles of management are outlined, and these may vary depending on the cause and severity of the raised intracranial pressure. Specific intervention is dealt with as appropriate in other chapters, according to the original cause of the hypertension. Medical management may include non-surgical and/or surgical methods in various combinations, e.g.

Rising intracranial pressure is suspected in a patient with a recent history of head injury. If intracranial pressure monitoring is in progress, a rapid assessment is performed of the recording system to check for faults. Any activities being performed which may be suspected as contributing to the hypertension are halted. If raised pressure still remains a tentative diagnosis, CT scanning is performed to establish a possible cause. Should a lesion be demonstrated, surgical intervention to relieve pressure may be indicated. Alternatively, if no obvious lesion is detected the use of non-surgical treatment will be initiated. Variations of this sequence of events will occur, depending upon circumstances.

Non-surgical management

Non-surgical management may be summarised as follows:

- drug therapy
- hyperventilation
- fluid restriction
- barbiturate coma
- hypothermia.

Drug therapy

Osmotic diuretics. These act by facilitating the removal of fluid from oedematous tissues. They do this by exploiting the principle of diffusion, in which water molecules will move in a random fashion from an area of high pressure to one of low, via a semi-permeable membrane. With the administration of a hyperosmolar agent (diuretic) removal of water from the brain tissue into the cerebral circulation is encouraged, as the tissue fluid is hypotonic in comparison with that of the medicated blood.

Mannitol (10% or 20%) is probably the most frequently used osmotic diuretic in the treatment of raised intracranial pressure. The usual dose is 1 g/kg of body weight, which works out in an average size adult as 100 ml of the 20% solution, administered over a period of 15 minutes. Mannitol acts quickly, and usually begins to work within 20 minutes of administration, its effect lasting for a variable length of time, between 3 and 6 hours. It is most often used as a holding mechanism, in order to transport the patient to a specialist centre for definitive treatment or to prepare a patient for emergency surgery, but it may also be used during the intra-operative period. Some centres advocate the use of a regime of repeated doses of mannitol over a period of time. This is not a universally accepted protocol as the results have been variable in terms of outcome and the administration of repeated large doses of mannitol is not without risk to the patient.

A large diuresis can be produced and with this rapid removal of extracellular fluid from the body; some disturbances of fluid balance and electrolytes can occur. A patient receiving mannitol therapy requires close monitoring of fluid balance; a urinary catheter is essential for an accurate measure of output, and regular estimations of serum electrolytes.

Other diuretics which may occasionally be used are urea and glycerol, although their popularity has now largely been superseded by mannitol. Urea can be given intravenously or via a nasogastric tube, as it is unpalatable. The effects are similar to mannitol and therefore its management follows the same principles. The side-effects and dangers are greater, and urea cannot be given to patients suffering from kidney or liver disease.

Corticosteroids. The administration of dexamethasone (Decadron), a powerful corticosteroid, may be indicated in patients with oedema associated with tumours and inflammatory lesions, but not in head injury. An initial dose of 8–16 mg, orally, intravenously or intramuscularly is usual, followed by maintenance therapy of 4 mg, 6 hourly. Other weaker corticosteriods may be used at the discretion of the medical staff.

The administration of corticosteroids can present problems and side-effects which may become dangerous include salt imbalance within the cells, leading to peripheral oedema and hypertension. Gastric irritation, which is countered by the administration of histamine-receptor antagonists, e.g. cimetidine (Tagamet) and/or an antacid, may also occur. The patient's immune system will also be depressed. When therapy is being discontinued, it needs to be performed gradually, otherwise the patient will suffer from adrenal insufficency.

Hyperventilation

Hypercapnia, as already demonstrated, leads to vasodilation of the cerebral blood vessels resulting in an increase in intracranial pressure. The normal range of arterial carbon dioxide levels is considered to be between 34 and 37 mmHg, and if this can be reduced to a level of 25–30 mmHg this reduces the chances of vasodilation occurring. This can be achieved by the administration of oxygen therapy to avoid hypoxia and by getting the patient to 'blow off' carbon dioxide by more rapid breathing. The most efficient way to achieve this is with intubation and controlled ventilation. Hyperventilation is often used during the intra-operative period. Estimation of the pCO_2 level is obtained by drawing arterial blood gases.

Fluid restriction

Patients with intracranial hypertension, may be prescribed a restriction of fluids in order to achieve a state of slight dehydration. The theory is that if intracellular fluids are decreased then any intracranial hypertension will also be reduced. A likely amount for an adult will be 1500–1750 ml over 24 hours.

Hypothermia

The use of hypothermia is not nearly so common as it once was. It involves cooling the patient's body temperature to around 32°C. As the temperature falls, the general metabolic processes within the body also decrease their activity. This produces a decrease in the production of waste products from all metabolism, one of which is carbon dioxide, a potent cerebral vasodilator. Perhaps what is of more significance nowadays is the maintenance of body temperature at normal levels (36–37°) and the treatment of any pyrexia. An increase in body temperature will speed up metabolic processes, consequently raising intracranial pressure, therefore treatment of the pyrexia and the use of local cooling measures should be instituted.

Barbiturate coma

The induction of a barbiturate coma may be considered in an effort to control resistant intracranial hypertension. It involves administering large doses of barbiturates intravenously to create a drug-induced coma. It can only be performed in specialist centres under very close observation. The patient will require the full support of meticulous nursing care, life support machinery and the associated technology which will, for example, continuously monitor blood pressure and intracranial pressure, full laboratory back up services and access to CT scanning. A bolus dose of pentobarbital 3–5 mg/kg of body weight is given intravenously followed by a maintenance dose of 150–250 mg, hourly in a continuous infusion. Serum barbiturate levels are closely monitored.

Surgical management

Surgical management may be viewed in terms of palliative treatment, as in the insertion of an external bypass system to drain off cerebrospinal fluid or on a more permanent basis, the removal of an offending space occupying lesion or insertion of an internal shunt to draw off cerebrospinal fluid.

Ventricular drainage

A catheter is placed in the right or left lateral ventricle and connected up via a capillary tubing system to a drainage reservoir. Once the reservoir is placed at head height any increase in intracranial pressure will force excess cerebrospinal fluid to drain out into the reservoir, thereby reducing intracranial pressure.

There are two risks associated with this technique, the first being infection. Entry of bacteria into the cerebrospinal fluid system is encouraged if a breach in the protective barrier occurs. The second risk involves the level of the reservoir. If it should drop below the prescribed level an excessive amount of cerebrospinal fluid will be drawn off leading to a low pressure state.

If the original cause of the raised intracranial pressure is inoperable a more permanent internal drainage system is required. Insertion of a ventriculo-atrial or peritoneal shunt would be performed. Elaboration of this technique is explained in Chapter 15.

Craniotomy

This may be performed to remove an expanding space occupying lesion, such as a haematoma or tumour. Further elaboration of the care involved can be found in Chapter 11. Occasionally healthy cerebral tissue has to be sacrificed in an internal decompression or alternatively, removal of a bone flap (external decompression) in order to accommodate the expanding lesion. By the time the patient reaches this stage it is unlikely that this type of surgery will help and therefore it is not performed very often now.

NURSING MANAGEMENT OF THE PATIENT WITH RAISED INTRACRANIAL PRESSURE

This is examined by looking at the relevant activities of living.

Maintaining a safe environment
Prevention of infection

An aseptic technique should be employed during the setting up of the monitoring/drainage system. Sterile, usually disposable, equipment is used and assembled by the doctor. The pressure transducer is also sterilised prior to the procedure. Any intentional breaches of the monitoring/drainage system are kept to an absolute minimum. If a breach is necessary, e.g. to withdraw cerebrospinal fluid or move the patient to another department, then this is performed under sterile conditions. The confused patient should be observed to ensure he does not interfere with the monitoring/drainage system. If a breach occurs, the tubing is clamped close to the head and the doctor informed. A new system will be required as soon as possible in order to reinstitute monitoring/drainage. If the system is being used for drainage, some additional points need to be noted. The reservoir must be kept at the prescribed level and changed every 24 hours with a note being taken of the amount of cerebrospinal fluid drained. Any alteration in the colour of the fluid should also be noted. Care must be taken that there are no kinks in the tubing and that it is clamped temporarily while transferring the patient from bed to trolley.

One of the functions of the dura mater is to act as a protective barrier for the brain. If this barrier is breached, as in intraventricular monitoring/drainage, then the patient's susceptibility to ventriculitis is increased. If the reservoir is not maintained at the prescribed level, the system will not operate as intended. If too high, cerebrospinal fluid will not drain; if too low, an excessive amount of fluid will be drained. The former will encourage intracranial pressure to rise higher and the latter will result in a low pressure state and the onset of headache. If cerebrospinal fluid appears cloudy this may be indicative of an infective process. Temporary clamping of the tubing during a potentially hazardous period, such as transferring the patient from bed to trolley, will ensure that if the system is breached, the patient is protected. Kinking of the tubing will block the system resulting in a rise in intracranial pressure.

Observation of intracranial pressure

The pressure transducer must be kept level with the patient's head. This can be achieved in different ways according to the equipment involved. The transducer may be attached to a variable height table or clamp and can be adjusted according to the height of the patient's head. The smaller lightweight transducer can be strapped to the patient's head eliminating the need to adjust its height each time the patient alters his head position.

The pressure transducer is calibrated for accurate monitoring once the system has been set up and should it move from this set position, false high or low readings will be produced.

The presence of waveforms or raised intracranial pressure and loss of the pulsatile waveform should be reported. The former may indicate a need for further investigation and/or surgical intervention and the latter indicates that a fault or leak has developed within the monitoring system and requires immediate investigation and correction.

Certain procedures, such as suctioning, will produce an artefact on the recording; in these instances a rise in intracranial pressure will occur but should, in the normal course of events, return to its previous level. When this occurs a note on the graph paper to indicate the artefact will alert other members of staff. This implies that those nursing procedures which are likely to produce intracranial hypertension should not be grouped together but spaced well apart.

A regular note is made of pressure readings; an appropriate place to do this could be the patient's conscious level chart.

Minimising the side-effects of corticosteroids

Administering the prescribed corticosteroids at the correct times and in the proper dosage is essential. An antacid or histamine receptor antagonist such as cimetidine (Tagamet) may also be prescribed for concurrent administration. Observation for oedema and hypertension is carried out and reported if necessary to the medical staff.

It is important that corticosteroids are given as prescribed for once the therapy has commenced omitting several doses would constitute sudden discontinuation and result in adrenal insufficiency. If side-effects are noted in the early stages, then effective treatment can be instituted to ameliorate the situation.

Communicating

Avoid verbal overstimulation. Excessive emotional stimuli which may upset the patient could result in a rise in blood pressure with a concomitant rise in intracranial pressure. The relatives should be encouraged to speak to the patient but to avoid topics which may provoke an emotional upset. Nurses should be guarded in their conversation while working with the patient.

Breathing

Maintaining a patent airway

Partial or complete obstruction of the airway will result in inadequate ventilation leading to a decrease in the oxygen supply and/or an increase in the carbon dioxide level. Such a situation produces a state of cerebral vasodilation causing intracranial pressure to rise.

The patient is closely observed for any signs of respiratory distress which will be apparent by a deterioration in his colour, alterations in the respiratory pattern (rate increased and breathing noisy and laboured) and the presence of retained secretions in the trachea and orolarynx. Noisy breathing is always indicative of an obstructed airway but a patient with an obstructed airway does not always breath noisily. Prescribed oxygen therapy should be administered and, if problems are encountered in achieving this, the doctor should be informed. Suctioning, using an aseptic technique, should be performed as required on an intermittent basis. The procedure should last no more than 15 seconds at any one time. Consider pre-oxygenation prior to suctioning if this is approved.

The patient's position is changed every 2 hours to encourage pulmonary drainage and toileting. Any patient with the slightest impair-

ment of conscious level should not be allowed to lie on his back for any reason lest he obstructs his airway with his tongue. The co-operative, alert patient can be encouraged to assist in efficient pulmonary function and chest physiotherapy. Where indicated, careful monitoring of the patient and his mechanical ventilator will be instituted. The above precautions regarding suctioning and position will apply and the safe working of the ventilator is ascertained by frequent checks on the apparatus. In some centres in the UK nurses are responsible for drawing blood gases from indwelling arterial catheters and the unit policy should be adhered to regarding this specialised procedure. If blood gases are drawn by the doctor using a direct stab it is imperative that pressure is applied over the puncture site for a minimum of 5 minutes to prevent haematoma formation.

Eating and drinking

Fluid intake

Some patients are permitted only a restricted intake as this may contribute to maintaining intracranial pressure within limits (remember that cerebral oedema can contribute to raised intracranial pressure). This implies that the nurse will have to maintain an accurate fluid balance. Calculations of intake include all routes of entry, i.e. oral, nasogastric, and intravenous, and output will include urine, cerebrospinal fluid, gastric aspirate and stool and an allowance for insensible loss. The administration of diuretics will demand stringent fluid balance. The nurse should check the strength of the solution against the prescription and ensure that the correct amount is infused safely. A urinary catheter should be inserted as a huge diuresis can be expected in most cases and this is the most effective and accurate method of measuring it.

If fluid balance is not closely monitored, we could inadvertently cause intracranial pressure to rise.

Eliminating

Prevention of constipation

The prevention of constipation by whatever means as dictated by local policy is necessary. The use of mild laxatives is preferable to enemas or suppositories. If a patient with raised intracranial pressure has to strain at stool this will induce further rises of intracranial pressure as a result of Valsalva's manoeuvre. This is induced when the patient exhales against a closed epiglottis producing a rise in intrathoracic pressure which in turn will impede venous outflow from the head resulting in a rise in intracranial pressure.

Monitoring fluid output

As already stated, knowledge of the patient's fluid balance is crucial, in order to maintain intracranial pressure as low as possible (see eating and drinking).

Personal cleansing and dressing

Aseptic wound dressing technique

For the relatively short period of time that intracranial pressure monitoring is in progress, it is not normally necessary to change the dressing. However, should the need arise this should be performed using an aseptic technique.

Monitoring for pressure sores

It has already been indicated that in order for accurate measurement of intracranial pressure to be performed, the patient is required to remain bedfast and lie still; this can increase the patient's chances of developing a pressure sore, particularly on the occiput. It is usually possible to avoid this by regular turning of the patient using sufficient numbers of nurses to preclude the patient's participation.

Controlling body temperature

As part of the observation process involved in monitoring for potential infection, the nurse must record and report any significant rises in body temperature.

Mobilising

The patient is nursed in a 10–30° head up tilt. This will encourage venous return which in turn will help to lower intracranial pressure by reducing congestion. Maintenance of the head in a neutral position and avoidance of flexion/extension movements of the neck, especially while turning the patient, are important. Body position is relevant; nursing the patient in the prone position or with his hips in extreme flexion would produce pressure over the abdomen and/or thorax. Mechanical obstruction of the blood vessels of the neck and/or raised intrathoracic or intra-abdominal pressure will produce a decrease in venous outflow from the head resulting in a rise in intracranial pressure.

Isometric activities should be avoided. An isometric exercise is one which involves contraction of a muscle resulting in tension without lengthening, e.g. a patient pushing down on the bed with his hands in order to turn over would be indulging in an isometric exercise. Isometric activities cause a rise in blood pressure which in turn will provoke a further rise in intracranial pressure. Patients should be assisted with turning and moving up and down in bed and encouraged not to push down on the footboard. Assistance with turning is given even although the patient is capable of turning himself. The alert patient should be requested to exhale while turning or moving up and down in bed in order to avoid initiating Valsalva's manoeuvre.

Passive range of movement exercises are not isometric and can be performed safely.

A patient who has spastic flexion (decortication) or extension (decerebration) of his limbs will mimic isometric activity, so the nurse should endeavour to avoid stimuli which will produce these responses. Medication is occasionally prescribed to diminish these responses.

Sleeping

Conscious level

Close observation and the use of gentle restraint will be necessary in the restless or confused patient. Agitation will worsen any existing intracranial hypertension, therefore the patient needs to be kept calm and quiet to avoid this.

Patients with a compromised conscious level will require the care necessary for such a situation depending upon the severity of loss of consciousness. This is discussed in more detail in Chapter 4.

Implementation of the use of a standardised coma scale, e.g. the Glasgow coma scale, would provide detailed and unambiguous information regarding the patient's conscious level. The frequency of the observations should be determined by the nurse in charge and/or the medical staff.

BIBLIOGRAPHY

Allan D 1982 Nursing aspects of artificial ventilation. Nursing Times 78(24):1006

Allan D 1984 Glasgow coma scale. Nursing Mirror 158(23):32

Bruya M A 1981 Planned periods of rest in the intensive care unit: nursing care activities and ICP. Journal of Neurosurgical Nursing 13(4):184

Grant L 1984 Hydrocephalus: an overview and update. Journal of Neurosurgical Nursing 16(6):313

Hausman K 1981 Nursing care of the patient with hydrocephalus. Journal of Neurosurgical Nursing 13(6):326

Hickey J 1986 The clinical practice of neurological and neurosurgical nursing, 2nd edn. J B Lippincott, Philadelphia

Hulme A, Cooper R 1976 The effect of head position and jugular vein compression on ICP. In: Beks J et al (eds) ICP III. Springer-Verlag, Berlin

Jackson P 1980 Ventriculo-peritoneal shunts. American Journal of Nursing 80(6):1104

Jennett B, Galbraith S 1983 An introduction to neurosurgery, 4th edn. Heinemann, London

Jennett B, Teasdale G 1981 Management of head injuries. F A Davis, Philadelphia

Johnson L 1983 If your patient has increased ICP, your goal should be no surprises. Nursing 13(6):58

Jones C, Crayard C 1982 Care of ICP monitoring devices: a nursing responsibility. Journal of Neurosurgical Nursing 14(5):255

Langfitt T W 1969 Increased ICP. Clinical Neurosurgery 16:436

Lipe H P, Mitchell P H 1980 Positioning the patient with intracranial hypertension: how turning and head rotation affect the internal jugular vein. Heart and Lung 9:1031

Marcotty S F, Levin A B 1984 A new approach in epidural ICP monitoring. Journal of Neurosurgical Nursing 16(1):54

McNamara M, Quinn C 1981 Epidural ICP monitoring: theory and clinical application. Journal of Neurosurgical Nursing 13(5):267

Miller J D 1978 ICP Monitoring. British Journal of Hospital Medicine 19(5):497

Miller J D, Becker D P, Ward J D 1977 Significance of intracranial hypertension in severe head injury. Journal of Neurosurgery 47:503

Mitchell P H 1980 Intracranial hypertension: implications of research for nursing care. Journal of Neurosurgical Nursing 12(3):145

Mitchell P H (1986) Intracranial hypertension: influence of nursing care activities. Nursing Clinics of North America 9 21(4):563

Mitchell P H 1982 In: Nikas D L (ed) The critically ill neurosurgical patient. Churchill Livingstone, New York

Mitchell P H, Mauss N K 1978 The relationship of patient and nurse activity to ICP variations. Nursing Research 27:4

Mitchell P H, Ozuna J, Lipe H 1981 Moving the patient in bed: effects on ICP. Nursing Research 30(4):212

Price M 1981 Significance of ICP waveforms. Journal of Neurosurgical Nursing 13(4):202

Purchese G, Allan D 1984 Neuromedical and neurosurgical nursing, 2nd edn. Baillière Tindall, London

Ross Russell R W, Wiles C M 1985 Neurology. Heinemann, London

Shapiro H M 1975 Intracranial hyptertension: therapeutic and anaesthetic considerations. Anaesthesiology 43:455

Snyder M 1983 Relation of nursing activities to increases in ICP. Journal of Advanced Nursing 8(4):273

Speers I 1981 Cerebral oedema. Journal of Neurosurgical Nursing 13(2): 102

Vogt G, Miller M, Esluer M 1985 Manual of neurological care. C V Mosby, St Louis

Young M S 1981 Understanding the signs of ICP: A bedside guide. Nursing 81 11(2):59

Zegeer L 1982 Nursing care of the patient with brain oedema. Journal of Neurosurgical Nursing 14(5):268

6

Craniotomy — pre-operative preparation

The pre-operative preparation for intracranial surgery begins after the patient is admitted to the ward, when investigations are carried out and before the operation day is finalised. The aim is to ensure the patient's optimal condition for surgery and for a successful recovery. This takes account of his physical needs, with attention to nutrition, sleep, rest and respiratory care, all of which influence his post-operative progress; his psychological needs, those for concern, support and time as well as those for explanation, instruction and reassurance; his spiritual needs and his needs relating to his family and cultural life. Nursing care is directed at both the patient and his family, of which he is an integral part; his needs cannot be separated from theirs.

It has been suggested by Hopps (1983) that there are four stages in the acceptance of cardiac surgery and these may also be applicable to neurosurgery. They are confrontation, self-reflection, resolution and countdown. If this is so, then the process and preparation also involves accurate timing, with the patient and his family being given support, guidance and information during the first two stages and the teaching and more active care commenced when it is more effective during the stage of resolution.

The preparation for surgery can be divided into three stages: the general and unobtrusive care before surgery becomes the definitive intention; the more specific care 'working up' to surgery, and the final pre-operative 'countdown'. The care throughout the whole pre-operative period should be planned, efficient and individualised. The content is important, as is the method of delivery and the timing.

Preparation for surgery is just one aspect of pre-operative care and it is this one aspect that is the main concern of this chapter.

GENERAL PRE-OPERATIVE CARE

The patient is admitted to a neurosurgical ward when there is a likelihood that surgery will prove the most suitable form of management. Until this is confirmed the nursing care of the patient can remain general and unimposing, though still preparatory in nature.

The aim is to develop a confident and supportive relationship between the staff and the family (including the patient), and to help the family members come to terms with the patient's illness and the possibility of surgery.

All the patients have a greater or lesser degree of raised intracranial pressure and their care includes measures for the prevention or early detection of any further, possibly disastrous, increases (see Ch. 5). Neurological and other deficits require the appropriate care and safety is important.

The patient's general physical state must be maintained or improved so that if surgery is decided upon, he reaches his optimum condition prior to the operation. Information and support are essential.

Routine investigations including computerised axial tomography and angiography are important both in diagnosis and in assessment of suitability for surgery and another aspect of care is the reduction of related anxiety, discomfort and complications.

If surgery is considered appropriate, then the more specific preparatory care can begin; if not, alternative care can be implemented.

Anxiety

All care is carried out against a background of anxiety. Surgery can be described as 'a combination of three major forms of immi-

nent danger — the possibility of suffering acute pain; of undergoing serious body damage and of dying' (Janis 1980).

This is a particularly apt description of neurosurgery; anxiety is a normal response and one common to the majority of patients and relatives. The level of anxiety and the way in which it is expressed is individual but in the assessment of the patient it should be remembered that many of the classical features of anxiety, e.g. facial expression, restlessness, increased muscle tone, can also be affected by neurological pathology.

Patients who display a moderate degree of anxiety pre-operatively have been shown to make a better postoperative recovery than those who display either high or low levels (Janis 1980).

A high level of anxiety, whether apparent or not, causes both biochemical and emotional changes (Hopps 1983) which result in an increase in both pain and nausea in the immediate postoperative period, and in the incidence of postoperative urine retention. A patient with a low level of anxiety may not expect, and so may find more frightening, the pain and discomfort that he experiences as an unavoidable consequence of surgery. Both experiences will influence the patient's feelings towards any future surgery that he may require and so also have long-term consequences.

A low anxiety level is seen in the minority of patients, for example those with personality disorders who may not perceive the impending operation as a threat and so do not experience an associated anxiety response. In others who are greatly stressed, May (1980) suggested that a similar freedom from anxiety may be experienced as a coping mechanism. These patients require realistic explanation and description of what surgery involves so that, at the least, the related discomfort may not be totally unexpected.

The majority of patients and relatives are, however, extremely anxious and the first stage in the process of reducing their anxiety is the development of a trusting and confident relationship between them and the hospital staff. The family must be convinced of both the credibility of the staff and of a genuine concern for their wellbeing. That being so, they will place more value on the teaching, advice and information offered and feel more able to discuss their feelings.

The major stressors that are causing the anxiety response in the patient and his family, i.e. his diagnosis, his operation and the uncertainty of his prognosis, cannot be removed. Many of the attendant stressors, however, can be reduced if they are identified, and studies have described many examples encompassing all aspects of care. Hayward (1975) found that 70% of patients were concerned about one or more aspects of general anaesthesia.

General uncertainties about the roles of 'patient', 'relative' or 'visitor' can be relieved and the nursing care can be adapted where possible and where beneficial. The patient, as a 'patient', experiences a loss of control over his life and it is important to minimise this feeling and as far as possible, allow him to retain that control.

However to identify those factors that are producing anxiety the patient and his family must feel able to express their feelings. 'Accepting' rather than 'comforting' responses are helpful as in the simple example where the patient expresses his concern over the forthcoming operation. The 'accepting' response 'Is there anything you would like me to do/explain?' may help to identify how he can be helped rather than the 'comforting' but dismissive 'I'm sure it'll be all right.'

As previously mentioned, information is essential to the patient and his family. Though it often helps to reduce anxiety levels, anxiety itself reduces the ability to concentrate and retain, and 50–60% of the information given to the hospital patient is forgotten (Franklin 1974). This percentage will be further increased in those patients whose memory or awareness is affected by their illness. Repetition and reinforcement then are of great value and feedback essential. Medical and nursing jargon is another barrier to communication and particular care has to be taken to ascertain that the patient or his relative understands the meanings and concepts involved in the vocabulary used. Communication must also be adapted to take account of any specific communication problem.

Consideration of these factors helps in the moderation of anxiety and this is the aim of care. Once this has been achieved the patient can be more easily and effectively motivated to co-operate with his pre-operative preparation.

The family

When the patient first becomes unwell he is supported and cared for within his family. When his health fails to return and his illness progresses he seeks medical assistance. Brain pathology and surgery are still viewed with a great deal of apprehension so when he and his family are confronted with this possibility the initial response, not surprisingly, includes shock and denial. It is a major upheaval within the family, with both short- and long-term implications. With the outcome of such intricate surgery being so variable, and with the persistence of ideas of gross personality changes and post-operative 'cabbages', the future must appear very uncertain. If the family are to cope with and adapt to this situation they require an accurate and realistic understanding of it. Information is essential and its provision is a priority for both the general practitioner and the hospital staff. Content, method of delivery and timing are all of importance in the attempt to meet their other needs as well as that for information.

Support of the patient and his family by both hospital and community staff is of great importance when aimed at maintaining the family's own supportive functions. These are strengthened by inclusion of the family in the patient's care and by the confidence derived from supportive relationships with others. Alternatively these normal family functions are threatened by the feeling of exclusion from the patient and his care and the resultant feelings of insecurity and lack of confidence. It is the family's own system of support that will be of greatest value to them in the long-term, so its maintenance or, if possible, strengthening should be a priority of care.

Each family differs in its methods of and ability to cope with the serious illness of its family member. Hospital staff, who have only a brief acquaintance with these families and always under difficult circumstances, cannot be expected to understand the dynamics of each one and of each individual relationship. It is sufficient to understand that each relationship or set of relationships is unique, real and important. The beliefs and traditions of different cultures or religions should also be accepted and catered for wherever possible. The priorities of the individual and the family are largely determined by these beliefs and so must often be accepted, perhaps without being fully understood. Greary (1979) states that each individual can exhibit various coping mechanisms. These can be defined as 'behaviour or mental processes used to attempt to come to terms with illness in the family'. Common coping mechanisms include minimisation, intellectualisation, repetition, acting strong and remaining near the patient. (Caplan 1964, Lipowski 1970, Greary 1979)

The care of the family, then, requires a sensitive and accepting approach. Family members require information and support, but also flexibility. Of great value in planning care are those studies that demonstrate the ability of relatives of seriously ill patients to identify their own needs and indeed rate them with respect to their importance (Hampe 1975, Molter 1979, Bouman 1984, Daley 1984, Stillwell 1984).

The two major categories of need were those 'for relief of anxiety' and 'for information' but there were many specific needs relevant to their care. Just one example relates to their visiting needs. Stillwell (1984) found a significant correlation between the perceived severity of the patient's condition and the importance of frequent visiting. And in all the studies referred to, the need to be with the patient was rated very highly. It is suggested that frequent visiting may help the family to come to terms with the patient's condition

and its effect on both personal and family life. Also of value is the finding that the ranking of needs does not correlate with demographic variables including age, sex, socioeconomic class, education, the type of unit or with the relationship to the patient, i.e. kin or significant other (Bouman 1984).

The nurse must remember that the relatives will have to experience their grief, that even the most gentle care cannot remove the situation that is the cause of it.

Communicating

Providing the most basic care requires some degree of effective communicating between the carer and the patient. Communicating is a two way process which aims to achieve specific objectives, e.g. instruction, and to provide social contact, company and support. There is a wide range of neurological factors that can reduce the patient's ability to communicate and when discussing the care, the explanation and the teaching required, the way in which this can be implemented must also be considered.

With regard to their communicating difficulties neurosurgical patients can be categorised as follows:

— conscious with a specific communication problem
— conscious but confused
— conscious with personality/mood changes
— unconscious
— conscious with unrelated focal symptoms.

In many cases a reasonable understanding by the patient of his surroundings and his illness is a realistic goal, although sometimes extremely difficult to achieve. In others only minimal understanding is possible and in a small minority even this is unrealistic.

Effective verbal communication involves several stages, as follows:

- ideas
- encoding
- word formation
- speech
- sound reception
- decoding
- ideas, response
- feedback

Examples of how neurodysfunction can affect each of these include:

— disorientation, confusion, personality/mood change
— expressive dysphasia
— dysarthria
— dysphonia
— hearing loss
— receptive dysphasia
— disorientation, confusion, personality/mood change
— altered conscious states.

General reasons for communication problems also apply to the neurosurgical patient, either separate from, or in conjunction with, the neurological causes. These include:

— anxiety or reduced concentration
— the patient's first or only language is not the spoken language of the hospital staff
— the patient does not like to bother the busy nurse or is embarrassed at asking stupid questions or is embarrassed at not being able to find the right words or is afraid of the answer
— lack of privacy
— hearing difficulties unrelated to the neurological pathology, e.g. a noisy environment
— use of medical/nursing jargon or unfamiliar terms
— difficulty in forming appropriate responses due to lack of knowledge, intimidation by doctor/patient or the nurse/patient relationship.

For simplicity, the five categories of patients are used here to illustrate appropriate care, although in reality a degree of overlap occurs.

Fully conscious with specific communication problems

Many of the signs and symptoms of neurological pathology interfere with the normal process of communication. For the patient who is fully orientated but who has lost some or all of his ability to communicate with others, it is not only frustrating but also isolating, particularly if he is treated as confused. Common examples associated with verbal communication include hearing loss, dysarthria and dysphasia — both expressive and receptive.

The patient's hearing difficulty may or may not be related to his neurological pathology. Where the 'nervous' component of hearing is involved, the clarity of sound may be affected as well as its perceived volume. In these cases increasing the volume, for example by louder speech or the use of a hearing aid, will not help the person to understand what is being said. He relies on non-verbal or visual and action-orientated communication. Accurate perception by these methods, including the accuracy of lipreading, whether an established or developing skill, can be adversely affected by the anxiety, depression and general fatigue associated with hospitalisation and impending major surgery. Feedback from the patient is essential to assess his knowledge and understanding.

The patient with expressive dysphasia may be able to find his words if given the time and encouragement, or he may have to use other means of self-expression. Pictures illustrating common situations or requests may be of use with both these and severely dysarthric patients.

Those with receptive problems require simplicity in the ideas, vocabulary and sentences of any attempted communications. Tasks and more complex ideas must be divided into smaller units, and the use of gestures or pantomime may help. Again feedback from the patient is essential to assess his level of understanding.

Problems that affect non-verbal communication can also be important but are often less handicapping. Examples include facial weakness where loss of facial expression makes it difficult to convey feelings; paresis with loss of gesturing; visual field impairment, and paraesthesia where a comforting touch may not be conceived as such.

Diplopia and nystagmus affect both verbal and non-verbal communication. It affects

Table 6.1 Summary of pre-operative preparation for intracranial surgery (according to Roper)

General care	Specific care (as categorised throughout the chapter)	Immediate pre-operative care
Maintaining a safe environment Environmental safety	Pre-operative teaching — limb and respiratory exercises	As checklist: Identity bands Removal of prostheses
Frequent neurological assessments		Removal or covering of jewellery
Understanding of specific neurological deficits	Information	Removal of make up
Reduction of risk of complications, e.g. — infection — sleep and rest — nutrition	Pre-operative visit — for identification of patient — for identification of priorities of postoperative care	Restriction on oral intake Check consent has been given Notes and X-rays Baseline neuro-assessment and vital signs Relevant information to Recovery staff
Communicating Attention to neurological and other barriers to verbal and non-verbal communication		
Breathing Assess condition of respiratory system — maintain or improve as necessary (teaching of respiratory exercises)		Reinforce previously taught respiratory exercises
Eating and drinking Maintenance or improvement of nutritional state Awareness of neurological factors predisposing to poor nutritional health		
High fibre diet to counteract constipating effect of codeine Awareness of history of GI ulceration (dexamethasone)		
Weight control — obesity increases the risks of general anaesthesia	Low fat diet on day prior to surgery	Food restriction Fluid restriction
Eliminating Assess any difficult of micturition Ascertain normal bowel habits Awareness of probability of constipation due to codeine		
Personal cleansing and dressing	Hair wash on day prior to head shave surgery	
Controlling body temperature Not generally a problem pre-operatively		
Mobilising	(Teach limb exercises)	Reinforcement of previously taught limb exercises

Table 6.1 (contd)

General care	Specific care (as categorised throughout the chapter)	Immediate pre-operative care
Working and playing Need for periods of activity alternating with periods of sleep and rest		
Expressing sexuality May be important in the husband-wife relationship, e.g. dress, appearance, make up	Psychological preparation for head shave	Depersonalisation during this stage may be distressing
Sleeping Need for alternating periods of sleep with rest and activity Sleep pattern often disturbed in hospital		
Dying Fear of dying 'accepting' rather than 'comforting' responses		May refuse surgery due to fear of dying

verbal communication by reducing the use of lipreading as a normal assistance to hearing.

With time, patience and skill, the nurse can often find ways of overcoming these barriers even though effective communication may remain very limited, and so both the patient and his family need a great deal of support and help from ward staff. The nursing objective with regard to his pre-operative preparation is maximum effective instruction, teaching, explanation and reassurance. Relatives can often be included in trying to reach these objectives and can often be more successful than hospital staff.

Fully conscious but confused

Each patient differs as to what he remembers, what he understands and in his perception of how it relates to him. The lack of reliable feedback makes this very difficult to assess and his individual needs difficult to ascertain.

An atmosphere of trust, safety and caring provides a good basis for attempted communication and simple ideas, e.g., of the patient's illness, of being in hospital and of his impending operation, may be remembered if not totally understood.

An understanding of unavoidable discomfort in the postoperative period may help to retain the feeling of trust throughout his hospital stay.

Although pre-operative learning generally requires some degree of awareness, the use of picture, imitation, repetition and reinforcement may be helpful in teaching specific ideas or physical activities, e.g. deep breathing exercises. The presence of a close relative may be very helpful in the patient's care.

Fully conscious with personality or mood changes

This patient may or may not perceive his situation and its severity so his reaction may not appear normal. A common example of this is the patient with frontal damage who does not perceive his impending operation as a threat and so does not experience an anxiety response. He may not be motivated to co-operate in pre-operative teaching and instruction. This personality change is pathological and not a façade, so it cannot be breached to reach the 'real ' person. His care must be adapted in order to get the maximum response from the 'new' personality.

The patient with altered consciousness

There have been several reported cases of patients who, having recovered consciousness, accurately relate details of conversation or of their care during their period of unconsciousness. This illustrates the difficulty in knowing the extent to which the unconscious patient is aware of different stimuli. Simple explanations to the patient of what is happening and what is going to happen are required. Again the feeling of caring and safety can be communicated by both verbal and non-verbal means. The family may be involved to a large extent in the patient's care and they should also know of his possible awareness and so avoid making discouraging comments in his presence.

Feedback may be possible from some patients but in general explanations and instructions must remain simple and supportive.

The conscious patient with unrelated focal symptoms

The conscious orientated patient who is found to have intracranial pathology cannot be regarded as having no communication problems. Anxiety, depression and fatigue may all constitute a less obvious barrier. Being in the same ward as people with neurological deficits, they may feel they have a lot to lose by surgery. They may feel tempted to put up with the minor symptoms rather than run the risk of further damage. In many of these straightforward elective cases the pace may be too fast for the patient, with the association between his symptoms and a 'brain problem' only being made clear a few days before his operation. The patient needs time to prepare himself and his family for this major surgery. Some may prefer to undergo surgery as soon as possible, others may prefer to return home for a short time and come to accept the need for surgery, within their familiar surroundings. The role of the nursing and medical staff is to provide support and information, to help the family towards acceptance.

A caring and efficient environment will reassure him and a well organised and individual pre-operative preparation may satisfy him that his welfare is of importance to the staff.

Physical preparation

The physical care includes the maintenance or improvement of the patient's nutritional state, the attempt to achieve a balance between sleep, rest and activity, and the provision of comfort, wellbeing and safety (see Table 6.1).

Eating and drinking

The body's metabolic responses to surgery is related to its response to stress, the degree of that response depending on the extent and severity of the injury. The increased production of glucocorticoid hormones at the time of surgery is responsible for an immediate catabolic effect which may last several days and during which there is extreme breakdown of body protein. The longer this catabolic phase, the greater the delay in wound healing and return to normal health and the greater the risks of post-operative complications.

The value of a high protein, high calorie diet in shortening this period is not yet established (Behrends 1982, Moghissi & Boore 1983) but it is generally agreed that a well nourished person can tolerate this period without serious consequences (Behrends 1982, Stotts 1982). The aim of pre-operative nutritional care is to optimise the patient's nutritional state.

Hill (1977) states that protein-calorie malnutrition is much more common amongst surgical patients than generally expected and furthermore a significant number of patients develop this type of malnutrition following their admission. Symptoms of the patient's neurological pathology can often help to identify whether he is nutritionally 'at risk', but the cause may be unrelated and it is apparent that the dietary intake of all patients should receive attention.

Examples of neurological factors which

Table 6.2 Examples of neurological factors which predispose to poor nutritional health

Altered level of consciousness	
Altered mentation — difficulty in concentration	
Depression or anxiety leading to loss of appetite or poor selection of food	All leading to reduced intake
Dysphagia or reduced gag or cough reflexes	
Motor dysfunction — skeletal muscles or muscles of mastication	
Vomiting due to raised intracranial pressure or posterior fossa involvement	Leads to reduced utilisation of ingested food
Increased activity due to anxiety	
Trauma	Leads to increased energy requirements
Pyrexia due to meningism following subarachnoid haemorrhage	

predispose to poor nutritional health are outlined in Table 6.2.

The type of operation the patient is due to undergo is also an important consideration as is the rate of post-operative complications. The disadvantage to the poorly nourished person often becomes apparent when complications occur and the patient has few nutritional reserves to draw on. The patient requiring posterior fossa surgery may be left with cranial nerve deficits that affect dietary intake. Those with an increased risk of post-operative fitting may do so, and have an extended period of fasting or reduced nutrition, if elective ventilation is instituted. The probable effect of surgery on the patient's nutritional health can be incorporated into his pre-operative care.

Sleeping

Sleep, rest and activity are all essential to the wellbeing of the individual. Although sleep and rest are often categorised together a daily need for alternative periods of each, and of activity, has been shown to exist (Bruya 1981). Where the balance is not maintained mental and physical discomfort result, obviously contrary to the general aims of pre-operative care.

In the hospital environment deprivation of both sleep and rest commonly occur (Narrow 1967, Murphy et al 1977). The sleep profile of the patient is disturbed by the hospital environment and routine, and the hours of sleep reduced (Murphy et al 1977). The early morning headache characteristic of raised intracranial pressure and pain are both factors, but so are the high levels of noise and the early start to the hospital day.

Narrow (1967) suggested that rest occurs when the individual is in control of his environment, is accepted by himself and others, understands his current situation, is free of physical or mental discomfort, is involved in purposeful activity and is aware that help is available, if needed. That the hospital patient is ever in this position is questionable and it is not surprising that the same author believes that 'providing it (rest), remains one of the most complex of all nursing problems.' Privacy, quiet and freedom from unnecessary interruption are also considered necessary for rest to take place and again this may be difficult to ensure within the ward situation.

Physical activity within the hospital is also to a certain extent restricted even for, or especially for, those who are physically able. Physiotherapy may be the only form of exercise available and as such is not only restricted but controlled in content. However activity is not confined to being active, it also includes 'doing something' and the great majority of patients are well enough to experience this need.

Sleep, rest and activity are often difficult to ensure within the constraints of the hospital, and a balance of the three must surely be impossible. However an appreciation of the problem can only increase its consideration in the future planning of the ward layout and the current planning of ward routine and patient care.

Maintaining a safe environment

It is the comfort, wellbeing and the safety of the patient that are most obvious to his family when they visit. Maximum comfort and a sense of wellbeing are generally achieved by good nursing care with practical understanding of the patient's deficits. Safety not only involves environmental safety but also safety of the patient's life. This is conveyed to the patient and his family by the diligence of the neurological observations and care, and by the professionalism of the staff. The family will be reassured that the nursing staff do know of measures to prevent further increases of intracranial pressure, and will incorporate them into their care.

These aspects of care are not specifically preparatory in nature but in her study Bouman (1984) found that the most important emotional need of the relatives seemed to be for the quality of the patient's care. She went on to suggest that this need took priority even over the need for information. Comfort and wellbeing in particular need no expert knowledge to assess and the confidence of the family in the quality of the patient's care must be related to their opinion of how these basic needs are being met.

SPECIFIC PRE-OPERATIVE CARE

Once surgery has been recommended and the patient and his family have reached the decision to accept the surgeon's advice the second stage of preparation can begin. The general care, discussed previously, continues, but as they come to terms with the prospect of surgery the most active preparation starts.

Pre-operative instruction is given by nursing, medical and paramedical staff and together they should meet the patient's need for information and for adequate preparation. This alone, according to Healey (1968), can reduce the length of hospital stay, the need for analgesia and the incidence of post-operative complications. The emotional state of the patient is important in determining his degree of motivation which in turn influences greatly his response to pre-operative education. New learning should be based on previous knowledge and experience, and participation, repetition and reinforcement help to increase its effectiveness. Evaluation is, of course, an integral part of the teaching process.

Pre-operative teaching of respiratory and limb exercises is aimed at preventing the related post-operative complications. The physiotherapist is usually responsible for this aspect of care but the nurse reinforces her teaching. Respiratory exercises facilitate the removal of retained secretions and so improve the degree of gaseous exchange and reduce the risk of post-anaesthetic chest infection. Because blood gas levels are of such great importance in the patient with raised intracranial pressure, respiratory care is essential both before and after surgery. Those patients particularly at risk include the elderly and the obese who tend to have a reduced chest expansion, and those with chronic obstructive airways disease (COAD) who have more secretions which easily become infected even under normal circumstances. Smokers are also at risk as the action of the tobacco is to paralyse the cilia which usually carry the secretions to the back of the throat from where they are removed by coughing. Ideally the patient should stop smoking for 6 weeks prior to surgery but in reality this is not often possible. The care of all these people has to be particularly diligent.

Patients with a history of respiratory disease, e.g. asthma, can be identified and reassured that the anaesthetist will be aware of their condition.

The rationale behind the practice of both respiratory and limb exercise should be explained to the patient to ensure that he understands their importance and to increase his motivation and co-operation.

In some centres a theatre or recovery nurse may visit the patient pre-operatively. Her role complements that of the ward nurse and not only allows for further patient education and continuity of care but also encourages interaction between the ward and theatre staff.

To the patient the operating theatre is 'unknown territory' and he is often grateful to meet a member of its staff, especially if he will meet her again when he is taken to theatre.

With the ward nurse having already described his preparation for surgery, the theatre nurse can explain pre- and postoperative procedures. She can ascertain the patient's previous experience of surgery and can perhaps understand better his feelings towards his impending operation. Misconceptions can be identified and corrected. She can explain arrangements for relatives to visit or contact the patient after his operation.

At the time of the visit the nurse can also gather information concerning the patient's neurological state and his pre-existing health problems. This knowledge, together with her psychological assessment, can help to identify the priorities of his postoperative care. Any needs that can be met by the nursing or medical staff of the ward can be communicated to them.

It is important that the patient be allowed time to express his feelings whether it is to the ward nurse or to the theatre/recovery nurse. This helps him to come to terms with surgery and can be encouraged by the use of open-ended questions and 'accepting' rather than 'comforting' responses. Again this helps to identify needs and priorities of care, and the same approach can be adopted with the relatives.

This is a particularly important time for the relatives who now must come to accept the reality of the patient's illness and the presence of both short- and long-term implications. As well as information about the patient and his operation and prognosis, they also need to understand the care he is receiving. Being with the patient can help overcome the persisting shock and denial, and flexibility in visiting arrangements is usually appreciated. Where individual visiting is practised, relatives state that they felt that their visiting needs were better met (Breu & Dracup 1978).

Another aspect of preparation that deserves to be mentioned is the psychological preparation for the head shave. In many centres shaving is performed under anaesthetic but in some it is still performed on the ward. Women especially, but increasingly men also are distressed by this necessity and are often given the alternative of total or partial head shave. Sikh patients have not only emotional but also religious reasons for their distress. However they can often be reassured that the head or remaining hair will be covered as soon as possible postoperatively, if not already covered by a head bandage.

Day of surgery

The priority for care immediately prior to surgery is the safety of the patient throughout and following his operation. The reduction of discomfort before and after surgery is also a major concern.

Ideally all the general preparation will be complete so that the minimum of new information needs to be given at this time. The 'countdown' to surgery should appear calm, efficient and supportive in order to reduce last minute doubts and confirm the patient's trust and confidence in the medical and nursing staff. Reinforcement of previously learnt or explained material rather than teaching of new ideas helps the patient to feel more in control of his situation and also demonstrates an organised and efficient approach to care.

A sedative premedication is rarely given in neurosurgery so this is a very anxious period for the patient. Each one copes with the impending surgery in his own way, but psychological needs remain a priority within the ward even after physical preparation is complete. If the patient wishes, it may be possible for a close relative to stay with him until he goes to theatre. This helps to provide the support that both patient and relative need at this time, and allows good psychological care even within a busy ward. The hospital chaplain is also available and can provide religious and/or spiritual support.

Physical preparation for surgery

The routine physical preparation for surgery is usually made easier by the use of a checklist (see Fig. 6.1). Although the inflexibility of the standard checklist has been criticised and

Ward _____ Room no./Theatre _____ Consultant _____ Date _____

Surname _____ Age _____ Unit no. _____

Other names _____

Proposed operation _____

Case notes	Identification
X-rays	Dentures removed
Drug & nursing Kardex	Allergies
Fluid chart	Prosthesis/contact lens
Fasted from	Jewellery
Premedication Time	Hearing aid

Anaesthetic and operation permission form completed

I certify that identification and documents are correct on leaving the ward.

Sister/charge nurse or deputies' signature _____

_____

Reception/theatre
Patient's documentation and identification = correct _____

Sister/charge nurse or deputy's signatures _____

_____

Postoperative information
Operation/procedure _____

_____

Surgeon _____

Catheters _____

Drain _____

Packs _____

Skin _____

Signature _____

Fig. 6.1 Recovery room and post operation form

indeed most items questioned as to their routine application, it remains a basic and safe preparation for surgery. However its use does tend to depersonalise the patient and care should be taken to minimise this effect.

In most centres fasting is required for 4 to 6 hours pre-operatively. This was traditionally the time taken for the stomach of a 'normal' person, having eaten a 'normal' meal, under 'normal' circumstances to be emptied of its contents. However, it is now known that gastric emptying can take up to 20 hours and that even adequate fasting does not empty the stomach of gastric secretions which may total up to 200 millilitres (Hamilton-Smith 1981).

This seems to indicate that the patient's diet on the day prior to surgery should be low in fat which is the constituent that slows gastric emptying to such an extent. It also indicates that such a strict enforcement of the nil orally rule is not appropriate and that small amounts of water would be acceptable up until 1 or 2 hours pre-operatively.

The removal of jewellery is also a standard pre-operative procedure that can be adapted to allow for the comfort of the patient. A patient's wedding ring is often a token of his chief supportive relationship and, even when covered in tape, the knowledge of its presence can be extremely reassuring as the impending surgery approaches. Even the confused patient may still derive support from a wedding ring and be distressed by its removal. Religious tokens usually worn by the patient can also be sent into theatre with the theatre sister's permission and her advice about safety.

Identity bands are used not only to identify the patient prior to surgery but also to allow prompt identification in the recovery area and prompt administration of analgesia. The wrist band may be removed in the anaesthetic room to allow intravenous or arterial cannula insertion so an additional ankle band is of great importance.

Transfer to theatre

The patient is transferred to the theatre suite on a trolley, ideally accompanied by a familiar ward nurse. Hers may be the only face that is real to him with the others not only unfamiliar and covered with masks, but also distorted due to the angle from which he views them. The presence of 'his' nurse is reassuring especially if she is able to stay until he is anaesthetised. If he is concerned about the repeated checking procedures it can be explained that they do not reflect uncertainty but are part of a routine which serves to protect him.

This is the point at which the patient's anxiety is greatest and the percentage of patients expressing fears is highest (Janis 1958). If he decides not to undergo surgery his decision must be accepted even though he has given written consent. Reassurance by the nurse or the surgeon may be sufficient to restore his confidence but it is unethical to pressure him for the sake of a smoothly running operation list. This situation is uncommon but sometimes a patient needs more explanation and more time to come to terms with his illness and to feel ready to submit himself to major surgery.

Preparation for recovery

A detailed and up-to-date neurological assessment should be recorded in the nursing records and forwarded to the recovery staff when the patient is taken into theatre. They may or may not have met the patient before but with accurate and complete records of his neurological and emotional states and his pre-existing health problems they are able to identify problem areas and priorities of care. A baseline set of vital signs should always be included, reflecting normal recordings rather than those related to high anxiety levels soon after admission or immediately prior to surgery. Any information that can enable problems to be anticipated and either prevented or quickly identified and treated, helps to make the patient's recovery safer and more comfortable and is of value to the recovery staff. Relevant information regarding the patient's family is also of use when they make enquiries.

If the patient is to remain in the recovery area for an extended period of time then any personal medication or property, for example, inhalers, dentures, glasses can be forwarded. This will also serve to reassure the patient that he is expected to survive surgery.

The family

This may be the most anxious time for the family, with total isolation from the patient, a complete lack of knowledge of the patient's condition during surgery, and concern over the risks of general anaesthesia (Kathol 1984). They need to be supported in their chosen method of coping and they need to understand the normal routines and procedures.

Once the patient has been taken to theatre the pre-operative care is complete. With the exception of some preparation, his post-operative care does not start until he returns to the ward. The care of the relatives, however, continues through this period and is a natural part of the relationship that has developed between themselves and the nursing staff since the patient's admission to the ward.

REFERENCES

Behrends, E A 1982 Nutrition in neurosciences. Journal of Neurosurgical Nursing 14(1):44

Bouman C 1984 Self perceived needs of family members of critically ill patients. Heart and Lung 13(3):294

Breu C, Dracup K 1978 Helping the spouses of critically ill patients. American Journal of Nursing 78(1):51

Bruya M 1981 Planned periods of rest in the ICU: nursing care activities and ICP. Journal of Neurosurgical Nursing 13(4):184

Caplan G 1964 Principles of preventative psychiatry. Basic Books, New York

Daley L 1984 The perceived immediate needs of families with relatives in the intensive care setting. Heart and Lung 13(3):231

Franklin BL 1974 Patient anxiety on admission to hospital. Royal College of Nursing, London

Greary M 1979 Supporting family coping. Supervisor Nurse 10(52):19

Hamilton-Smith S 1981 Nil by mouth? Royal College of Nursing, London

Hampe S O 1975 Needs of the grieving spouse in a hospital setting. Nursing Research 24(2):113

Hayward J 1975 Information — a prescription against pain. Royal College of Nursing, London

Healey K M 1968 Does pre-operative instruction make a difference? American Journal of Nursing 68(1):62

Hill G L 1977 Malnutrition in surgical patients. Lancet: 1 689

Hopps L 1983 A case for patient teaching. Nursing Times 79(48):42

Janis I L 1958 Psychological stress. Wiley, Chichester

Janis I L 1980 In: Phippen M L (ed) Nursing assessment of pre-operative anxiety. American Association of Operating Room Nurses Journal 31(6):1019

Kathol D 1984 Anxiety in surgical patient's families. American Association of Operating Room Nurses Journal 40(1):131

Lipowski Z 1970 Physical illness, the individual and the coping process. Psychiatry in Medicine 1:91

May R 1980 In: Phippen M L (ed) Nursing assessment of pre-operative anxiety. American Association of Operating Room Nurses Journal 31(6):1019

Moghissi K, Boore J 1983 Parenteral and enteral nutrition for nurses. Heinemann, London

Molter N C 1979 Needs of relatives of critically ill patients, a descriptive study. Heart and Lung 8:332

Murphy F et al 1977 Sleep deprivation in patients undergoing operation: a factor in the stress of surgery. British Medical Journal 2:1522

Narrow B 1967 Rest is. . . American Journal of Nursing 67:1646

Stillwell S B 1984 Importance of visiting needs as perceived by family members in the ICU. Heart and Lung 13(3):238

Stotts N 1982 Nutritional assessment before surgery. American Association of Operating Room Nurses Journal 35(2):207

7

Care of the patient with a head injury

Head injury is a common cause of morbidity and mortality in children and young adults, and presents a serious problem in the developed nations. Over 100 000 people are admitted to hospitals in the UK each year following a head injury, although only 4% are transferred to neurosurgical units. Among the survivors discharged from hospital, physical and mental dysfunction will prevent half of them returning to work. As the average age of head injured patients is 30 years this can cause great financial, economic and social problems. At present there are 70 000 severely head injured people in the UK.

There is difficulty with the analysis of the effects of head injury for various reasons.

1. A lack of agreement about the definition of what constitutes a 'head injury'.
2. The variety of sources from which the statistics on head injury are drawn.
3. The fact that 'head injury' does not appear as a separate entity in the International Classification of Diseases (ICD).

However, it is the brain damage, primary or secondary which is important, as scalp and skull can be damaged without cerebral trauma. In 1977, a Scottish survey gave rise to the practical definition of 'cranio-cerebral trauma' as being synonymous with head injury. The term has proved useful and must include one or more of the following factors:

— a definite history of a blow to the head
— laceration of the scalp or forehead

— an altered conscious level, no matter how brief.

This does not include facial lacerations, fractures of the lower jaw, foreign bodies in the eyes, nose or ears, unless associated with one of the above features.

CAUSES OF HEAD INJURY

Road traffic accidents and vehicle/pedestrian accidents account for 60% of all severe and fatal head injuries, with alcohol intoxication implicated in a large number of cases. Many assaults and falls are also alcohol-related. Industrial and sports injuries are less common (7%) and include falls from roofs, scaffolding, mountains and horses.

Most peacetime injuries are 'blunt' (or 'non-penetrating' or 'closed') injuries. A penetrating injury occurs when weaponry such as an axe, knife, handgun or rifle is involved and the damage can be extensive.

MECHANISM OF HEAD INJURY

Blunt injury (closed head injury)

This is caused by either of two events:

1. a moving object striking the stationary head, such as a brick or a hammer
2. the moving head striking a static surface, such as the road or a wall.

Primary brain damage is caused by the acceleration force imparted when the stationary head is struck, and the rapid deceleration when the moving head comes to an abrupt halt. Also rotational forces contribute greatly to the overall damage, due to the greater potential for shearing and tearing of brain tissue.

Penetrating injury

In conventional war 95% of penetrating head injuries are the result of blast and shrapnel, and 5% are caused by bullets. In urban guer-

illa warfare up to 80% are due to bullets. The extent of brain damage depends on the kinetic energy of the missile which increases with the square of the velocity. 'Low velocity' is less than 1000 feet per second (FPS), e.g. handgun, whereas high velocity is greater than 1000 FPS, e.g. rifle. The entrance wound will be small, the exit wound (if any) large. The damage caused is extensive due to the explosion, implosion and cavitation effects. The injury is further complicated by retained missile or bony fragments and a high likelihood of haematoma formation and infection. This type of injury is not common in normal hospital practice.

Skull fracture

The scalp plays a major role in protecting the skull from fracture. Approximately 900 lb per square inch (PSI) is the pressure required to cause a fracture with an intact scalp, as opposed to only 40 PSI without scalp. The rigid skull is composed of three layers: the outer table, the diploe and the inner table which is grooved by arteries and venous sinuses. The vault is smooth in comparison with the irregular base with its sharp ridges, prominences and fossae. Approximately 70% of skull fractures are linear and tend to cross points of weakness, e.g. frontal sinuses and orbital roof, temporal, parietal and occipital squamous areas. If an underlying blood vessel is torn, an intracranial haematoma can form. Linear fractures can extend from the vault into the skull base causing a tear in the dura mater which may allow CSF to leak out or air to get in.

Depressed fracture

This mainly occurs due to localised violence and the damage to the brain is much reduced, e.g. a hammer blow to the head. However, the severity can vary from a simple depression of a fragment of bone below the normal skull contour with no scalp laceration, to fragmentation of inner table, torn dura and in-driven fragments of bone (compound).

Primary brain damage

The primary brain damage is caused by the initial impact forces acting on the brain, i.e. acceleration–deceleration and rotational acceleration forces, and severe or fatal brain injury can occur even in the absence of scalp injury and fracture of the skull. Due to the brain's consistency it is easily deformed but highly incompressible. During rapid movement tearing and shearing of brain tissue occurs particularly between areas of different density such as grey and white matter. Further direct damage occurs when the brain is forced against the irregular skull base, and the sharp edges of the falx and tentorium.

It is now believed that in every head injury which causes even brief loss of consciousness (as in concussion) there is structural brain damage. At the other end of the scale is the head injured person who may survive in a 'vegetative state' for weeks or months, due to widespread severe cortical and brain stem shearing lesions.

Concussion

There may be a brief loss of consciousness with post-traumatic amnesia. For several months the person may complain of headache, poor memory and concentration, visual difficulties, irritability, anxiety, depression, poor judgement and reduced libido. There is an organic basis for these symptoms in the form of microscopic damage to axons and blood vessels. Recovery does occasionally occur quickly following settlement of compensation claims indicating that some people exaggerate their symptoms because of financial reasons.

Contusion

Each of us carries our own 'built-in dashboard' against which the vulnerable brain collides. The irregular and rough sphenoidal ridges and orbital bones present an unyielding and damaging surface to the brain. Wherever the impact on the head, contusions are most often found on the undersurfaces of the frontal lobes, and around the temporal poles on the crests of the cortical gyri. They are usually bilateral, but may be more severe on one side. Rarely, they occur in the occipital lobes, corpus callosum and medial surfaces of the hemispheres.

Blood vessels are often torn leading to subarachnoid haemorrhage or to intracerebral clot formation. Cerebral oedema surrounding these coarse lesions can greatly increase the 'cerebral mass effect' and herniation syndromes can rapidly occur, particularly where the contusions are in bifrontal areas.

Laceration

Contusion and laceration often occur together in closed head injury, the distinction between them being related to severity. Lacerations involve tearing of the cortical surface caused by movement of the brain over the irregular skull base, or underlying a compound depressed fracture (an 'open' injury).

Diffuse white matter injury

This is the commonest form of damage after severe blunt injury to the head. Due to rotational forces imparted to the brain, shearing stresses are set up, particularly between areas of differing density such as grey and white matter. Axons are stretched and torn, small haemorrhages occur, often in the corpus callosum and in or adjacent to the superior cerebellar peduncle.

INITIAL MANAGEMENT AND ADMISSION CRITERIA

The majority of people who present at hospital with a head injury will make an uneventful recovery. A few will develop intracranial complications, such as haematoma or meningitis, and careful examination and assessment should identify those at risk. Realistic assessment reduces the number of people with minor head injuries who are admitted, and also helps to prevent under-estimation of the severity of some head injuries, where confusion may be attributed to another cause (e.g. alcohol) or skull fracture is not detected. This can lead to delayed diagnosis of complications.

Guidelines have been devised by a group of British neurosurgeons which take account of the availability of facilities and geographical location of specialist centres. These guidelines suggest that skull X-ray should be performed after recent head injury in the patient with:

— Loss of consciousness or amnesia at any time
— Neurological symptoms or signs
— CSF or blood from the nose or ears
— Suspected penetrating injury
— Scalp bruising or swelling
— Difficulty in assessing the patient, i.e. alcohol intoxication, epilepsy, children.

The guidelines also suggest admission to a primary hospital is necessary if there is evidence of:

— Confusion or any other depression of the level of consciousness at the time of examination
— Skull fracture
— Neurological symptoms or signs
— Difficulty in assessing the patient, as above
— Other medical conditions e.g. haemophilia
— The patient's social conditions are such that there is no responsible adult or relative to observe him.

If a patient is sent home he or his next of kin should receive written advice to return immediately if any of the following occur:
• Severe headache
• Blurred vision
• Vomiting
• Extreme drowsiness or dizziness.

Criteria have also been established as to when head injured patients should be referred for treatment to a specialised neuro-surgical unit. These are:

1. The presence of a fractured skull with:
   a. confusion or deterioration in level of consciousness

   b. focal neurological signs
   c. seizure activity
   d. any other neurological symptom or sign
2. Coma continuing after resuscitation (even if no skull fracture is present)
3. Deterioration in the level of conscious-ness or other neurological signs
4. Confusion or other neurological disturb-ances persisting for more than 6–8 hours, even if there is no skull fracture
5. Compound depressed fracture of the skull vault
6. Suspected fracture of the base of the skull or other penetrating injury.

It is recommended that patients in categories 1–3 are referred urgently.

Severe head injury

The main objectives in initial resuscitation are:

— To establish and maintain a clear airway
— To secure and maintain a normal blood pressure
— To assess conscious level and understand the significance of changes (i.e. devel-oping secondary complication)
— To assess other life-threatening injuries, e.g. flail segments in the chest wall, ruptured spleen
— To attend to any scalp wound.

If the airway is compromised by improper positioning so that the tongue falls back or vomit, blood or saliva is inhaled, then an unconscious patient's prognosis is immedi-ately worsened. During the ambulance journey, on admission and during investigations the patient must be on his side so that the jaw and tongue are forward and any potential aspirate will drain out of the mouth, rather than into the lungs. A disposable plastic airway will not help if the patient is lying on his back, as aspiration can still occur. The presence of an airway or endotracheal tube can greatly facili-tate mechanical suctioning to clear secretions. An orogastric tube should be passed and the stomach contents aspirated, to prevent their inhalation. Once the airway is clear, oxygen is administered to prevent hypoxia, and adequate ventilation must be ensured to prevent hypercapnia and the resultant cerebral vasodilatation which increases the intracranial pressure (ICP).

Many studies have shown that hypoxia and/or hypotension are the two most common insults associated with an unfavourable outcome in patients with an acute head injury. It is not unusual to find an improved level of responsiveness in a head-injured patient once inadequate ventilation has been corrected and arterial blood pressure restored to within normal limits.

Continuous monitoring of the conscious level is necessary to detect changes, either improvement due to treatment or that occurring naturally, or deterioration due to a secondary complication. It is necessary to use a well designed neurological observation chart, which shows clearly the patient's condition and progress. The Glasgow Coma Scale using three modes of behaviour — eye opening, verbal response and motor response — is one which is used worldwide, and designed for use by all grades of nursing and medical staff. It is also essential to understand the significance of any change in conscious level, or motor response pattern; then the appropriate investigation and treatment can be instituted.

Chest injuries, such as multiple rib fractures, pneumothorax or flail segments can cause hypoxia and lead to rapid neurological deterioration. Airway obstruction may be caused by facial or mandibular fractures and the swelling or haemorrhage associated with these.

Blood loss from scalp wounds, ruptured spleen or long-bone fracture can cause hypotension leading to reduced cerebral perfusion, ischaemia and infarction if not treated promptly with intravenous fluids, plasma and/or blood transfusion followed by appropriate surgical intervention.

Investigations

Skull X-ray may be carried out in the referral hospital, or in an emergency should be delayed until resuscitation is complete. In very seriously injured patients only chest and cervical spine X-rays need be done. A cranial vault linear fracture is fairly easy to detect radiologically and the majority require no specific treatment. However, combined with impaired conscious level it does indicate the increased risk of intracranial haematoma formation (1 in 4).

Basal fractures or those involving the air sinuses are difficult to see on plain films but are indicated by:

— CSF otorrhoea and/or rhinorrhoea
— Mastoid bruising (Battle's sign) or symmetrical bilateral periorbital bruising (Racoon's eyes)
— CT scan finding of an aerocele (or abscess developing later)
— Development of meningitis (if no fracture seen on X-ray) or if the tympanic membrane is intact.
— Other findings due to cranial nerve damage, e.g. unilateral deafness or anosmia.

At least two views, including a tangential view, should be taken when a depressed fracture is suspected, to show the extent of depression. Lateral shift of a calcified pineal gland indicates an expanding mass lesion and is best seen on a high quality anterior view skull X-ray. CT scan is an invaluable aid to diagnosis and management of the head-injured patient as it can demonstrate and localise intracranial haematoma, air, foreign bodies, contusion, oedema, infarction, intraventricular or cisternal blood and white matter damage where the patient is comatose or neurologically deteriorating.

Angiography and echoencephalography are seldom used now in head injury, due to widespread easier access to CT scan equipment.

ICP monitoring (see Ch. 5)

Opinion varies regarding the value of ICP monitoring, and the method employed, in diagnosis, prognosis and assessing treatment in head-injured patients.

Intracranial pressure monitoring *may* be carried out following a head injury where:

— CT scan has shown no haematoma but the patient is deeply unconscious and is being mechanically ventilated. A rise in ICP can then reflect respiratory dysfunction and abnormal blood gases or brain swelling

— CT scan has shown a haematoma and ICP monitoring may be helpful in determining the need for surgery (if pressure > 30 mmHg)

— CT scan has shown severe contusions and the patient is at risk of developing brain shift and tentorial herniation

— To act as an early warning system post operatively to detect re-collection of an evacuated haematoma.

A report from Miller (1978) showed that more than 80% of head injured patients in coma had raised intracranial pressure (over 11 mmHg). It is now thought by neurosurgeons that lowering high ICP, unless by evacuation of an expanding lesion, does not affect eventual outcome.

Secondary events

Intracranial haematoma

Traumatic intracranial haemorrhage is a common complication of 'blunt' head injury. Haemorrhage may start within minutes of injury, but it may be hours or even days before the signs of an expanding lesion are evident. The majority of cases have an associated skull fracture.

Extradural haematoma (acute). This usually occurs in the temporal region due to a tear in the underlying middle meningeal artery. Blood accumulates between the dura and the skull and the dura is stripped from the skull to accommodate the expanding lesion. Other less common sites for extradural haematoma are frontal and parietal lobes and the posterior fossa. These are usually due to haemorrhage from venous sinuses or diploic veins and may be termed subacute or chronic if signs and symptoms are delayed.

The classic sequence of developing extradural haematoma is described as loss of consciousness followed by a lucid interval prior to lapse into coma with hemiplegia and ipsilateral dilated pupil. In fact this occurs in less than a third of adults (and 50% of childhood extradurals).

Deterioration in conscious level is the most consistent and important sign, with developing hemiparesis following later. Pupillary dilatation, if it occurs, and extensor rigidity are late signs indicative of tentorial herniation.

Subdural haematoma. This refers to bleeding between the dura and arachnoid mater, from rupture of small bridging vessels and/or contused areas of the brain.

Acute subdural haematoma. This is usually associated with severe cerebral trauma. There is often a combination of subdural and intracerebral clot — the 'burst lobe', and usually there is associated brain swelling. Compression signs develop quickly, coma deepens, focal signs increase and brain stem distortion may occur leading to changes in respiratory rate, blood pressure and pulse.

Subacute subdural haematoma. The clinical picture is less dramatic; signs and symptoms may not present for 1 or 2 weeks. Sometimes there is a 'failure to improve' rather than a deterioration in conscious level.

Chronic subdural haematoma. This is more common in the elderly person, sometimes with a history of a trivial bump on the head, but more often with no such history. Due to cerebral atrophy which accompanies the ageing process, compression effects from an expanding clot are not apparent until pressure-volume compensation can no longer occur. Typically signs fluctuate; there is memory impairment, confusion, headache, drowsiness and hemiparesis which may be present one day, only to resolve the next day, before recurring again.

Infantile subdural haematoma. The two main causes are birth trauma and non-accidental injury and the majority of infants are less than 6 months old. Vomiting, convulsions, a tense anterior fontanelle and retinal haemorrhages are the usual signs.

Subdural hygroma. This condition may follow a relatively minor head injury, where a tear of the arachnoid mater allows CSF and blood to accumulate in the subdural space. The fluid is clear, yellowish or pinkish. Symptoms and signs are similar to that of a slowly developing subdural haematoma.

Intracerebral haematoma

This is a common complication of moderate to severe injury where cerebral laceration and contusion have affected the surface of the frontal or temporal lobes. It can also occur in the hemispheres due to shearing stresses and rupture of deep blood vessels. There is often a mixed intracerebral and subdural haematoma.

Traumatic subarachnoid haemorrhage

Following severe head injury blood is often present in the subarachnoid space and/or ventricles. If consciousness returns the patient may complain of headache, stiff neck and sensitivity to bright light, just like patients with spontaneous subarachnoid haemorrhage.

Brain swelling

This is defined as 'an increase in the volume of the brain as a result of the increase in the brain water content'. Brain swelling in head injury is a response to the insult, just as other tissues respond to trauma. The oedema may be localised or diffuse.

Several types of oedema exist: vasogenic, cytotoxic, hydrostatic, interstitial and hypoosmotic. In head injury, two types predominate: vasogenic and cytotoxic oedema.

Vasogenic. With contusion and haemorrhage there is increased permeability in the capillaries allowing water and some proteins to escape into the extravascular compartment of the brain. It is often localised and can contribute towards brain shift and herniation.

Cytotoxic. The common cause of this is hypoxia which causes neurones and glial cells to swell up with retained water.

Both forms of oedema lead to raised ICP, decreased cerebral blood flow, further cellular ischaemia and the continued development of oedema. A cycle develops as the biochemical and vascular changes lead towards a further rise in ICP until irreversible pressure-volume decompensation occurs, resulting in tentorial or foraminal coning and death due to brain stem compression.

In order to reduce the effects of cerebral oedema, some advocate the use of mannitol, an osmotic diuretic. However, its use is now usually restricted to short-term use, i.e. to transfer the patient or while awaiting the preparation of theatre.

Further elaboration of the mechanics in the development of oedema can be found in Chapter 5.

Infection

The risk of infection is present with all injuries where the dura is torn. This occurs because of fracture of the vault or base of skull and fractures involving the air sinuses or cribriform plate. Linear vault fractures may extend into the skull base and meningitis can occur where rhinorrhoea and/or otorrhoea is present due to open access to bacteria. Abscess is rare but can occur following depressed fractures or missile injury due to in-driven fragments of bone, hair or foreign bodies. Prophylactic antibiotics are administered, and penicillin is the most effective.

Extracranial complications

Hypoxia and hypotension

The effect of hypoxaemia (leading to cell hypoxia) and hypotension 'are frequently underestimated by the less experienced'. Continuing education of medical and nursing staff to make them aware of these dangers is absolutely crucial. The likelihood of a favourable outcome is lessened by adding hypoxic and hypotensive insults to the already injured brain.

Hypoxia ($PaO_2 < 60$ mmHg) and hypercapnia occur together when ventilation is inadequate (either due to respiratory obstruction or chest injury) and cause particularly adverse effects when the brain has been recently injured, as normal pressure-volume compensatory mechanisms are impaired. Cerebral vasodilatation (due to hypercapnia) and the resultant raised ICP leads to a fall in cerebral perfusion pressure, reduced cerebral blood flow and further cell hypoxia.

Hypotension (BP<95 mmHg systolic) following a head injury is usually due to other major injuries such as occult intra-abdominal haemorrhage.

Fat embolism

This can be due to a fracture of a marrow bone which causes emboli of fat to be carried to the brain, lungs, kidneys, etc. It can give rise to drowsiness, confusion and seizures, with dyspnoea, tachypnoea, tachycardia and pyrexia. The characteristic petechial rash over the chest, shoulders and base of the neck appears on the 2nd or 3rd day. Fat droplets may be present in the urine. This complication occurs rarely.

Other disorders

Hyperpyrexia

In the head-injured patient fever can be a sign of infection, commonly in the respiratory tract, or it may indicate upper brain stem or hypothalamic damage. Hyperpyrexia can cause a dangerous rise in ICP, cerebral metabolic needs are increased and ischaemia may result.

Hyperventilation

This is caused by brain stem damage and leads to a fall in $PaCO_2$ and increase in the PaO_2. Respirations are deep, rapid and regular and may result in alkalosis.

Metabolic disturbances

The metabolic changes which occur as a result of head injury are probably caused by damage to the hypothalamic and pituitary regions.

Hyponatraemia (Na < 130 mEq/l). This is a specific post-traumatic event. A mild hypona-

traemia is caused by salt and water retention after injury, with a greater retention of water than sodium. It may be worsened by excessive fluid intake, or sometimes inappropriate excessive secretion of anti-diuretic hormone (ADH) may be responsible, particularly in patients with basal fractures. It can cause further impairment of cerebral function.

Hypernatraemia. There are several explanations for hypernatraemia, the most common being an inadequate fluid intake, often because the patient is confused and uncooperative and will not swallow fluids or tolerate an intragastric tube.

Occasionally, hypernatraemia is due to diabetes insipidus developing as a result of the head injury, and excessive amounts of urine are passed due to lack of ADH. The conscious patient may complain of thirst, or be seen to be drinking large amounts of fluids whereas the patient in coma may rapidly become dehydrated and uraemic.

Glycosuria. There is occasionally glucose intolerance following head injury, and hyperglycaemia may occur if large amounts of carbohydrate are given once gastric feeding is established. Glycosuria will be found and insulin may be required temporarily to correct the hyperglycaemia.

Haematological disorder

In a study by Van der Sande et al (1978) coagulation tests were found to be abnormal in 40% of the patients following head injury, although only 8% were thought to be significant. Disseminated intravascular coagulation may cause bleeding tendencies or obstruction in the microcirculation from fibrin deposition, leading to pulmonary, renal and cerebral dysfunction. It may also be an important component of fat embolism.

Gastric erosion

Severe gastric bleeding may occur in up to 10% of severely head injured patients, possibly as a result of damage to the third ventricle/hypothalamic areas. It is thought to be a stress reaction as it can also occur with other injuries, and severe burns, and not solely as a direct result of head injury.

Surgical management

Operation for intracranial haematoma

Large acute haematomas should be evacuated via craniotomy, the approach depending on CT scan location of the lesion. If CT scanning is not available, the clinical signs alone can localise the haematoma in some. If the patient has a dilated pupil, the haematoma will be on the same side in 90% of cases, and if a skull fracture is also present on the same side as the dilated pupil, this probability is strengthened.

The aim of surgery is to remove the mass lesion and to seal the bleeding points, and is seldom a simple procedure. When there is time, blood should be taken for grouping and cross-matching, especially with children where the total blood loss requires immediate replacement.

A detailed explanation of the procedure of craniotomy is given in Chapter 11. The main points are:

— a generous skin flap, either 'question mark' or 'horseshoe' in shape, over the site of the haematoma
— removal of all the blood clot and extradural haemostasis where an extradural haematoma is present; when the haematoma is intradural (i.e. subdural or intracerebral) removal of all the blood clot and soft necrotic tissue
— whenever possible, the dura is closed and the bone flap replaced.

Chronic subdural haematoma

Burr holes alone, at least two, are used to drain chronic subdural haematomas which are usually liquefied. The area is thoroughly irrigated with normal saline, and some surgeons prefer to leave a drain in situ to prevent re-collection of the haematoma before the brain re-expands. Occasionally, in less than 20% of cases, bilateral haematomas exist, requiring bilateral exploration.

Posterior fossa exploration

Cerebellar signs and cranial nerve palsies arise from a haematoma in this unusual position, although an acute presentation results in rapid deterioration, foraminal impaction and respiratory arrest. Midline or paramedian craniectomy is appropriate to explore this compartment and evacuate the clot.

Compound depressed fracture

There is usually no immediate urgency to elevate the bony fragments providing that the scalp wound is cleaned and sutured, surrounding hair shaved and prophylactic antibiotic therapy commenced. At operation, the bone fragments are sometimes replaced in their normal position, the dural tear (the dura is torn in 50% of cases) sutured or patched and bleeding points sealed.

Recovery is normally uneventful in the absence of focal brain damage, although there is a 5% risk of epilepsy in the first week, which increases when either the dura is torn or there is a haematoma.

Base of skull fracture

Patients with persistent CSF rhinorrhoea require surgery to repair the dural tear otherwise meningitis may develop. (CSF rhinorrhoea stops spontaneously within 14 days in 70% of patients.) Neurosurgeon and maxillofacial surgeon operate together when facial bones and air sinuses are involved.

At operation, dural tears should be repaired with either temporal fascia, periosteum or lyodura. Suturing can be very difficult in this area and occasionally tissue glues are used.

IMMEDIATE POSTOPERATIVE MANAGEMENT

Following major surgery, patients will be transferred to the neurosurgical ITU for at least 24 hours, or if this facility is not available, to an easily observed area of the neurosurgical ward.

The important aspects of nursing management during this critical period are:

- airway
- breathing
- circulation.

The patient should be nursed on his side following surgery and may have a disposable airway in situ, or he may still be intubated because chest or facial injuries are compromising his breathing. Once the nurse receiving the patient from theatre has ensured that he is breathing properly and that his skin colour is normal, i.e. no cyanosis or undue pallor, she should ascertain what operation has been performed, the operative findings and the postoperative instructions regarding oxygen therapy, rate of infusion of i.v. fluids and presence of any monitoring equipment. Respiratory rate, rhythm and depth should be observed. Any abnormalities such as a change in pattern or rate, or development of breathing difficulties should be dealt with immediately by attention to the patient's position, by mechanical suctioning to clear secretions and by ensuring that the correct oxygen percentage is being administered. The anaesthetist should be informed of any problems which are not resolved after careful attention to these basic considerations, as hypoxia is a common cause of neurological deterioration.

The patient should be nursed in a good light to assess central and peripheral circulation; pallor or cyanosis may indicate blood loss or hypoxia. Blood pressure and heart rate are recorded and charted every 15 minutes until the patient's condition stabilises.

Assessment of conscious level

An accurate initial recording of the level of responsiveness provides a baseline for identifying subsequent improvement or deterioration after surgery and can give early warning of impending complications. With care and experience a trained nurse can sometimes detect a slight change before an appreciable difference is seen on the observation chart.

Postoperatively the patient will have an i.v. infusion, arterial line, wound drain, intragastric tube, urinary catheter and possibly be connected to cardiac and respiratory monitoring equipment. These should all be observed and their function checked regularly.

The patient's ICP may be measured also to act as an early warning system of intracerebral complications such as recollection of a haematoma. This will be indicated by a rise in pressure.

Wound care

The head bandage should be checked frequently for excessive blood staining or evidence of CSF leakage.

Other injuries

As many severely head-injured patients have other injuries too, such as limb fractures and lacerations, these must also be attended to promptly although they may not be life-threatening, as they can give rise to complications or disability in the future.

Control of pain

The patient's ability to feel pain may be underestimated because of an impaired conscious level. Although the patient cannot state that he is in pain or discomfort, he may become restless, or very tense, or groan when moved and these are often reliable signs. Regular administration of non-opiate drugs is frequently effective in relieving these indicators of pain. Codeine phosphate is often prescribed.

General nursing care

The patient's general needs, such as attention to personal hygiene, care of eyes and mouth, 2 hourly positional changes, passive limb movement, feeding and eliminating, will be met, or aided, by nursing staff. It is often during the time spent with the patient carrying out basic care that slight changes in condition are noticed. Care must be taken to include the patient in conversation at the bedside, and to avoid talking over him. The patient must be treated as if he can hear and not shouted at, although he appears to be in coma.

This early stage is an extremely anxious and difficult time for the family as often their questions cannot be answered easily, as so many factors can influence recovery. This uncertainty adds to their distress. If possible, the relatives should be spoken to regularly by the same surgeon and nursing sister so that there is continuity of information given to them. Information usually has to be repeated, as often the close family are so upset that they do not retain much of what they have been told. They may feel helpless sitting at the bedside, unsure of what to do or say and it will help them if there are ways in which they can contribute to their relative's care, by simply talking about everyday familiar things, holding a hand or helping to wash a child's hands and face. They should also be reminded not to say anything that could distress their relative.

POSTOPERATIVE COMPLICATIONS

Rarely, an extradural or subdural haematoma may recur in the first 48 hours, indicated by a deteriorating conscious level, developing hemiplegia, and progressive dilatation of the ipsilateral pupil. Postoperative monitoring of ICP may be valuable in distinguishing between deterioration due to haematoma recollection and that due to brain swelling. Swelling of one or both hemispheres due to oedema may cause persisting elevation of ICP following surgery.

Approximately 5% of head injured patients will have a fit during the first week following injury. The incidence is increased if the patient has a very severe injury, depressed fracture or haematoma. most commonly the fits are focal rather than generalised.

Following evacuation of a chronic subdural haematoma CSF pressure is often low and the brain may not re-expand immediately following removal of the haematoma. To avoid re-collection, some surgeons recommend that the patient is nursed in a head down position with adequate hydration to encourage the brain to 'come up' while others see no benefit in this and allow the patient to be mobilised as soon as he is able. A subdural drain is usually left in situ for 24 hours. If a subdural haematoma recollects, the fluid can often be aspirated through the burr hole under local anaesthetic.

Most patients will make an uneventful recovery from elevation of a depressed fracture but a few may develop some of the following complications:

— Infection due to inadequate debridement which may lead to meningitis or abscess formation.
— Intracerebral haematoma may develop if the fracture has involved one of the venous sinuses, and severe haemorrhage has occurred. The risk of epilepsy increases when the dura is torn or there is a haematoma. The incidence of epilepsy during the first week after injury is 5%.

Difficulty with swallowing, coughing, facial paralysis, dysarthria, ataxic gait and vertigo may be experienced after posterior fossa exploration for the removal of a haematoma. More dramatically, rapid deterioration and respiratory arrest may occur due to oedema or haematoma re-collection.

ONGOING CARE

Following the immediate postoperative intensive observation and care, a care plan incorporating the activities of living should be created according to the patient's condition and progress which can be extremely varied, from rapid recovery following elevation of a depressed fracture to the tragic non-recovery of a patient who remains in a persistent vegetative state.

For the majority who do improve, the main aim is a return to independence and this should be strongly enforced. It must be emphasised that recovery can take a long time, 2 years or longer before the head injured person may reach his maximum potential. The patient will often need lots of encouragement and reassurance from nursing staff, who must constantly strive to help him regain independence. It may be quicker, kinder and easier for a nurse to spoon feed a patient rather than encourage him to feed himself, but she will not be helping him gain independence. Planned stimulation should be practised by every member of the nursing team, despite opposition from the patient, who very often wishes to be left alone to sleep, and, as well as physically resisting the nurses, will say so in very certain terms.

When physical condition and any deficits allow, the patient should be nursed out of bed, assisted in immersion bathing or showering himself, taken for short walks, encouraged to feed himself and take an active role in his own care. The physiotherapist, occupational therapist and speech therapist may all have major roles to play in the sometimes long road to recovery. A planned programme of activity should also allow for periods of rest and sleep.

All technical equipment should be removed as soon as safely possible. Many head-injured patients strongly dislike i.v. lines, wound drains, urinary catheters and intragastric tubes, and unless supervised, or 'boxing gloves' applied, will remove them before the nursing staff plan to, during this restless uncooperative stage of recovery which many pass through. The nurse must ensure that there is not also severe headache, thirst, a full bladder or rectum, or hypoxia from a respiratory tract infection exacerbating the restlessness and aggression. In extreme cases, for safety it is better to nurse the patient on mattresses on the floor when not sitting safely supported in a chair, e.g. the Buxton tilt-back type. Raised cot sides on a bed frequently lead only to a confused and restless patient falling from a greater height in his attempt to get out of bed, by climbing up over them. Their use with head-injured patients is questionable; if necessary, a garment such as the 'Posey' waistcoat restrainer is safer, and although perhaps distressing for relatives to see, a sympathetic explanation will help them to understand. The nurse attending a confused aggressive patient must always try to speak and act calmly and not be offended by insults (and sometimes objects) hurled at her. The patient will remember none of his disorganised behaviour. Memory loss is common, the period of post-traumatic amnesia (PTA) depending on the severity of the injury. Problems with speech or understanding of the spoken word (expressive or receptive dysphasia) may worsen the patient's confused state by adding frustration to the communication difficulties.

Continuous assessment of the patient's difficulties and the methods used to help him overcome or adapt to them, will hopefully improve his day to day living when or if he eventually returns home.

The length of time spent in a neurosurgical ward prior to transfer back to the primary hospital or home depends on several factors including the rate of recovery from head and other injuries, facilities at the primary referring hospital, family and home circumstances. Even when the head-injured person is well enough to be at home, many problems can still beset the family in the future.

NON-RECOVERY

When, due to severe diffuse white matter damage suffered at the initial impact, the victim does not progress beyond spontaneous eye opening (not sentient) alone, with no purposeful limb movement or attempts to speak, and this state is prolonged, it is termed the persistent vegetative state. Fortunately it only occurs in around 10% of all severe head injuries, usually due to diffuse axonal injury or basal ganglia haematoma.

There is often evidence of a sleep/wake cycle, but the cerebral cortex is believed to be inactive, the patient surviving on brain stem function, breathing independently, awake at times but not aware of his environment. In these tragic circumstances, all the patient's needs are met by nursing staff. After 1 year, approximately 50% of them will have died.

PREDICTING OUTCOME

Coma score using the Glasgow coma scale appears to be one of the best predictors of general outcome after severe head injury. Outcome can be predicted with considerable accuracy in the first 24 hours, although other factors have to be taken into consideration. As an initial prediction can affect management decisions it is essential to form a reliable method of assessment. An MRC study in Glasgow in 1984, based on 2700 head-injured patients and their outcomes since 1969, formed the basis for computer assisted predictions, which in practice seems to be as good as the most experienced neurosurgeons at predicting outcomes, if not better. The computer does not allow for extracranial complications and is inclined to be optimistic, which in itself dispels fears that the computer prediction might lead to a scaling down of intensive care. The six indicators required to form a data base are age, coma score and pupil reactivity plus motor response pattern change (improving or deteriorating), and eye signs such as spontaneous movement, oculo-cephalic and oculo–vestibular reflexes. It has been shown that further information does not improve computer accuracy.

In future, computer predictions will be made at 24 hours, 3 days and 7 days from the onset of coma and this information will be made available to both medical and nursing staff. This is intended to help the neurosurgeon and the nurse provide relatives with an accurate prognosis as soon as possible and to act as an aid in the rational use of resources and to confirm that a particular course of action is appropriate. Computer predictions can also be used in the assessment of new treatments.

Assessment of outcome

Whatever the actual physical or mental sequelae, it is useful to categorise the overall social outcome. The Glasgow Outcome Scale serves this purpose. It comprises four categories for surviving patients, as follows:

1. **Vegetative state**: the patient shows no evidence of meaningful responsiveness. They breathe spontaneously and have periods of eye opening. Described as a non-sentient state.
2. **Severe disability**: the patient is conscious but needs the assistance of another person for some activities of daily living, every day.
3. **Moderate disability**: the patient is able to look after himself although some previous activities may no longer be possible. May be described as 'independent but disabled'.
4. **Good recovery**: despite possible minor physical or mental deficits the patient may or may not resume normal occupational or social activities.

The majority of patients have reached their final outcome category within 3 months of injury.

The physical deficits which can persist as a result of severe injury include hemiplegia, dysphasia, cranial nerve deficits and epilepsy. Some patients also develop delayed complications such as meningitis, osteomyelitis, carotico-cavernous fistula (rare), late traumatic epilepsy and hydrocephalus.

Hemiplegia (or paresis) combined with dysphasia can cause difficulties with all the activities of living: washing, dressing, mobilising, communicating, eating, drinking and eliminating, may not be achieved without help or supervision. Because of physical deficits, the head-injured person often will lose his job which will have a marked effect on his morale and quality of life. Cranial nerve deficits may also persist. The olfactory nerve is most commonly damaged causing anosmia. It is often due to a fracture of the thin cribriform plate or ethmoid bone. Anterior fossa and orbital plate fractures can also damage the optic and oculomotor nerves resulting in impaired eye movement, visual field defects or blindness. Temporal bone and middle fossa fractures can injure the facial and auditory nerves.

Post-traumatic epilepsy

Early epilepsy occurs in the first week and in 60% of patients the first (and sometimes only) fit occurs in the first 24 hours of injury. Early epilepsy is significant when it occurs soon after injury because:

— it may indicate an intracranial complication
— it may cause additional brain damage due to hypoxia if not adequately controlled
— it increases the risk of late epilepsy (by four times).

Generally, it is more common in patients with a prolonged PTA, depressed fracture or intracranial haematoma but in young children it can complicate a trivial injury. The fits can be either focal or generalised.

Several anticonvulsants are used in the treatment of early epilepsy. The regime will depend upon the type of seizure.

Following an initial fit, phenytoin sodium 300 mg is often given, followed by the same dose on a daily basis, for an average sized adult. If fits are frequent then a high serum level must be attained within 24 hours, i.e. phenytoin sodium 500 mg, intravenously and then depending on the patient's condition, 250 mg in each of the next two 6 hour periods, i.e. 1 g in the first 24 hours. The so-called 'therapeutic serum level' is the level at which the fits are controlled, not a specific blood level.

Status epilepticus

This happens more frequently in children, and is potentially fatal if not controlled immediately due to hypoxic damage. There is a series of generalised seizures without a recovery of consciousness between each one. The adverse effects are cumulative, with cerebral venous congestion and hypoxia during the periods of apnoea causing further brain damage.

Status epilepticus used to be treated with diazepam however, because of the associated dangers of depressed respirations and hypotension, phenytoin sodium is now preferred. Again, 500 mg is given by slow intravenous injection, followed 30 minutes later with a repeat dose if the fits are not controlled. This may be repeated again after another 30 minutes, if necessary. If this regime fails, barbiturate anaesthesia and ventilation is begun for 24–48 hours while maintaining the phenytoin therapy. Alternative drugs which may be used to control status epilepticus include clonazepam or chlormethiazole. These are given intravenously and the dose is titrated against the clinical response.

Delayed complications

Meningitis can occur several weeks after injury, if a basal dural defect has been plugged by brain tissue. CSF rhinorrhoea may have stopped spontaneously but bacteria can still enter through the dural tear.

Osteomyelitis, (infection of the bone flap), which leads to a chronic discharging scalp sinus, may occur weeks or months after surgery. This requires removal of the whole bone flap which often has a moth-eaten appearance on plain X-ray. No attempt at cranioplasty should be made until the wound has been free of inflammation and infection for 6–12 months.

Occasionally, following even mild blunt head injury, fractured base of skull or penetrating eye injury, the patient becomes aware of a noise in his head, a pulsating 'swishing' sound, with pain and development of a proptosis. The underlying cause is a fistulous opening from the carotid artery into the cavernous sinus (carotico-cavernous fistula) causing a bruit, diplopia due to ocular nerve damage and protrusion of the eyeball as the orbital veins distend. Chemosis and conjunctivitis may arise. The bruit can be heard on auscultation over the affected eye and may be abolished or reduced by direct carotid artery compression on the neck. Carotid angiography will confirm the diagnosis and successful treatment can be achieved with balloon embolisation under radiological control.

Post-traumatic hydrocephalus is divided into three types:

— that caused by wasting of the white matter following severe injury (hydrocephalus ex vacuo)
— obstructive hydrocephalus probably caused by adhesions in the CSF pathways secondary to haemorrhage
— intermittent pressure (or communicating hydrocephalus):

some of these patients may be asymptomatic while others may have developed headache and vomiting, or mental impairment, ataxic gait and incontinence.

Patients with evidence of raised ICP will usually improve after a shunt is inserted. There is a variable response to shunting operations in patients with intermittent pressure hydrocephalus. Hydrocephalus secondary to white matter loss or atrophy does not respond at all to CSF shunting.

The most common of the delayed complications is late traumatic epilepsy. The risk is higher in those patients who have had an intracranial haematoma, a depressed fracture or an early fit. About 70% of the patients have generalised seizures; few have focal motor seizures and temporal lobe seizures affect about 20%. Half of the patients who will suffer from epilepsy will do so in the first year. Each patient is unique in regard to his pattern and frequency of seizures, reaction to drug therapy and compliance with treatment. There are many anticonvulsants in use, and drug treatment often needs to be adjusted to meet the requirements of individual patients, in terms of choice of drug and dosage.

Mental sequelae

By far the most devastating feature of severe head injury is the mental sequelae, which may be the sole handicap. Studies have shown that mental disability contributes more significantly to the ultimate handicap than does physical disability.

Where there is a physical deficit such as hemiplegia, the head-injured person and his family can learn to cope with, accept and adapt to the limitations that it imposes. Mental disability naturally interferes with this process, as the capability of the head-injured person to reason, accept and cope are reduced. The family structure is disrupted and relationships suffer as stress increases.

Personality change, aggression, memory loss, irresponsible behaviour, loss of social tact and inhibition, reduced intellectual and reasoning powers, apathy, lack of motivation and initiative are the factors which often destroy the head-injured family's relationships. In addition to this the person with the head injury is likely to be unaware of how different he is.

Severe head injury is three times more common in men than women, and the majority are under 30 years old. In practical terms this often means that the survivors will be looked after by wives and mothers for many years. A degree of recovery often takes place in the first 2 or 3 years following the injury, but seldom enough to change the outcome category. Improvement is often as a result of adjustment and adaptation by the family members rather than a change in a relatively static disability.

The family

Apart from the victim of the head injury, the main sufferers are naturally the family members who in most cases experience shock, fear, disbelief and distress much greater than that of the head-injured husband, wife or child, who fortunately will probably not remember the trauma. As well as the distress caused by the actual injury and prolonged morbidity, social, legal and financial problems often beset the family. In the early stages, hostility and aggression due to anxiety are often encountered by nursing staff, and although it can be very difficult to cope with, the nurses should try to remain relaxed and handle the family kindly and with understanding. Where possible, different members of the family should be discouraged from asking several nurses the same questions, as differing opinions may create an atmosphere of distrust. Instead of feeling relief when their relative is transferred from ITU to the ward, the family are often alarmed because there are so many other patients for the nurses to attend to as well, and because he does not have a nurse at his bedside all the time. They will need reassurance that the 'intensive care' and observation can now be relaxed a bit, as their relative has either improved or his condition is now stable.

In retrospect, immediate family members are consistent in points of criticism during the initial stages, and these arise frequently during discussion:

— The surgeon was not available as often as they felt would have been helpful to give authoritative and experienced opinion of outcome.
— That they, the family, and future carers, were not adequately prepared for the disabilities and the long road to recovery, if indeed recovery is possible.

Research, however, has proved that very little information is retained regarding the events of the first 24 hours, who spoke to them and what they were told, so this information must be reinforced several times. Also, disbelief and denial of the possible severe effects of the injury may 'blank' out this 'bad news'. At this stage wives are often emphatic that their husbands will recover and be as they were before.

Later, anger and resentment are caused by several factors:

1. Following excellent initial care and early rehabilitation in the 'acute' stage, this is seldom continued in the primary referring hospital, partly due to lack of specialist knowledge, and partly due to financial constraints. However, as the recovery process is usually slow, this may exaggerate relatives' feelings that not enough is being done. When morbidity is prolonged, the victim of the head injury may eventually be nursed in totally inappropriate extended care facilities, such as geriatric or psychiatric wards, as there is an almost total lack of appropriate rehabilitation units in most regions.

2. The paucity of social and community resources available to provide help and advice once their relative is well enough to be at home.

3. Isolation and loneliness; wives and mothers feel they have been abandoned to cope alone with what may seem at times to be totally insurmountable problems. Friends and other relatives tend to visit less frequently, outside support gradually ceases and the constant stress of caring and supervising 24 hours a day results in eventual failure to cope. Tension and family strife worsen, and eventual breakdown of the family unit occurs, despite genuine attempts to cope. Each family is different with differing roles and responsibilities, social and financial background, differing emotional, intellectual and psychological make-up, and must be evaluated separately in their responses to caring for a head-injured person. A sympathetic, knowledgeable social worker can offer much in terms of practical assistance, advice, and information on available resources.

Headway

The National Head Injuries Association (Headway), a support group for the 'head-injured family' has achieved much since its inception in 1979. Its predecessor, Headline, continues to thrive in Bristol and remains affiliated to Headway. New groups are forming regularly, aided by interested members of the social work department, nursing staff, therapists and doctors who are aware of the need for improved after care and rehabilitation.

The aims of the groups are:

To offer objective, but caring support and advice. The burden of caring can often be lightened by listening to other people who are in a similar situation or who have already experienced the problems which can arise.

To provide information on a practical level, by inviting speakers from the Epilepsy Association, Welfare Rights Group, Legal Advisory Service and individual members of the hospital team such as a neurosurgeon, psychologist or psychiatrist.

To increase professional and media awareness and understanding of the very serious psychosocial aspects of severe head injury.

To help exert pressure where appropriate and beneficial, so that rehabilitation units designed specifically for the head-injured will one day be the norm, rather than the exception. In this day of advanced neurosurgical techniques and improved mortality rates, it is inconsistent that rehabilitation facilities are often non-existent following excellent intensive treatment, surgery and nursing care. More and more assault and accident victims are denied the right of programmed rehabilitation designed to maximise their potential for recovery. As there are at present 70 000 severely head-injured people in the UK (1 in 800, 1 in 300 families) and more added to this number each day, this need must be fulfilled.

It is probable that head injuries will continue to be a common cause of death and disability in young adults, though their numbers may be contained or even reduced by preventative and therapeutic measures. There are three stages of prevention, as follows:

— forestalling the accident
— minimising the damage sustained on impact
— reducing the risk of damage as a result of secondary events.

The majority of head injuries are potentially avoidable, but as cars, buses, high buildings, weapons and alcohol are part of our daily lives, accident prevention involves increasing public awareness of the dangers in relation to these irremovable hazards.

Since the introduction in 1983 of the legislation on compulsory wearing of seat belts in cars in the UK, fatal and severe injury in head-on collisions has been reduced by 25%, although the incidence of neck injury due to 'whiplash' and cracked ribs has increased. However, some dispute still remains with regard to the effectiveness of this legislation. The implication of alcohol and the change in drinking patterns during the same period may account for part of the reduction in these figures.

Reduction in road speed limit has been proven to reduce the number of fatal accidents, as shown by statistical analysis of the accident rate in Britain during the period November 1973 to July 1975, when the road speed limit was reduced from 70 mph to 50 mph because of the oil crisis.

The value of protective headgear in industry and in appropriate sports has been well established.

There is currently much publicity aimed at younger people to increase their awareness of alcohol related problems, and certainly in Scotland alcohol intoxication is more often associated with falls and assaults than with road accidents.

However, when a head injury has occurred the aim of management must be to try to prevent those avoidable factors which can contribute to mortality and morbidity.

BIBLIOGRAPHY

Allan D 1986 Management of the head injured patient. Nursing Times 82(25):36

Barlow P, Teasdale G, Jennett B, Murray L, Duff C, Murray G 1984 Computer assisted prediction of outcome of severely head-injured patients. Journal of Microcomputer Applications 7:271

Brooks N 1979 Psychological deficits after severe blunt head injury: their significance and rehabilitation. In: Oborne A B, Gruneberg C D, Eiser E F (eds) Research in psychology and medicine II:469. Academic Press, London

Brooks N 1984 Closed head injury: psychological, social and family consequences. Oxford University Press, Oxford

Galbraith S L 1976 Acute traumatic intracranial haematoma. M.D. thesis

Gentleman D, Jennett B 1981 Hazards of inter-hospital transfer of comatose head injured patients. Lancet 2:853

Gurdjian E S 1975 Impact head injury: mechanistics, clinical and preventative correlations. Charles C Thomas, Springfield

Hayes M 1985 The medical effects of seat belt legislation in the UK. DHSS, London

Hickey J 1986 The clinical practice of neurosurgical and neurological nursing, 2nd edn. Lippincott, Philadelphia

Jennett B 1979 Defining brain damage after head injury. Journal of Royal College of Physicians of London 13(4):197

Jennett B 1983 Medical aspects of head injury. Medical Education (International), 1(30):1415

Jennett B, Galbraith S 1983 An introduction to neurosurgery, 4th edn. Heinemann, London

Jennett B, Snoek J, Bond M R, Brooks N 1981 Disability after severe head injury: observations on the use of the Glasgow Outcome Scale. Journal of Neurology, Neurosurgery and Psychiatry 44:285

Jennett B et al 1984 Guidelines for the initial management after head injury in adults. British Medical Journal 288:983

Kohi Y M , Mendelow A D, Teasdale G, Allardice G M 1984 Extracranial insults and outcome in patients with acute head injury: relationship to the Glasgow Coma Scale. Injury-British Journal of Accident Surgery 16(1):25

Konikow N S 1982 Head injury: core packet. University of Washington, Seattle

Mendelow A D, Teasdale G 1983 Pathophysiology of head injuries. British Journal of Surgery 70:641

Miller J D 1978 Intracranial pressure monitoring. British Journal of Hospital Medicine 19:497

Miller J D, Becker D P 1982 Secondary insults to the injured brain. Journal of the Royal College of Surgeons of Edinburgh 27(5):292

North B 1984 Jamieson's first notebook of head injury 3rd edn. Butterworth, London

Pownall M 1985 Clunk-clink. Nursing Times 81 (48):14

Purchese G, Allan D 1984 Neuromedical and neurosurgical nursing, 2nd edn. Baillière Tindall, London

Russell W R 1971 The traumatic amnesias. Oxford University Press, Oxford

Teasdale G, Mendelow A D 1986 Management of head injuries. Nursing Times 82(20):59

Teasdale G, Galbraith S, Murray L, Ward P, Gentleman D, McKean M 1982 Management of traumatic intracranial haematoma. British Medical Journal. 285:1695

Van der Sande J J, Veltkamp J J, Boekhout-Mussert R J 1978 Head injury and coagulation disorders. Journal of Neurosurgery 49:357

Williams J M 1984 Predicting outcome from closed head injury by early assessment of trauma severity. Journal of Neurosurgery 61:581

Yanko J 1984 Head injuries. Journal of Neurosurgical Nursing 16(4):173

Young J A 1981 Head injury: advances in care during the last decade. Nursing Times 77(18):766

8

Care of the patient with an intracranial tumour

The nursing care of the patient with a brain tumour is one of the most difficult and demanding experiences which can face a nurse. The pessimistic outlook often attached to the diagnosis is, unfortunately, appropriate for some patients. However, major advances in medicine and nursing care over the last 20 years have considerably improved the prognosis and many patients now achieve a worthwhile recovery, to varying degrees.

Many studies have attempted to identify the true incidence of intracranial tumours and a worldwide incidence of 5 per 100 000 of the population has been calculated although a study carried out in the UK produced a higher figure of 11.7 per 100 000. Each year approximately 2250 people die in the UK as a result of a brain tumour.

Two major age peaks of incidence are noted; one in children under 10 years of age and the second in the 40 to 60 years age group. Intracranial tumours, with the exception of meningiomas and neurilemmomas, demonstrate a slight male preponderance. No definite cause has been established, although many theories have been postulated including toxoplasma infection, head injury and exposure to certain types of industrial pollutants. A possible link has been established with therapeutic irradiation of the head.

The clinical presentation of a brain tissue can vary greatly from one individual to another, depending on numerous prevailing factors such as the pathology, size and lo-

125

cation of the tumour. The number of neurological signs and symptoms can be as few as one, e.g. late onset epilepsy, or the patient may present with a complex combination of several symptoms affecting not only the nervous system but other body systems, e.g. hormone imbalances involving the endocrine system.

When considering signs and symptoms of cerebral tumours it is useful to seek an explanation of how they are caused and we can achieve this by examining the pathophysiology.

Tumours will grow in one of two ways: they will remain encapsulated (meningioma) or will spread and infiltrate neighbouring normal tissue (anaplastic astrocytoma). The cell growth may be slow or rapid. Either way this will produce an effect on the normal functioning of that area, e.g. a tumour in the frontal lobe may produce a change in the patient's personality.

The concepts to consider which are affected by abnormal pathophysiological phenomena are:

- cerebral oedema
- raised intracranial pressure (ICP)
- focal neurological deficits
- seizure activity
- pituitary function
- cerebrospinal fluid flow obstruction.

CEREBRAL OEDEMA

This is an invariable ocurrence within the surrounding cerebral tissue in the presence of a brain tumour and can often exacerbate existing signs and symptoms (due to a further rise in ICP). Presence of oedema will act to increase the overall mass effect of the original space occupying lesion. There are at least four different mechanisms by which oedema occurs. The one which is thought to occur in the brain is due to an increase in the capillary permeability. The capillary pores of the endothelial tissue, which constitute the white matter, become enlarged or their integrity is destroyed so that plasma proteins and other

similar osmotically active materials to leak out into the extracellular spaces, resulting in oedema. This response is initiated by the presence of the tumour and its compression of the surrounding tissue. This is known as vasogenic oedema. A second type, cytotoxic oedema, is also thought to occur.

RAISED INTRACRANIAL PRESSURE

ICP is the measurable pressure exerted by the brain tissue, blood and cerebrospinal fluid within the rigid bony skull. It is automatically maintained within a set of normal limits until abnormal pathology interferes to upset the balance, e.g. the presence of a brain tumour. The rate of growth of the tumour will determine the progress of the resultant signs and symptoms; some very slow growing tumours such as a meningioma can take several years to develop therefore they allow greater compensation to occur within the cranial cavity than do rapidly growing tumours. Most adult tumours are located supratentorially, causing the associated herniation syndromes to occur. As already stated, the occurrence of cerebral oedema will serve to hasten the increase in ICP. For detailed elaboration of the concepts of raised ICP, see the appropriate chapter.

FOCAL NEUROLOGICAL DEFICITS

Focal deficits are produced by:

— direct compression of specific areas of cerebral tissue or neuronal pathways
— interference in the functioning of certain cranial nerves
— compression of blood vessels supplying the cerebral tissue.

It is difficult to say with any degree of accuracy which of the above mechanisms in any patient with a cerebral tumour have been affected, in which order or to what degree. A combination of one or more of them will add to the complexity of the situation.

Direct compression on a specific area may result in the related neurological deficit, e.g. a tumour in the prefrontal area producing a communication disorder. The interconnecting neuronal pathways might also be affected resulting in failure to function properly. Likewise, interference in the function of the cranial nerves will result in an alteration from the normal response, e.g. the oculomotor nerve (3rd), if affected, would result in a failure of the pupil to react to light when tested. The vital blood supply to the brain can be compromised as a result of invasion from a neighbouring brain tumour. Compression of the vessels would result in ischaemia as the brain would be denied its supply of oxygen and glucose at a time when it critically needs it.

SEIZURE ACTIVITY

Seizure activity, either focal or generalised, can occur in the patient with a brain tumour. It is due to the altered neuronal excitability resulting in abnormal electrical discharges throughout the cellular level of the brain. It is the presenting symptom in about two-thirds of the cases of astrocytoma and meningioma. An adult in the middle years of life who presents with a sudden onset of even an isolated seizure should be suspected of having a brain tumour. Generalised seizures usually indicate a lesion of the frontal or temporal lobes, although this is not always the case. Focal seizures provide a better indication of the location of a tumour, e.g. corticospinal excitation in the motor cortex leads to a Jacksonian seizure, in which a small part of one side of the body is affected without loss of consciousness.

ALTERATION IN PITUITARY FUNCTION

The pituitary gland is situated at the base of the brain connected to the hypothalamus via the hypophyseal stalk. It secretes several hormones which are all concerned with metabolic functions within the body; therefore, if a tumour is present this will manifest itself by producing a hormone imbalance along with visual and/or neurological dysfunction. These will cause conditions such as acromegaly and Cushing's disease. The types of tumour seen are pituitary adenomas, craniopharyngiomas and certain types of meningioma although metastases, cholesteatoma, chordoma, mucocele, teratoma, third ventricle tumour, optic nerve glioma and the empty sella syndrome are other remote possibilities.

CEREBROSPINAL FLUID FLOW OBSTRUCTION

An expanding tumour, either fast or slow growing, may encroach upon the CSF pathways to cause an obstruction in their flow. This results in the development of hydrocephalus, which will in turn also add to the increase in ICP which may already be present. This type of hydrocephalus, which is common with childhood tumours, used to be termed as obstructive but the terminology of noncommunicating is preferred. Hydrocephalus is more likely to occur due to obstruction in the confined posterior fossa.

CLASSIFICATION OF TUMOURS (Table 8.1)

Classification of cerebral tumours has undergone many revisions over the last decade in an effort to simplify a complex system. The following classification is based on that recommended by the World Health Organization in 1979 and is based on histological features and clinical experience. It should also be noted that the grading of malignancy of a brain tumour is different from that of a neoplasm elsewhere in the body. A tumour, irrespective of histology, present within the rigid bony skull can prove fatal due entirely to its space-occupying effect and the subsequent increase in pressure. Likewise a small benign tumour located at a crucial site within the cranium can also prove fatal.

Table 8.1 Classification of tumours

Tumour	Description	Usual sites	Incidence % of total	Remarks
Tumours of neuro-epithelial tissue				
Astrocytoma Grade 1	Well differentiated, insidiously invasive, relatively benign	Cerebral hemispheres of adults; most commonly the frontal lobes followed by the temporal and parietal sites (Occipital lobe astrocytoma is rare.)	10%	A cystic type of astrocytoma is sometimes located in the cerebellum. A childhood tumour of the first decade of life
Intermediate astrocytoma Grades II & III	Will possess some of the characteristics of Grade 1 astrocytomas but cell differentiation less well defined			
Glioblastoma multiforme (anaplastic astrocytoma) Grade IV	Rapidly growing, undifferentiated cells, extremely malignant, and highly vascular. Infiltrates brain tissue extensively. Peak age is 48–52 years with a male bias. Can produce extensive brain swelling while still relatively small in size	Grade IV shown, to spread into the white matter of both hemispheres via the anterior corpus callosum	18%	
Oligodendro-glioma	Rare, slow growing tumour, age of onset = 40 years. Relatively benign — minor signs and symptoms can be present for a number of years before diagnosis is confirmed. Shows a marked tendency to calcify. (May be seen on skull X-ray.)	Demonstrates a predilection to grow in close proximity to the ventricular wall and commisural midline structures in the frontal region of the cerebral hemispheres. Can also be found in the temporal lobes	4%	Can 'mimic' a meningioma upon presentation. Unlike many tumours, raised ICP is a late sign in the patient with an oligodendroglioma. Sudden deterioration can occur, thought to be due to spontaneous haemorrhage and cystic degeneration within the tumour body.
Ependymoma	Rare undifferentiated slow growing glioma. Often seen in childhood and young adult	Arises from the ependymal layer of the ventricular system, therefore may be found in any of four lobes	5%	Due to involvement of the CSF pathways hydrocephalus and raised ICP are early common features
Optic nerve glioma	Occurs mainly before the age of 20 years. Follows a relatively benign course, remaining localised to the optic nerve and chiasma	Optic nerve and chiasma	4%	Approximately 60% of patients have an associated neurofibromatosis called a spongioblastoma
Medulloblastoma	Rapidly growing, malignant tumour of childhood. Composed of round, undifferentiated cells. Commonest intracranial neoplasm of childhood. Usually occurs before the age of 10 years	Cerebellar vermis or 4th ventricle roof	3%	Can 'seed' throughout the subarachnoid space. Slight male bias. Hydrocephalus is common

Table 8.1 (contd)

Tumours of nerve sheath cells

Neurilemma/ schwannoma	Slow growing, benign tumour. Well encapsulated. Usually unilateral, predilection for females, occurs in the middle years of life	The Schwann cell sheath of cranial nerves 8, 5 & 7 located within the confined cerebello-pontine angle		A tumour of the sheath of the eighth nerve. Referred to as an acoustic neuroma. Other tumour types may be seen in this location, e.g. meningioma, but a differential diagnosis may not be made till surgery
Neuroma (Neurofibroma)	A complex familial disorder characterised by widespread benign tumours throughout the nervous system. Inherited as an autosomal dominant trait. Known as Recklinghausen's disease. Manifests itself in young adulthood	The neurilemma of nerves, therefore tumours may appear intracranially, i.e. 7th nerve, acoustic neuroma or extra-cranially, i.e. spinal roots and peripheral nerves	10%	Patient will present with cutaneous pigmentation of the skin termed 'café au lait' spots. Some of these patients will also have a meningioma or glioma as well

Tumours of meningeal and related tissues

Meningioma	Benign, slow growing tumour arising from the arachnoid cells of the arachnoid villi. An irregular single mass usually well encapsulated.	Intracranial venous sinuses — most common, superior sagittal sinus known as a parasagittal meningioma. Other sites include sphenoid ridge convexity of hemispheres and suprasellar region and olfactory groove	15%	Can become very large before signs and symptoms appear. Predilection for females in 40–60 year age group. Do not show any malignant change

Tumours of blood vessel origin

Haemangio-blastoma	Slow growing, vascular tumour of developmental origin. Single or multiple lesions occur. Manifests in children and young adults, male bias. May be familial	Cerebellar hemisphere	2%	May be associated angiomatosis of the retina or abnormal organs. von Hippel-Lindau disease

Germ cell tumours

Teratoma	Rare tumour of childhood and young adulthood	Pineal parenchymal cells therefore located around the pineal gland		Terms pinealoma and teratoma are often interchanged

Table 8.1 (contd)

Other malformative tumours

Craniopharyn-gioma	A tumour of developmental origin, may be cystic or solid. Does not usually present until adolescence. May calcify	Arises from embryological remnants of the cranio-pharyngeal duct (Rathke's pouch) into the suprasellar region and the posterior fossa.	3%	Sometimes referred to as a cholesteatoma
Epidermoid cyst	Congenital fluid-filled cyst of the ectodermal layer. May contain keratin and cholesterol. Occurs in childhood	Posterior fossa		
Dermoid cyst	Similar to epidermoid cyst; arises from the ectodermal layer but contains more solid material such as hair, sebaceous glands or even teeth	Posterior fossa		Difficult to differentiate from other posterior fossa tumours until direct visualisation at surgery
Colloid cyst of the third ventricle	Rounded cystic tumour of childhood	Choroid plexus within the third ventricle		Often presents with an acute, sometimes intermittent hydrocephalus

Vascular malformations

Angioma	Arterial and/or venous congenital abnormality comprising enlarged and tortuous vessels. Usually have a 'feeder' artery and a 'draining' vein	Anywhere in the cerebral cortex, most commonly in the region of the middle cerebral artery		A unilateral capillary-venous malformation and the presence of a facial naevus is termed the Sturge-Weber syndrome. Hamartomas are small vascular malformations
Angioblastoma	Cystic tumour comprised of angioblasts	Cerebellum		The patient may also exhibit, an angioblastoma of the retina

Tumour of the anterior pituitary

Pituitary adenoma	Benign, slow growing, well encapsulated tumour. Classified by the clinical syndrome, i.e. the hormone produced. Three types of hypersecreting adenomas: prolactin secreting (prolactinoma); excess growth hormone (acromegaly); ACTH secreting (Cushing's disease). Hyposecreting tumours are very rare	Anterior lobe of the pituitary gland.	8%	Hyposecreting tumours will produce panhypopituitarism and chiasmal compression

Table 8.1 (contd)

Local extensions from regional tumours				
Chordoma	Soft tumour with a jelly like consistency	Arise extra-durally at the base of the skull		
Metastatic tumours				
Metastatic tumour	Well defined, usually multiple secondary deposits of a primary growth elsewhere in the body. Common primary sites are bronchus and breast	As lesions are often multiple, can occur anywhere in the cerebrum or cerebellum	12%	The symptoms and signs of a secondary intracranial growth may precede those of the original growth

SIGNS AND SYMPTOMS OF BRAIN TUMOURS

Headache

Initially, this is intermittent and of a brief dull duration but as the tumour expands, it becomes constant. It is usually described as throbbing or bursting and is at its worse in the early morning and during the night. This is thought to be due to the decreased venous return from the head (brought about by lying flat in bed) which is experienced with raised ICP. When the patient wakens in the morning and rises from his bed, the headache characteristically disappears as the elevated ICP is relieved. Likewise the headache will be worsened during manoeuvres which will raise ICP, such as coughing or sneezing. There is a difference of opinion as to the localising value of the headache; some patients will present with a headache which they can fairly accurately pinpoint to one side or to the front or back of their head while in others the headache is described as diffuse. It would be reasonable to assume that a patient with a posterior fossa tumour is more likely to feel pain at the back of the head and neck.

Vomiting

The pattern of vomiting is similar to that of headache, in that it occurs at night and in the early morning when ICP is at its highest. It is described as effortless and may also be projectile. It is believed to occur as a result of direct stimulation of the vomiting centre in the medulla (a manifestation of raised ICP).

Papilloedema

This is a swelling of the optic disc and can only be detected with direct ophthalmoscopy. Raised ICP is one of the commonest causes of papilloedema; the increase in pressure within the cranial cavity is transmitted down the optic nerve to produce the characteristic changes of oedema and hyperaemia of the disc. It is not a sign often seen in the early stages although it will become apparent as the disease progresses. The patient may complain of a visual disturbance such as diplopia or attacks of transient blindness. Occasionally it may be a visual disturbance which prompts the patient to seek medical advice.

Mental deterioration

This is manifested in two different ways:

— the patient presents with drowsiness, lethargy and mental confusion and if left untreated, will lapse into coma
— the patient undergoes a personality change; involving impairment of memory, disinhibition and loss of intellectual capacity. This is an insidious process and it is often the patient's family who notices the subtle changes before the patient himself.

Epilepsy

This may be focal or generalised, and can sometimes occur months or years before any other signs or symptoms manifest themselves. Approximately 30% of adults with brain tumours develop some type of seizure.

Focal symptoms

These are variable and are due either to direct pressure on, or infiltration of, the area of the brain responsible for the normal function of a part of the body. Similarly, pressure may be exerted on one of the nerve tracts (including the cranial nerves) which acts as a communication link between the brain and the rest of the body. These focal symptoms include ocular problems, such as failing vision, loss of the visual field and diplopia. These could arise as a result of a lesion in or around the optic chiasma or in a tumour of the temporal, parietal or occipital lobes. Deafness may occur, as the result of interference in the functioning of the 8th cranial nerve (vestibulocochlear) such as when a schwannoma grows from the sheath of the nerve. Ataxia would be indicative of a lesion of the cerebellum and language problems can be localised to the pre-frontal and temporal lobes. Weakness and numbness in any part of the body will be caused by destruction of the corresponding corticospinal tract fibres.

Pituitary dysfunction

Tumours in and around the pituitary fossa may cause endocrine, visual and/or neurological dysfunction. Occasionally other cranial nerves may be affected, or hydrocephalus develops due to obstruction of cerebrospinal fluid flow through the interventricular foramina (foramina of Munro).

SIGNS AND SYMPTOMS RELATED TO SPECIFIC AREAS

As different areas of the brain are responsible for different functions within the body, it follows that a tumour's presence may be localised by the dysfunction which it is producing. The range and severity of a deficit will vary according to the location, size, rate of growth and type of tumour responsible. Some tumours will spread from one area to another producing a complex set of symptoms and in some instances, it is possible to produce a set of false localising symptoms. This is brought about as a result of mechanical displacement and distortion of remote structures by a cerebral tumour. An example of this is the production of a VIth cranial nerve (abducens) palsy as a result of interference of the function of the cerebral hemispheres through hydrocephalus.

Only the signs and symptoms peculiar to the regions are given below as these will occur in addition to some of the general signs and symptoms already outlined.

Frontal region

A wide range of mental symptoms can occur including inappropriate behaviour, loss of the ability to concentrate, emotional lability, loss of social control (which in turn can lead to incontinence) and impairment of recent memory. The relatives might simply state that the patient has changed or that he is not the same person as he was before. As the motor speech area (Broca's area) is located within the frontal region, the patient may present with expressive dysphasia. There may be generalised seizures. Other symptoms include frontal headache, and contralateral hemiplegia or hemiparesis.

Parietal region

Sensory discrimination is impaired. The patient may complain of a wide range of sensory related deficits such as paraesthesia, loss of two point discrimination, astereognosis and hyperaesthesia. As the region is responsible for accommodating the association areas for body orientation, vision and language, the patient may experience loss of right-left discrimination, agraphia, anosognosia or disorientation of the external environmental space. Other symptoms include seizure activity, particularly Jacksonian; visual deficits, e.g. homonymous hemianopia; receptive speech problems.

Temporal region

— temporal lobe epilepsy, which is characterised by a disturbance of the content of consciousness, e.g. sensory hallucinations
— receptive aphasia
— visual deficits, e.g. an upper quadrant hemianopia.

Occipital region

— visual deficits, consisting of a hemianopia
— focal or generalised seizures.

Brain stem

— cerebellar dysfunction, i.e. ataxia, unco-ordination
— eye symptoms, i.e. diplopia and paresis of conjugate ocular deviation
— dysphagia
— vomiting.

Mid-brain

— hydrocephalus
— ocular abnormalities, ptosis and diminished light reflexes
— cerebellar symptoms, i.e. ataxia, unco-ordination, nystagmus and tremor.

Cerebellum

— cerebellar symptoms, more marked on standing and usually ipsilateral
— raised ICP; headache, vomiting and papilloedema
— hydrocephalus.
— disturbances of cranial nerves, the 5th, 6th and 7th are most commonly affected.

Pituitary region

— headache

— visual disturbances
— hormonal disturbances.

Ventricular region

Tumours in or around any of the ventricles will lead to obstruction of cerebrospinal fluid flow.

DIAGNOSIS

A wide range of sophisticated investigative procedures is now available to assist in the diagnosis of a suspected tumour. Facilities will vary depending upon the size of the unit and availability of the necessary equipment to perform these studies.

Prior to proceeding to formal investigative studies the patient will have had a full neurological and general examination performed by the doctor. Signs and symptoms indicative of a possible tumour cannot, in many cases, be confirmed until sophisticated diagnostic studies are performed, as there are a wide range of differential diagnoses which may account for the symptoms. These may include subdural haematoma, abscess, hydrocephalus, hypertension, atheroma, epilepsy and migraine.

Investigation

A detailed neurological and general examination of the patient. In adults, the occurrence of late onset epilepsy, signs and symptoms of raised ICP, focal signs and behavioural changes all raise suspicion.

Skull X-ray. Characteristic changes may be seen in the patient with chronically raised ICP; erosion of the dorsum sellae in adults or a 'beaten brass' appearance in children, who may also have widening of the skull sutures. Calcification of the pineal gland and shift from the midline may also be demonstrated.

Computerised tomography (CT scan). When available, CT is probably the most useful and definitive investigation available. It can reveal detailed information of the size, location and possible pathology of the tumour. Prior to the advent of CT scanning, and in those centres without this facility, patients may undergo lumbar air encephalography, ventriculography or isotope scanning to outline the tumour. These investigations are not as precise as a CT scan and carry some dangers for the patient. Some tumours may be enhanced on the CT scan by administering intravenous contrast. Associated problems such as cerebral oedema and hydrocephalus will also be demonstrated. Newer developments include CT directed biopsies and pre-operative CT scanning at craniotomy.

Electroencephalography (EEG). This is a non-invasive technique which has been superseded by CT scanning. It may be performed in a primary hospital prior to referring the patient to a specialist centre. It will only localise a focal lesion, which could be one of a number of different pathologies.

Cerebral angiography. This technique is used in some instances to demonstrate displacement of blood vessels or an abnormal circulation indicative of certain types of lesions, e.g. angiomas.

Magnetic resonance imaging (MRI). A new sophisticated imaging technique, available in only a few centres, MRI is useful in diagnosing tumours of the posterior fossa.

Chest X-ray. A patient with a secondary brain tumour could have a primary lesion in the lungs, which will be detected by chest X-ray.

Lumbar puncture. Although this is unlikely to be performed because of the danger of herniation, it may be useful for obtaining cerebrospinal fluid for examination. Carcinomatosis infiltration of the cerebrospinal fluid may prove diagnostic.

Specialist investigation. Certain additional investigative techniques may include:

— endocrine evaluation involving examination of serum and urinary hormonal levels
— visual fields
— audiometric studies.

MEDICAL TREATMENT

The approach to the treatment of brain tumours will vary for each individual. A typical course of events might include:

— initial investigation and tentative diagnosis.
— commencement of steroids and possibly anticonvulsant drug therapy (if not already started)
— burr-hole biopsy
— surgical removal (if possible) via a craniotomy, posterior fossa craniectomy or transphenoidal approach
— where indicated, either shunting procedure for hydrocephalus and/or radiotherapy

Each of these stages is now described in more detail.

Drug therapy

Steroids. Dexamethasone (a synthetic glucocorticoid) is the one favoured by most neurosurgeons. It is often commenced as soon as the presence of an intracranial tumour is suspected and acts by decreasing the amount of cerebral oedema and thereby reduces the untoward effects of raised ICP. A loading dose of 12 mg i.v. is given, followed by 4 mg orally every 6 hours; the dosage being reduced in children. The usual precautions employed when administering steroids should be observed. Many patients will demonstrate a marked improvement following the administration of dexamethasone even to the extent of reversing apparently profound neurological deficits.

Anticonvulsants. Patients who present with a history of seizure activity will receive anticonvulsant therapy immediately. Phenytoin 300 mg daily (adults) is often used. In some cases, even those patients who did not have any pre-operative seizures might be started on prophylactic anti-convulsant therapy as they are placed at an increased risk following certain types of craniotomy. This policy will vary greatly according to the surgeon's preference, as no standard agreement appears to exist.

Burr-hole biopsy

This involves obtaining a small sample of

cerebral tissue for examination by the pathologist. It is only used in supratentorial intracerebral lesions where a differential diagnosis might include abscess or infarct. The accuracy of diagnosis is very much dependent upon the skill of the surgeon to obtain a sample of tissue which is reasonably histologically representative of the lesion. However, this can be an extremely useful tool in the diagnostic process as it can determine whether to proceed to further prolonged treatment.

Surgical removal

If this is indicated and the patient agrees, then all or as much as possible of the tumour will be resected. A supratentorial lesion would involve a craniotomy, while a tumour located in the posterior fossa would require a craniectomy. Occasionally, a partial lobectomy will also be performed. If the tumour is in the pituitary gland, then it is removed via the trans-sphenoidal route, which involves a sublabial approach. More comprehensive information on these operative techniques can be found in Chapter 15.

Shunting. Redirection of the flow of the cerebrospinal fluid via a ventriculo-peritoneal shunt may be required, particularly in tumours of the posterior fossa which may have blocked the pathway. This procedure may be performed in either the pre- or postoperative period.

Radiotherapy

This may be used alone or as an adjuvant to surgery. It appears to be of some use in malignant gliomas, meningiomas and pituitary adenomas. Whether radiotherapy is used will depend upon the surgeon's preference and, in many cases, ethical considerations are raised in view of the modest results.

NURSING CARE OF PATIENTS WITH INTRACRANIAL TUMOURS

The patient will be admitted to a specialist unit for investigations and treatment and may be aware of the possible diagnosis prior to this. It is essential that the nurse is aware of the extent of the information already given to the patient and his level of understanding. This is an emotionally traumatic period for the patient and his family and it is imperative that the nurse provides realistic and useful support. The patient is assisted by the nurse to prepare for his investigations by the provision of information in respect of the procedure involved, when and where it will be performed and what is expected of the patient. This will be in addition, where appropriate, to the information given by the doctor when obtaining consent.

The patient may have been started on steroids and/or anticonvulsants and it is the nurse's responsibility to ensure that the medications are administered correctly and via the appropriate route. It is essential that the nurse is aware of the therapeutic effect of the drugs involved and any possible side-effects or reactions.

Steroids can pose particular problems. Dexamethasone is often used and side-effects may include adrenocortical insufficiency, electrolyte imbalance and Cushing's syndrome. As part of the routine nursing care an accurate record of the patient's fluid balance should be maintained along with monitoring of serum electrolyte levels. Blood pressure should also be routinely checked. An increase in gastric acidity is often produced, causing exacerbation of an existing ulcer. Administration of an antacid or cimetidine along with routine monitoring of the patient's stool for blood will help to minimise this. As dexamethasone will depress the normal production of the hormone by the adrenal cortex, it is imperative that the patient receives the correct dosage as sudden discontinuation would result in an adrenal crisis.

The most frequently prescribed anticonvulsant is phenytoin sodium and this is normally well tolerated in the short-term. The usual dose for an adult is 300 mg daily orally (the drug is poorly absorbed intramuscularly). Intravenous administration should be used with extreme caution.

Maintaining a safe environment

Some neurological deficits may be evident and nursing care will need to be modified in the light of these. The patient with a balance problem as a result of ataxia due to a cerebellar tumour or hemiplegia will present safety problems. In turn mobility will also be affected. The patient with a frontal lobe tumour may present with confusion or disinhibition and the nurse will need to exercise tact and diplomacy when dealing with this. A very confused patient may not understand why he is in hospital and attempt to leave, posing a threat to his own safety. Relatives, understandably, can be very upset to see the patient behave in this way and they will need constant reassurance and support.

A third group of symptoms which may pose problems involve those leading to difficulties associated with sensory loss or impairment. This may include a visual loss, due to the encroachment of the optic chiasma by a pituitary tumour or a hearing loss due to the presence of an acoustic neuroma. Loss of sensation over a particular part of the body, depending on the location of the tumour, will lead to the inability of the patient to distinguish hot from cold, rough from smooth and so on. The nurse should provide facilities and exercise techniques to counter these deficiencies while allowing the patient to continue to do as much as he can for himself.

Communicating

The inability to communicate can be very distressing. The patient with dysphasia/aphasia or a hearing loss will have difficulty making himself understood and/or being understood by the carer. Various alternative methods may need to be used in order to minimise the problem. These may range from providing the patient with pencil and paper to the use of sophisticated electronic communication aids. Body language and facial expression are important components of the ability to communicate and the patient with a facial palsy or impaired mobility due to, for example, the existence of a hemiplegia will be deprived of the ability to communicate nonverbally. It is important that the nurse recognises this and employs different techniques to overcome this problem. If the patient is confined to a chair or bed, the nurse should communicate with him at a similar level, in order to encourage eye contact rather than standing over him. The use of touch is often employed during verbal exchanges and if the patient has a loss of sensation in a particular part of the body it may be that he is unaware of a reassuring hand touching him.

Eating and drinking

Several problems can present themselves when the patient attempts to eat or drink. The presence of physical problems such as a hemiplegia will deprive the patient of the use of one hand so that he is unable to cut up his food, or a facial palsy which may preclude the patient from chewing his food properly. In addition to this, the swallowing reflex may be impaired, exposing the patient to the danger of choking and/or possibly aspirating the gastric contents into the respiratory tract. The nurse should be aware of these possibilities and be ready to adapt to the individual patient's needs. Special cutlery and associated feeding accessories such as non-slip mats may be useful. Alternatively the patient may need his food to be cut up even though he may be able to feed himself satisfactorily. Careful oral hygiene in the patient with a facial palsy is necessary as food debris is often left in the mouth following a meal. A modified diet may be indicated for these patients and also for the patient with a swallowing deficiency. If a modified diet is not adequately tolerated, it may be necessary to feed the patient via a nasogastric tube. For details of procedure and regimes see Chapter 3.

The patient with intracranial hypertension may be feeling nauseated (particularly at breakfast time) or may be vomiting. A prescription of anti-emetics and the provision of a late, light breakfast may assist in alleviating the problem.

Should surgery be performed the nursing care involved is that outlined for the post-operative care of a patient following craniotomy (Ch. 11).

The patient with a possible diagnosis of brain tumour faces an uncertain future while diagnosis is ongoing and prognosis is being established. This is, for most patients, a crucial episode in their life and it is at this time when they are at their most vulnerable and scared. The role of the nurse during this period cannot be underestimated and she will have many demands made upon a wide range of skills including counselling, comforting, reassuring, supporting, communicating and co-ordinating the patient's care.

BIBLIOGRAPHY

Allan D 1978 A patient with an acoustic neuroma. Nursing Times 74(49):2015

Anchie T 1980 Acoustic neuroma: a benign tumour. Journal of Neurosurgical Nursing 12(1):11

Bannister R 1985 Brain's clinical neurology 6th edn. Oxford University Press, London

Blanco K M 1981 Acoustic neuroma: postoperative nursing care and rehabilitation. Journal of Neurosurgical Nursing 13(3):153

Cleavland M J 1982 Nursing care in childhood cancer: brain tumour. American Journal of Nursing 82(3):422

Damon J, Taylor L 1980 Brain tumours in children. Nursing Clinics of North America 15(1):99

Gehrke M 1980 Identifying brain tumours. Journal of Neurosurgical Nursing 12(2):90

Hickey J 1986 The clinical practice of neurological and neurosurgical nursing. J B Lippincott, Philadelphia

Larson E 1980 Epidemiology of primary brain tumours. Journal of Neurosurgical Nursing 12(3):121

Lowther J 1984 Mandy's story. Nursing Mirror 158(13):43

Macrae A 1984 Cerebral tumours. Nursing Mirror 158(17):36

McInerney M 1981 Prolactin producing pituitary adenomas. Journal of Neurosurgical Nursing 13(1):15

Mitchem H L 1984 A CT guided stereotactic apparatus: new approach to biopsy and removal of brain tumours. Journal of Neurosurgical Nursing 16(5):231

Nemeroff D R 1981 Transphenoidal hypophysectomy: an overview. Journal of Neurosurgical Nursing 13(6):303

Purchese G, Allan D 1984 Neuromedical and neurosurgical nursing, 2nd edn. Baillière Tindall, London

Stewart C 1980 Current concepts of chemotherapy for brain tumours. Journal of Neurosurgical Nursing 12(2):97

Stillman M J 1981 Transphenoidal hypophysectomy for pituitary tumours. Journal of Neurosurgical Nursing 13(3):117

Tortorelli B A 1981 Acoustic neuroma: An overview of the disorder and nursing care for these patients. Journal of Neurosurgical Nursing 13(4):170

Thomas D G T 1983 Brain tumours. British Journal of Hospital Medicine 29(2):148

Thomas D G T, Graham D I 1980 Brain tumours: scientific basis, clinical investigation and current therapy. Butterworths, London

Walton J 1982 Essentials of neurology. Pitman, London

Wheeler P 1977 Care of the patient with a cerebellar tumour. American Journal of Nursing 77(2):263

Zulch K J 1979 Histological typing of tumours of the central nervous system. World Health Organization, Geneva

9

Care of the patient with a malformation of the cerebrovascular system

Of the large number of people who suffer a haemorrhagic 'stroke' or develop other neurological signs and symptoms, some are found to have an operable lesion. The main vascular abnormalities are cerebral aneurysm, and arteriovenous malformation (angioma, AVM). Sturge-Weber syndrome and vein of Galen anomaly are rare.

Around 12 per 100 000 of the population in the UK each year are affected by subarachnoid haemorrhage (SAH) most commonly from a ruptured aneurysm on a major cerebral blood vessel (around 60–70%). In comparison, only 5% are from rupture of an AVM; other rarer causes of SAH are tumour, infection, trauma or blood disorder. In up to 25% of cases of proven SAH, no cause is demonstrated during angiography. This is thought to be due to a very small aneurysm, a micro-aneurysm which obliterates itself during rupture and recurrence is rare.

Ruptured aneurysm affects people in the age range 25–60 and is uncommon in children. Coarctation of the aorta and the resulting high arterial pressure in the carotico-vertebral system can cause rupture of an aneurysm at an early age.

The majority of cerebral aneurysms are referred to as congenital, but it is only the tendency to form saccular or berry aneurysms at the junctions on the circle of Willis that appears to be developmentally determined. They often arise at the bifurcations where the muscle layer of the artery is weakest, and when combined with local stresses, e.g. systemic hypertension and degenerative arterial disease, rupture can occur. Through time a small vascular bulge can develop into a formed aneurysm which, at 5 mm or more in size, may burst, causing haemorrhage into the subarachnoid space and cerebral tissue.

The incidence of anatomical variation in the circle of Willis and local haemodynamic factors point to a correlation with aneurysm development. 10–15% of patients have bilateral or multiple aneurysms (thought by some to be linked with polycystic kidney disease) and rarely, a giant aneurysm has formed.

Most aneurysms form on the anterior half of the circle of Willis which derives its blood supply from the internal carotid arteries. The commonest sites are:

— anterior cerebral artery
— anterior communicating artery
— origin of posterior communicating artery
— terminal bifurcation (carotid)
— ophthalmic artery
— cavernous sinus.

Middle cerebral artery aneurysms are less common, and even more rare are those on the pericallosal, posterior inferior cerebellar, posterior cerebral and basilar arteries.

Aneurysms can present by sudden rupture, or by symptoms leading to a diagnosis of unruptured syndrome.

RUPTURED ANEURYSM

Often there is no precipitating factor causing rupture and haemorrhage, which can occur during exercise or at rest. Occasionally, there has been a similar, though much milder, episode in the preceding weeks — a 'warning' leak of a tiny amount of blood.

If the haemorrhage is large, the victim loses consciousness rapidly and may die within a short time (minutes or hours). A smaller bleed will cause sudden, very severe headache,

often occipital. It then radiates to the forehead, accompanied or followed by nausea and vomiting. Conscious level varies from slight 'clouding' of consciousness to deep coma. The presence of a neurological deficit may help to localise the site of the haemorrhage, e.g. hemiplegia and dysphasia due to contralateral middle cerebral artery aneurysm; 3rd nerve palsy due to a posterior communicating artery aneurysm; confusion and disinhibition due to an anterior artery bleed. However, these signs are not wholly reliable as they can also arise from 'brain shift' if an intracerebral haematoma has formed causing compression and ischaemia.

Photophobia may develop and neck stiffness occurs on the 2nd or 3rd day post-bleed. Other signs and symptoms are variable, e.g. mild pyrexia, systemic hypertension, bradycardia, transient glycosuria, abdominal pain and focal or generalised seizures. Vasovagal signs are thought to be due to catecholamine release; an ECG may show transient arrhythmias, Q wave and ST segment depression or T wave inversion. Hypothalamic injury can cause biochemical disturbance resulting in hyponatraemia.

UNRUPTURED SYNDROMES

Within the cavernous sinus

This gives rise to trigeminal pain, followed by sensory loss and ocular palsies, occurring often in middle-aged women. The symptoms may indicate tumour initially. Erosion of the clinoids is shown on skull X-ray.

At internal carotid bifurcation

Aneurysms here are often directed forward mimicking signs of pituitary region tumour. Skull X-ray shows erosion of the sella turcica.

At origin of posterior communicating artery

Unilateral ptosis and a dilated pupil is caused by 3rd nerve compression as the aneurysm is often directed backward.

ARTERIOVENOUS MALFORMATION (AVM, angioma)

An AVM commonly ruptures in young people in the 10–25 age group. It arises from a tiny arteriovenous fistula and can vary in size. It is comprised of a bundle of veins and arteries without the normal capillary system and can occur almost anywhere in the brain, involving the dura or tentorium, the basal ganglia or brain stem but more often occurs in the parietal or occipital lobes. It is frequently cone-shaped with the apex pointing inward and the base towards the surface. It is thought that it may enlarge through time, shunting more arterial blood from other areas of the brain, causing ischaemia and infarction. (Compression effects of the AVM can cause neurological deficits, headache and seizures.)

A quarter of the patients present with focal seizure, often sensory, when the parietal lobe is involved. There may be a history of a variety of signs and symptoms: syncope, migrainous headache, hemianopia, cranial bruit or dementia. The majority present with sub-arachnoid haemorrhage, although the outlook is better as recurrent bleeding is less common. The initial symptoms are similar: headache, neck stiffness, nausea and vomiting, but as bleeding is venous the effects are less severe. A 'bruit' may be heard, due to abnormal blood flow.

Sturge-Weber syndrome (facial and leptomeningeal angiomatosis)

This disease which often presents in infancy and childhood with seizure activity is also a rare cause of subarachnoid haemorrhage. It consists of a capillary angioma of the meninges associated with a superficial characteristic 'port wine' naevus on the face. The underlying cortex may undergo gliosis and calcification.

Vein of Galen anomaly

An aneurysm of the vein of Galen, occurring in neonates, can obstruct the ventricular system causing non-communicating hydrocephalus. Cardiac hypertrophy and congestive heart failure can ensue, if a large amount of blood is passing through the anomaly, due to the demands put upon the cardiovascular system. Treatment of the vein of Galen aneurysm is surgical.

INVESTIGATIONS

History and examination

The abrupt onset of headache followed by vomiting should arouse suspicion that a haemorrhage has occurred, even in the absence of focal neurological signs. On examination the patient may be fully alert and orientated, with no deficit, or display varying degrees of neurological dysfunction i.e. dysphasia, hemiplegia, confusion and drowsiness or a solitary 3rd nerve palsy (following a moderate haemorrhage).

Lumbar puncture

Examination of the cerebrospinal fluid should be done early after admission to hospital, the exception being patients who are suspected of having an intracerebral haematoma with raised intracranial pressure. Three consecutive specimens of CSF are obtained and if the red cell count is similar in each (i.e. uniformly bloodstained), the diagnosis is confirmed. After 9 days, red cells disappear from the CSF. Xanthochromia appears after 24 hours and may persist for several days, enabling a retrospective diagnosis to be made. Meningitis can also be excluded by bacteriological culture.

CT scanning

After a moderate sized bleed, blood will usually show in the basal cisterns, ventricles or Sylvian fissure indicating the site of an aneurysm and a focus for future angiography. The presence of an intracerebral haematoma or acute hydrocephalus in a comatose or neurologically deteriorating patient may be an indication for urgent surgery to evacuate the clot or to insert a ventricular shunt. If, however, despite CT scan findings of haematoma or hydrocephalus, the patient's clinical state is stable, close observation is sufficient. Removal of a haematoma may improve conscious level, but has no effect on focal deficits. CT scan should be performed before lumbar puncture if a haematoma is suspected, as the risk of 'coning' is present.

Even small AVMs will be defined with CT scan and contrast enhancement.

Cerebral angiography

If the patient is in coma, is confused or has severe neurological deficit, angiography will be delayed until a degree of recovery has occurred, as there is always the risk that deterioration may be precipitated by this procedure. When the patient is alert and orientated, angiography should be performed without delay, and if an aneurysm or AVM is demonstrated, surgery should be carried out as soon as possible, to minimise the risk of further haemorrhage (most likely in the first 2 weeks following initial 'bleed'). Total angiography (4-vessel) is performed if the aneurysmal site is unknown, or if the surgeon wishes to operate on each aneurysm where the patient has multiple aneurysms. More limited (i.e. unilateral carotid) angiography can be carried out if only the ruptured aneurysm is to be clipped, the site having been previously localised by CT scan. Similarly, even tiny AVMs can be demonstrated by angiography; the degree of vasospasm, if present, can be seen affecting blood vessels adjacent to the aneurysm.

With an AVM there are three distinct phases seen during angiography:

arterial phase — the abnormal arteries fill with contrast sooner than the normal arteries in the rest of the brain

venous phase — by the time the normal brain capillaries are being filled the contrast is already seen in the abnormal draining veins

capillary phase — when the capillaries are filled, contrast is already in the large venous sinuses.

This rapid circulation is characteristic of an AVM.

Magnetic Resonance Imaging (MRI) scan

A Magnetic resonance imaging scan can be useful following initial CT scan, where results are inconclusive. It produces a very accurate, almost anatomically reproduced, 'picture', using radio frequency waves.

NURSING MANAGEMENT

General

The broad aims of nursing care throughout this investigative period are:

— to support the patient and his family through this stressful time
— to give simple explanations of the various procedures and ensure they are understood
— to reinforce information given by the medical staff
— to listen, and enlist services of others in the multidisciplinary team, as problems arise
— to prepare the patient, emotionally and physically, for the investigation.

Naturally it is impossible to predict outcome, but the relatives should always be made aware of the true gravity of the condition, and the uncertain prognosis.

The priorities of nursing management are:

• to minimise the risk of secondary bleed by avoiding procedures or events which may cause a surge of increased BP
• to minimise headache, vomiting and distress
• to observe and record neurological status and vital signs and understand significance of changes which can indicate a complication arising.

Specific

Initially, where headache, nausea and vomiting are severe, bed rest in a quiet darkened environment is beneficial, with exertion kept to a minimum.

A patient in coma will have all nursing care performed for him (see Ch. 4). As the initial symptoms subside, the patient can begin to participate in his own care and mobilise as he feels able, and any deficits allow.

The frequency of recording neurological observations will be decided by the nurse-in-charge in accordance with the patient's condition. Any changes in conscious level, neurological deficit or vital signs will be reported to medical staff immediately and any appropriate investigation or treatment initiated.

Accurate 'fluid balance' recording is essential in all SAH patients, as good hydration must be maintained to prevent dehydration, electrolyte imbalance and lowering of arterial blood pressure which can lead to reduced cerebral perfusion, ischaemia and infarction. If insufficient fluids are taken orally perhaps due to nausea, or disturbed conscious level, then an intravenous regime should be commenced. A difference of opinion presently exists in relation to fluid intake; some surgeons advocate a 2–3 litres per day intake while others prefer only 1 litre in the 24 hour period.

Occasionally transient 'diabetes insipidus' is diagnosed where the patient has bled near the hypothalamus, and excessive amounts of dilute urine are voided. Conversely, inappropriate ADH secretion may lead to excess fluid being retained in the circulation and hyponatraemia develops. These disturbances are usually transient and easily remedied. Daily blood samples should be obtained to estimate urea, electrolyte and osmolality levels, and a urine specimen for osmolality. A light nourishing diet, with sufficient dietary fibre should be offered, or dietary supplements if appetite is poor. Stool softeners, e.g. Lactulose, may be prescribed to help the patient avoid constipation and the accompanying 'straining' at stool, which increases intracranial pressure.

Headache can be quite difficult to relieve as stronger narcotic drugs are often withheld in case they mask signs of a deteriorating conscious level. Codeine phosphate 60 mg administered i.m on a regular basis is commonly prescribed.

Troublesome nausea and vomiting can be prevented with the use of a regular anti-emetic, e.g. prochlorperazine 12.5 mg

Occasionally, cerebral ischaemia and infarction develop early after the haemorrhage, perhaps correlated to arterial spasm, and the patient becomes more drowsy, and confused and may develop a hemiparesis or gradual onset of hemiplegia. As it is thought to be dangerous to administer a large fluid load or plasma expanders to increase BP, in case it precipitates a secondary haemorrhage, treatment can only be conservative until the patient improves spontaneously.

Conservative management

For those patients who are frail, very ill, deteriorating, have pre-existing disease or decline surgery, management is conservative.

In the initial stages, the patient will be nursed on complete bed rest followed by gradual ambulation and a return to his usual activities of living, aided by drug therapy, e.g. analgesics and anti-emetics.

Surgical management

Opinion varies regarding the optimum time lapse between the initial haemorrhage and surgical intervention, although the condition of the patient is often the main deciding factor. Some surgeons prefer to operate within 3 or 4 days, others prefer to wait 10–14 days. Both carry risks, i.e. intra-operative morbidity due to 'vasospasm' or the risk of re-bleeding prior to delayed surgery.

The patient and his family will be informed about the operative procedure and expected results and should be made aware of the risks and possible residual deficits.

Newer techniques, however, have lessened operative risks with the use of the operating microscope, and controlled hypotension and respiration during dissection and clipping of the aneurysm.

Pre-operative care (see also Ch. 6)

In brief, the pre-operative management must include complete physical examination, full blood count, ECG, chest X-ray, blood type and cross match, urea and electrolyte estimation, and informed consent. The theatre check list is carefully completed. In most centres the patient's hair is shaved off after the anaesthetic has been administered to avoid added distress.

The aneurysm can be dealt with either directly as in 'clipping' or 'wrapping', or indirectly by carotid ligation where clipping is impossible or inadvisable. The 'pterional' approach is used for aneurysms on the anterior part of the circle, and either subtemporal or pterional for those on the posterior part, including the basilar artery aneurysms.

The most effective method is to place a clip across the neck of the aneurysm, thereby isolating it from the parent artery. The majority can be dealt with this way, although it can be very difficult and hazardous during dissection of a recently ruptured aneurysm, where adjacent tissue is friable due to haemorrhage. Occasionally the aneurysm ruptures and subsequent bleeding may only be controlled by clipping the parent artery temporarily which can lead to permanent deficit.

If it is impossible to 'clip' the aneurysm either because the neck is too wide or inaccessible, then the sac can be 'wrapped' with muscle, fibrin foam or Terylene gauze to prevent further rupture.

This procedure is useful with patients where major surgery is contra-indicated and who have an aneurysm arising directly from the internal carotid artery. Blood flow and pressure are reduced by ligation, often of the common carotid artery. This immediately lessens the risk of a second rupture of the aneurysm, particularly in the first 6 months. Angiography has shown occasionally that the aneurysm disappears probably due to thrombosis within the sac where the blood has become stagnant. However, ligation of the artery can cause adverse effects of hemisphere ischaemia. There are various methods of assessing collateral circulation, pre-operative and intra-operative: e.g. percutaneous carotid compression, EEG or angiography during trial occlusion of the ipsilateral artery, but none is totally reliable. Even when a satisfactory collateral circulation is demonstrated, hemiplegia may develop postoperatively due to postural hypotension. The patient is therefore nursed in bed for several days, with frequent recording of blood pressure.

A cavernous sinus aneurysm can be dealt with by 'trapping', i.e. ligating the artery at the distal and proximal ends.

There are various methods of 'removing' an AVM: embolisation during angiography which may be followed by surgical excision; surgical excision after clipping the 'feeding' vessels; radiotherapy; cryosurgery and stereotaxy. Surgical excision is the most effective, although does not influence epilepsy, and will only be undertaken if the AVM lies in a relatively silent area of the brain.

Postoperative management (see Ch. 11)

After craniotomy, most patients will be nursed in an ITU or high dependency area for at least 24 hours where continual monitoring of neurological status and vital signs is essential. There are no rigid rules regarding recovery rate- and rehabilitation. As the clinical condition stabilises and the patient feels well enough on return to the ward, oral fluids, diet, and mobilisation are re-commenced. Urinary catheter, i.v. lines, wound drain, oxygen therapy are all removed or discontinued when deemed unnecessary. An individualised care plan for each patient should ensure an uneventful return to independence. Wound clips or sutures are removed between 3–7 days post-surgery depending on unit policy, and the patient selects a suitable wig.

POSTOPERATIVE COMPLICATIONS

Along with general complications which can

arise, i.e. chest or bladder infection and deep venous thrombosis, there are other hazards specific to aneurysm surgery, the most important of these being delayed cerebral ischaemia which can occur during the first 3 to 4 days after surgery. The mechanism is largely unknown but may depend on many factors, including

— the presence of an intracerebral haematoma
— cerebral vasospasm
— hypotension and hypoxia
— disturbance of fluid balance, e.g. dehydration, hyponatraemia
— hydrocephalus
— surgery.

All of the above can lead to infarction and neurological deficit. Deteriorating conscious level and development of focal neurological signs are an indication of delayed ischaemia if CT scan excludes the presence of haematoma or hydrocephalus.

One of the drug treatments presently recommended is dopamine, used in the 'Glasgow hypertension regime' and is commenced by infusion via a central line once the diagnosis has been made. The initial rate of infusion is gradually increased until a systolic blood pressure of 180 mmHg is attained, and this is maintained with the lowest dose possible. DDAVP (synthetic ADH) 4 micrograms i.m. and 500 ml dextran 40 (a plasma expander) are administered daily. If blood pressure does fall nevertheless, 1 unit of plasma protein solution (PPS) is given quickly intravenously. Overall daily intake must be at least 3 litres and daily estimation of haemoglobin, urea and electrolytes is performed.

The Glasgow hypertension regime is very gradually withdrawn, depending upon blood pressure, and can take 3 to 4 days. During this time PPS can be given p.r.n. to sustain BP above 100–120 mmHg, and fluorocortisone 2 mg b.d. is also administered. Initial results of this treatment appear to be encouraging.

Some drug treatments and protocols preferred by surgeons include the use of steroids, mannitol and dextran during and following surgery. Research is also being carried out on drugs to prevent delayed ischaemia, including nimodipine, a cerebral vasodilator.

Hydrocephalus

This condition may develop gradually postoperatively, and if symptomatic, further surgery may be scheduled to insert a ventriculoperitoneal shunt (or ventriculo-arterial). This usually improves conscious level and general rate of recovery if no focal deficits were already present.

Focal neurological deficits

Permanent deficits may occur, both physical and mental, following successful aneurysm 'clipping', due to intra-operative rupture or delayed ischaemia. The residual physical disability may be a hemiplegia (with or without dysphasia) causing many problems, social, emotional and economic affecting the patient and the family. The mental changes, however, may be the most distressing for the family, most often occurring where the haemorrhage has damaged the frontal lobes. There can be confusion, inappropriate mood, tactlessness, loss of concentration and normal social inhibitions. The severity can vary, some patients showing great improvement within 3 months, others remaining demented.

Epilepsy may also be a distressing side-effect but can be well controlled with drug therapy.

During intensive rehabilitation many members of the multidisciplinary team may be involved, e.g. occupational therapist, physiotherapist, speech therapist, clinical psychologist and medical social worker all working towards similar objectives, i.e. to assess and improve physical and mental capacity, to help the patient and his family cope and adapt to the problem with a view to eventual discharge home and return to employment.

The recovery time, if indeed recovery is possible, is very individual, and often improvement occurs as a result of social adaptation rather than recovery of function.

The primary aim of surgery is to prevent fatal recurrent haemorrhage, 80% of which occurs in the 8 weeks after the first haemorrhage. Much difficulty has been experienced in assessing the exact value of surgery. Many factors have to be taken into consideration when comparing survival rates following surgical and conservative management including clinical 'grade': the patient's age, the size, site and shape of the aneurysm, presence of vasospasm and the number of haemorrhages which have occurred. Morbidity and mortality rates vary tremendously, e.g. from 2–3% in patients with unruptured syndromes to 20–30% in grade III patients.

BIBLIOGRAPHY

Chase M, Whelan-Decker D 1984 Nursing management of patient with a subarachnoid haemorrhage. Journal of Neurosurgical Nursing 16(1):23

De Jong R N, Currier R D 1983 The year book of neurology and neurosurgery. Year Book Medical Publishers, Chicago

Fode N A 1984 Cerebral arteriovenous malformations: update for neurosciences nurses. Journal of Neurosurgical Nursing 16 (6):319

Galbraith S L 1979 Management of patient with subarachnoid haemorrhage. Nursing Times 75(43):1857

Guidetti B, Delitala A 1980 Intracranial arteriovenous malformation: conservative and surgical treatment. Journal of Neurosurgery 53:149

Hayashi M, Nasakiyo S, Sunitada H 1984 Cerebral blood flow and intracranial pressure patterns in patients with communicating hydrocephalus after aneurysm rupture. Journal of Neurosurgery 61:30

Hickey J 1986 The clinical practice of neurological and neurosurgical nursing. J B Lippincott, Philadelphia

Jennett B, Galbraith S L 1983 An introduction to neurosurgery. Heinemann, London

Kayembe K N T et al 1984 Cerebral aneurysms and variations in the circle of Willis. Stroke 15(5):846

McPhee M 1984 Like being hit by a hammer (SAH). Nursing Mirror 158(22):31

Purchese G, Allan D 1984 Neuromedical and neurosurgical nursing, 2nd edn. Baillière Tindall, London

Rosen I 1984 Neurophysiological evaluation of a case with secondary epileptogenesis, successfully treated with lobectomy. Hippokrates (Verlag-Berlin) 15:95

Wilkins R H 1980 Attempted prevention or treatment of intracranial arterial spasm. Journal of Neurosurgery 6:198

Williams M H 1985 Arteriovenous malformations: complications of surgical intervention and implications for nurses. Journal of Neurosurgical Nursing 17(1):14

10

Care of the patient with a stroke

INTRODUCTION

'Cerebrovascular accident' (CVA), or the preferred term 'stroke', covers a multitude of conditions associated with the vascular supply to the brain. Neurones depend upon a constant supply of oxygen, which is carried in the bloodstream. Should the blood supply to the brain be interrupted, even for a few seconds, damage to the neurones can occur. If the blood supply is completely obstructed to an area of the brain for more than 4 to 6 minutes, the neurones are unable to survive.

Severe forms of vascular disturbance to the brain result in a sudden collapse, associated with loss of consciousness — 'cut down at a stroke'. This description gave rise to the term 'stroke', although, in reality, it is not the most common manifestation. Cerebrovascular accidents may range from a 'stroke in evolution', which takes up to 6 hours to reach its peak, to a 'completed stroke', which is more acute and persists.

A definition of stroke by the World Health Organization (WHO 1971) is '. . . a focal neurological deficit due to a local disturbance in the blood supply to the brain: its onset is usually abrupt but may extend over a few hours or longer'.

INCIDENCE AND OUTCOME OF STROKE

Strokes are a frequent cause of death —

particularly in developed countries — and are superseded only by heart disease and cancer in the mortality rates. Of those people who survive a stroke, many have residual neurological deficits, which may vary from mild to severe. The incidence of stroke greatly increases with age, the majority occurring in people aged 65 years or over. This is a factor likely to be of great significance in coming years, as more people are surviving beyond 65 years. Younger victims of stroke are also increasing in numbers.

The annual incidence in Great Britain is not accurately documented. It is said to be about 2 per 1000 of the total population, but, in reality, is probably much higher. There is a higher incidence in females, as they tend to live longer than males, and hypertension adds to the risk.

About 50% of stroke victims die within the first 2 to 3 weeks of the onset — many of them in the first few days. Of the remaining 50% who survive, more than half die in less than 5 years. The remainder — about 20% of the total initial victims — tend to fall fairly evenly into one of two categories. They may be fully independent (with slight deficits such as incomplete use of the hand) or they may be dependent on others for help (having more severe handicaps and mental dysfunction).

The burden on the health services, families of the victims, and the victims themselves is high. Little work has been done to determine methods which will help in the prevention of strokes. However, a report by the 'European Working Party on High Blood Pressure in the Elderly' (Amery et al 1985) indicates that a reduction in mortality and a significant reduction in morbidity in cerebrovascular events can be achieved. The study was carried out on elderly patients (over 60 years of age) with a minimum systolic/diastolic blood pressure of 160/90 mmHg, using a combination of triamterine and hydrochlorothiazide. The study report concluded that non-terminating cerebrovascular events were reduced by 52% and fatal cerebrovascular events were reduced by 43% (the latter being a non-significant decrease).

CAUSES OF STROKE

There are many factors which predispose to cerebrovascular impairment, including stress, overwork, obesity, advancing age, diabetes mellitus and hypertension. An accumulation of some of these factors may eventually culminate in a stroke. Increasing age and hypertension are high risk factors, but strokes can occur in young people. The predisposing factors in younger victims vary, but include congenital abnormalities such as cerebral aneurysm and arteriovenous malformation (angioma). Conditions such as cerebral tumours, infection (e.g., arteritis, meningitis) and systemic diseases also have some significance.

The actual causes of stroke can be classified into three main groups:

- cerebral thrombosis
- cerebral haemorrhage
- cerebral embolism.

Cerebral thrombosis

Thrombosis most commonly occurs in the internal carotid and vertebral arteries, and is mainly due to atheroma. Stenosis (narrowing) or complete occlusion of the artery may occur. The majority of strokes — probably as many as 80% — are due to cerebral thrombosis.

Cerebral haemorrhage

Bleeding may occur into the brain tissue — *intracerebral haematoma* — or into the subarachnoid space — *subarachnoid haemorrhage*. There are many causes of haemorrhage, including trauma, congenital abnormalities (where there is a weakness of blood vessels) and systemic diseases (blood clotting disorders).

Congenital abnormalities which may result in cerebrovascular impairment include those mentioned above, i.e., aneurysm and arteriovenous malformation.

An *aneurysm* is a sac-like protrusion of the

blood vessel wall. It commonly occurs at the bifurcation of blood vessels, where the wall is weaker, because there is less muscle and elastic tissue in the tunica media. Aneurysms may take the form of a saccular bulge, or be attached to the blood vessel by a narrow neck. The latter are known as 'berry aneurysms'. Single or multiple aneurysms may be present. These congenital weaknesses are found in many people (at post-mortem) but may never have caused any problems. In some cases, however, an aneurysm may leak or rupture, with severe consequences. A ruptured aneurysm is a common cause of subarachnoid haemorrhage — especially in the 25 to 50 year age group. Sometimes, an intracerebral haematoma may form, resulting in a raised intracranial pressure.

A cerebral *arteriovenous malformation* (*angioma*) is an abnormal growth of blood vessels. These tend to increase in size, with age, and act as space-occupying lesions. They may be associated with an external angioma of the face or scalp. The malformation is usually fed by one or more arteries and drained by several large veins. Venous blood from the malformation is at a higher pressure than normal, and it is usually a vein which ruptures, resulting in a subarachnoid haemorrhage. This most commonly occurs in the 10 to 25 year age group. Most arteriovenous malformations arise in the parietal and occipital lobes of the cerebral hemispheres. If they do not rupture, they may be detected because of symptoms such as migraine, epilepsy or dementia (see also Ch. 9).

Cerebral embolism

Emboli which migrate to the cerebral circulation usually arise in the atheromatous vessels of the neck (carotid arteries) or in the lining of the heart. Most emboli lodge in the smaller middle cerebral artery, after passing through the internal carotid artery. Occasionally, emboli may pass through the vertebral arteries and become lodged in the basilar artery. If small, they may continue to travel to one of the posterior cerebral arteries.

TRANSIENT ISCHAEMIC ATTACKS (TIAs)

Transient ischaemic attacks, or 'little strokes', are temporary disturbances of neurological function, which may last up to 24 hours. They are considered as a warning of a completed stroke, which usually results within 5 years of the onset of the TIAs, if untreated. Symptoms of TIAs may include numbness or weakness of a hand or one side of the face, dysphasia, or partial or complete blindness of one eye. These are due to carotid artery embolism. If the vertebral artery is affected, vertigo and ataxia may occur.

MANIFESTATIONS OF STROKE

Just as the predisposing factors and causes of stroke vary, so does the outcome in individual patients. Generally, the effect of a diminished blood supply to part of the brain — *ischaemia* — is an impairment of cell function. Complete occlusion of an artery, as in cerebral thrombosis, results in an *infarction* of tissue. The part of the brain normally supplied by that artery is deprived of its oxygen and nutrients and dies. Functions normally controlled by that particular area of the brain are either impaired or completely lost, depending upon how much tissue is damaged.

The outcome of a stroke also depends upon whether a small or large artery is involved, and whether or not a collateral circulation can be quickly established.

When brain tissue is damaged, the surrounding area becomes oedematous. Some initial neurological dysfunction may be due to the cerebral oedema, which settles in time and a subsequent recovery may occur. Depending upon which cerebral hemisphere is affected, *hemiparesis* (weakness) or *hemiplegia* (paralysis) arises on the opposite side of the body. Other disorders may occur according to whether or not the damage is in the dominant hemisphere. Symptoms also vary to some extent depending upon which artery is occluded. Some of these manifestations are detailed below.

Internal carotid artery

Transient ischaemic attacks may occur as a warning of diseased internal carotid arteries. When a completed stroke occurs, the patient may be confused or lose consciousness. Hemiplegia (loss of motor function), hemi-anaesthesia (loss of sensation) and hemi-anopia (loss of vision) are present. If the dominant cerebral hemisphere is affected, expressive and receptive dysphasia will result. There is a good chance of a collateral circulation being established, therefore some recovery from the initial presenting symptoms is to be expected.

Middle cerebral artery

If this artery is occluded, hemiplegia and hemianaesthesia occur; the face, tongue and arm are particularly affected, and dysphagia is common. Mobility is usually quite good, as the leg is not severely affected. The symptoms are more severe if the artery is occluded near to its origin at the internal carotid artery.

Anterior cerebral artery

The lower limb tends to be the more severely affected if this artery is occluded. Dysphasia and apraxia (forgetting simple, learned activities) may occur. Urinary incontinence is common and tends to persist, even though there may be recovery from other symptoms. There is often a lack of concern about incontinence on the patient's part.

Posterior cerebral artery

This artery supplies various parts of the hemisphere therefore symptoms can vary depending upon which area of the brain is affected. Some of the problems which may arise are hemiplegia, blindness, visual agnosia, spontaneous pain and confusion. Recovery is usually poor and mortality is high.

Basilar artery

A variety of symptoms can arise, such as disturbances of balance, hearing and cranial nerve function. There may be motor and sensory loss. If the vital centres in the brain stem are deprived of blood, the outcome is rapidly fatal. Signs of this are rapid loss of consciousness, Cheyne-Stokes respiration, small and fixed pupils, tremors and severely impaired swallowing reflex.

MANIFESTATIONS OF HEMISPHERE INVOLVEMENT

When the non-dominant cerebral hemisphere is deprived of blood, severe hemiplegia and hemianopia may occur on the opposite side of the body. The patient may develop *anosognosia* — a failure to recognise the affected side. It is important to approach the patient from the unaffected side, as he will not be aware of anything or anyone on his affected side.

Speech problems usually arise when the dominant hemisphere is affected, i.e., in most right-handed people, the left hemisphere is the dominant one.

Damage to the right parietal lobe may result in difficulties with perception. The patient will be disorientated, lose his way (even in familiar surroundings), be unable to dress correctly (e.g., put on clothing back to front) and fail to recognise familiar faces and objects. These symptoms may be mistaken for dementia, especially in the elderly patient. The patient will have difficulty in carrying out skills which are demonstrated to him, but can usually understand verbal and written instructions. Slow, clear instructions should be given to the patient rather than trying to show him how to do something. The patient should be encouraged to do things slowly, as he will tend to carry out activities quickly and become frustrated at his difficulties.

When the left hemisphere is damaged, slow performance of activities tends to result. Conceptual functions — e.g., logic and ideas — are disrupted. There is usually difficulty in understanding verbal or written instructions, but demonstrations are effective.

IMPLICATIONS FOR THE NURSE AND THE PATIENT

If the nurse understands the disabilities of the patient, she can assess him more accurately and help him, as far as possible, towards independence. Both patient and nurse will be less frustrated, and there will be more of an opportunity to develop a positive approach to the problems encountered.

Rehabilitation of the patient will depend upon his particular disabilities and whether or not some recovery is expected. Patients who have suffered a sudden collapse, with recovery of consciousness but some residual neurological impairment, may find it difficult to accept that their recovery may take a long time. Patience, perseverance and encouragement are vital on the part of the nurse. The patient whose co-operation is gained, and who has a determined attitude, is more likely to benefit and achieve some independence.

Depression is a common feature in stroke patients, especially in those who have moderate or severe handicaps. It is important for the nurse to set short-term, achievable goals with her patient, when planning care. Praise for small achievements can go a long way towards helping the patient to independence within his capabilities.

Paramedical staff, such as the physiotherapist, speech therapist and occupational therapist, have an important role in the rehabilitation of the stroke patient. Liaison between all those involved is important, so that the patient does not become confused with different instructions.

Relatives of the patient need to be involved. Obviously, they will require information about the patient and his condition, and should be updated with progress (or deterioration). Initially, they may feel at a loss — some relatives like to help with the basic care of the patient, if encouraged to do so. The relatives who are going to support the patient at home, when he is discharged from hospital, need to know how best to help him. Sometimes this may be doing less than they thought, i.e., encouraging the patient to be as independent as possible, rather than being overprotective and treating him as an invalid. Adequate community support services should be provided, where needed, and the advice and help of such people as the social worker, community nurse liaison officer and occupational therapist should be sought.

MANAGEMENT OF STROKE

The overall aim in caring for stroke victims is rehabilitation, where recovery is seen or expected. It is essential to maximise independence, within the patient's limitations. There are several ways of managing and treating stroke patients, just as there are several causes and a variety of problems. As the greatest number of stroke patients are elderly, they tend to be cared for in geriatric or general medical wards, rather than specialised units. This, of course, depends upon the health authority protocol and the facilities available. Not all stroke patients will be admitted to hospital, e.g., if symptoms are minimal and home circumstances are suitable.

A few specialised 'stroke units' have been established, but these are not widely situated. In many cases, patients will receive medical treatment, but some may benefit from surgery. Neuro-science units can take only a small percentage of patients, owing to limited numbers of beds. Selection criteria may vary from place to place, but it is often the younger patients who are selected for admission to a specialised unit. Neurosurgery is offered when there is an identifiable cause which is likely to benefit from surgical intervention.

A number of specialised tests and investigations can be undertaken, but facilities for these tend to be concentrated in the regional centres. Most of the tests and investigations involve the use of expensive equipment, which is not widely available. It has to be accepted that what happens to a patient is often a matter of 'chance', e.g., the place to which he is referred and the facilities available.

As mentioned earlier, the younger, rather than the older patient usually takes precedence for more intensive investigation and treatment. A subjective explanation of this is that it is more of a risk to subject the elderly to a number of investigations and to surgery. However, many of the modern investigative techniques are less invasive than those used in the past, and anaesthesia can be controlled to reduce risk to the patient.

There is a need to make more facilities available for stroke patients which, of course, carries large financial implications. Alternatively, resources could be allocated to more research into the prevention of strokes, and in the implementation of favourable preventative measures.

INVESTIGATIONS

A summary of some of the investigations, which may be carried out in relation to the stroke patient, is included here. Details of the investigative techniques can be found in the relevant chapter.

1. **A history and examination** of the patient are essential starting points — e.g., does the patient present with transient ischaemic attacks, a stroke in evolution or a completed stroke? Is there any neurological dysfunction? Is there any relevant history, such as hypertension?

2. **Cerebral angiography** (arteriography), including carotid and/or vertebral arteries, is carried out where appropriate.

3. **Computerised axial tomography** (CT scan) is often the investigation of choice, where facilities are available. This has largely superseded ventriculography and air encephalography, which are unpleasant for the patient.

4. **Radioisotope scanning.**

5. **Magnetic Resonance Imaging scanning** (MRI) — not widely available, at present.

6. **Lumbar puncture,** to detect blood-stained cerebrospinal fluid.

7. **Electroencephalography.**

8. **Other investigations** relating to known, or to determine, underlying systemic disease — e.g., blood and urine tests.

TREATMENT OF STROKE

Mention has already been made of the different ways in which stroke patients may be treated — i.e., the two main categories are medical and surgical management.

Medical management varies depending upon the age and condition of the patient and the neurologist's/physician's preferences. Elderly patients admitted to a geriatric unit are mobilised early if their condition allows. Younger patients tend to be treated more conservatively, i.e., with a longer period of bedrest. Supportive care is the main area of management, the nurse having an important role in this. Other staff, too, have an important part to play, e.g., physiotherapist, as the main aim is to rehabilitate the patient when possible. Drugs, such as hypotensive agents, may be used where appropriate.

Surgical treatment is aimed mainly at those patients with intracranial aneurysms and arteriovenous malformations (although some of the latter are too large for successful removal). Other surgical techniques, such as carotid endarterectomy and temporal-cerebral vessel anastamosis, may be of benefit to some patients.

Patients who present with transient ischaemic attacks may be prevented from developing a completed stroke. Conservative treatment may involve the use of drugs such as aspirin or anticoagulant therapy. Surgical treatment may be by means of carotid endarterectomy if atheroma is causing carotid stenosis. (This is performed by vascular surgeons in some hospitals.) Stenosis of the internal carotid artery or middle cerebral artery may be treated by anastamosis. The superior temporal artery is joined to the middle cerebral artery to provide a bypass circulation. This is usually undertaken in patients who have no permanent neurological deficits.

Surgical drainage of intracerebral haematoma may be undertaken in a patient whose level of consciousness continues to deteriorate. However, neurological deficits which have already occurred cannot be corrected, and severe disabilities usually ensue. The aim is to relieve intracranial pressure, but damage to the brain tissue has occurred at the time of the initial haemorrhage and does not resolve.

NURSING CARE OF THE STROKE PATIENT

It can be seen from the preceding information that patients present in and are treated in various ways. Generally, the nurse's role is important in supportive care of the patient. Specific aspects of nursing care in relation to neurosurgical techniques are dealt with in other chapters. However, the nurse must assess each individual patient's needs, and plan care according to these. A detailed account of aspects of caring for a patient with a cerebrovascular disorder is included here. This is based on a fictitious case study and related to needs arising from aspects of daily living activities.

The plan of care contains relevant information and explanations, which aim to give some of the reasons underlying the nursing care. A care plan used in practice would, obviously, not be so detailed.

Patient history

Mrs Lynn Brooks is a 38-year-old married woman, who works part-time in a baker's shop. She is 1.58 m tall and weighs 65 kilograms. For the past 10 years she has been taking oral contraceptives, following the birth of her second child.

In her spare time, Lynn likes to read novels, to cultivate house plants and to sew (she is right-handed). She likes cooking, and her husband and children are helpful in the home. Lynn smokes 10 to 15 cigarettes a day.

After sudden collapse at work, Lynn is admitted to hospital. She is unconscious and has a right-sided paralysis. Upon her arrival in the neurological unit, Lynn is placed on a bed in a semi-prone position. A nursing assessment is made to identify her immediate needs and to plan the relevant nursing care. (These are explained later in the text.)

Dealing with the immediate needs of the patient's husband

Mr Brooks has been contacted by Lynn's employer and is on his way to the hospital. The nurses, therefore, must anticipate his arrival and prepare to deal with his anxiety about the situation. After the doctor has assessed Lynn's condition, arrangements should be made for Mr Brooks to see the doctor.

Support for the family is essential at this traumatic time, and Mr Brooks may require some help with the care of the two children. If necessary, the social worker can be contacted for advice.

When Mr Brooks arrives and his immediate worries have been dealt with in a sympathetic manner, he will probably want to see his wife. The admitting nurse can then explain the need to obtain further details from him to help with the assessment of Lynn's needs. This is best done in a comfortable environment where Mr Brooks can be offered a chair and a cup of tea or coffee. Privacy is important, and so is the assurance that he can see Lynn again before he leaves. He should be offered reassurance and advised about visiting and telephoning the ward. The nurse should check that details of how and where to contact Mr Brooks are obtained, should the need arise.

Nursing care of Lynn

The overall aim in caring for Lynn, following her admission, is to maintain her safety, to monitor her for any changes in condition and to prevent further complications. A nursing care plan, based on a model of nursing related to activities of daily living, is used here. As explained earlier in the text, this is a detailed plan including reasons for Lynn's problems and care. A care plan used in practice would be much briefer. The details include care related to Lynn's immediate problems (priorities of care on admission) and continuing care. Each problem is identified, the goal (or aim) is stated along with the nursing care to be implemented. In practice, it is important to evaluate the nursing care and to reassess the patient's condition at regular intervals.

Immediate problems

Breathing. She is unable to maintain her own airway due to loss of consciousness; damage to brain tissue and raised intracranial pressure inhibit the respiratory centre, resulting in difficulty in breathing and inadequate ventilation; if compression of the medulla oblongata occurs, coughing and swallowing reflexes are inhibited, with potential obstruction of the airway.

Nursing goal
- To maintain a clear airway and ensure that there is adequate ventilation; hypoxia results in increasing damage to brain tissue and increasing intracranial pressure; anoxia results in death of brain cells and permanent neurological deficits — and death of the patient if not rectified quickly.

Nursing care
- Place Lynn in a semi-prone, or well supported lateral position, to prevent obstruction of pharynx by her tongue; she will be less likely to inhale saliva or vomit in this position.
- Remove any dentures, loose teeth or debris from her mouth to prevent inhalation, and note any capped or crowned teeth which could be dislodged.
- Place an oropharyngeal airway in her mouth, if necessary, to prevent obstruction.
- Provide suction, as required, to remove secretions.
- Administer oxygen, if prescribed by the doctor (or if the emergency need arises), via a humidifier, to ensure an adequate supply.
- Observe and record the rate, rhythm and depth of her respirations frequently, to monitor any changes in her condition. Skin colour should also be noted, e.g., any cyanosis.
- Change Lynn's position to alternate sides, e.g., every 2 hours, to aid lung expansion, ventilation and drainage of any secretions.
- Provide care associated with specific techniques, if required, such as tracheostomy or positive pressure ventilation.

Maintaining a safe environment. She may be unaware of her surroundings and unable to respond to stimuli, due to loss of consciousness; she may have diminished sensation and loss of protective reflexes, and be at risk of further cerebral damage if ischaemia or bleeding occurs.

Nursing goal
- To provide a safe environment, with minimal risk to Lynn, and to monitor her condition closely in order to detect any changes.

Nursing care
- Provide constant supervision and observe her general condition; padded cot-sides may be used to prevent her from falling out of bed if she becomes restless.
- Prevent damage to skin or other injuries by handling her gently and positioning her correctly.
- Observe and record her vital signs and neurological status, as frequently as necessary:

— respiration (as mentioned previously)
— pulse — a slowing pulse rate indicates rising intracranial pressure (ICP)
— blood pressure — a rising blood pressure indicates increasing ICP
— temperature — hyperpyrexia could indicate damage to the hypothalamus
— level of consciousness, response to verbal/painful stimuli — to detect stability, improvement or deterioration in her condition
— pupil size and reaction to light — unequal pupils, dilatation or sluggish response indicates pressure on the oculomotor nerve

— limb movements — spontaneous/ response to painful stimuli/abnormal movements. Note any paralysis and type (spastic or flaccid), or paresis; right side of body affected, therefore lesion is in left cerebral hemisphere.

Initial observations will provide a baseline for future recordings, and any changes should be reported to the nurse in charge or the doctor.

Communicating. Lynn is unable to communicate due to loss of consciousness.

Nursing goal
- To anticipate her needs and communicate with her verbally and by touch.

Nursing care
- Observe Lynn carefully in order to identify her needs e.g., restlessness may indicate pain or a desire to eliminate urine/faeces.
- Stimulate Lynn by verbal communication and gentle handling during procedures, and note any responses
- Establish a good nurse–patient relationship by having a minimum number of nurses caring for her, rather than a variety of different nurses which could be more distressing for her.
- Give clear explanations and information, talk in a purposeful way, keep her orientated, reassure her and do not say anything you would not want her to hear — although she is unconscious, she may be able to hear even if she does not respond to the spoken word.

The three problems identified above are the most crucial areas and should be seen as priorities of care. Other immediate problems relate to the care of an unconscious patient, as Lynn is admitted in an unconscious state (see Ch. 4). The continuing care of Lynn depends upon any changes in her condition. A nursing care plan, suggesting care when she recovers consciousness within 24 hours of her admission to the unit, is included below. Lynn's right-sided hemiplegia begins to show some recovery, but she has dysphasia.

Aspects of care relating to special investigations and to surgery are not detailed here. Lynn could undergo these procedures, in view of her age, and the reader should refer to the relevant chapters which give information on these subjects.

Continuing problems

Breathing. Return to consciousness should put Lynn at less risk of breathing difficulties or an obstructed airway but coughing and swallowing reflexes could remain impaired for some time. There is still a risk of further cerebral damage if haemorrhaging recurs.

Nursing goal
- As identified in the immediate breathing problems, i.e., to maintain an unobstructed airway and to ensure adequate ventilation.

Nursing care
- Nurse Lynn in a lateral position, which is changed at least 2 hourly to aid ventilation and drainage of secretions; support her back with pillows to prevent her from rolling onto her back or face; she may be allowed to have a pillow under her head, as this is usually more comfortable: as her condition improves, she is able to sit up more.
- Observe for the return of coughing and swallowing reflexes; keep her mouth, nose and pharynx clear of any debris and secretions by applying suction, if required — to prevent inhalation/obstruction.
- Continue to provide humidified oxygen, if prescribed.
- Continue to provide care associated with specific needs, such as tracheostomy or aided ventilation, as required.
- Offer explanations and reassurance to alleviate her anxieties, especially if any procedures which are unfamiliar to Lynn are instituted; her breathing will be easier if she is calm and relaxed.
- Continue to observe and record respirations as frequently as necessary, in order to monitor any changes in her condition.

- Liaise with the physiotherapist with regard to any procedures relating to aiding chest drainage and lung expansion; encourage Lynn to breathe deeply and to expectorate secretions when cough reflex is present.
- Provide tissues and a sputum carton if Lynn has excessive sputum; assist her with coughing, if necessary, and remove used tissues/cartons.
- Advise Lynn not to smoke, if she expresses the desire to do so, giving reasons — e.g., it may have contributed to her illness and could cause further problems, safety aspects while she is in bed (especially if oxygen equipment in use).
- Administer antibiotics if prescribed by the doctor as a prophylactic measure against chest infection.

Maintaining a safe environment. There is a risk of injury on Lynn's return to consciousness, as she is in an unfamiliar environment and may not be aware of her neurological dysfunctions immediately; impaired movement and sensation of the right-hand side of her body results in a loss of independence; there is the possibility of impairment of special senses, such as vision, e.g., hemianopia; Lynn could have amnesia when consciousness returns; she remains at risk of further cerebral damage if haemorrhaging recurs; she has problems in communicating her needs due to dysphasia (this area is dealt with in the next section).

Nursing goal
- As stated in the immediate problems, i.e., to provide and maintain a safe environment.

Nursing care
- Continue to observe Lynn's general condition and supervise as necessary; monitor her awareness, memory and special senses.
- Continue to observe and record her vital signs and neurological status as frequently as necessary, and report any changes in her condition.

- Orientate her to her environment and educate her about her limitations i.e., impaired movement and sensation; take care with hot fluids and items which could damage her skin.
- Change her position frequently in order to prevent pressure sores; provide aids, if required, to assist in the prevention of pressure. (Detail in section on Personal cleansing and dressing.)
- Maintain safe practices/policies when administering any prescribed medications, and note effects/side effects of any drugs given to Lynn.
- Maintain hygiene and aseptic procedures in order to reduce the risk of infection.
- Alleviate any pain by ensuring that Lynn is as comfortable as possible and that analgesia (if prescribed by the doctor) is given as appropriate.
- Offer explanations and information to help to decrease any anxieties, and maintain a calm, quiet environment for Lynn; reassure her about her loss of independence.

Communicating. Lynn has dysphasia due to damage to speech centres in the left cerebral hemisphere (her dominant hemisphere, as she is right-handed); she has difficulty in communicating her needs and feelings, and in responding verbally to others; people unaware of the reasons for her dysphasia may think that her intelligence/reasoning is impaired.

Nursing goal
- To establish suitable ways of communicating and to encourage Lynn to communicate her needs and feelings; to educate others about her problems and encourage them to communicate with Lynn.

Nursing care
- Establish and maintain good nurse-patient relationships, by demonstrating an understanding of her problems; be prepared to spend time with her and have a patient and tactful approach.
- Give clear explanations, information and instructions about any procedures.

- Orientate her to her new environment and to time, date and other people; initially she may have difficulties in recognising familiar people/things.
- Offer her reassurance and help to prevent her from feeling isolated or stigmatised.
- Try to anticipate her needs and feelings, but encourage Lynn to express these; help her to deal with any frustrations about her difficulties in communicating.
- Observe for any specific difficulties which impair communication, e.g., expressive/receptive dysphasia, impaired vision or hearing — and find the best methods to overcome these.
- Liaise with the speech therapist, using aids to communication, and encourage Lynn to carry out any exercises which will help her to speak clearly.
- Inform relatives, visitors and others involved in her care about her problem; encourage them to communicate with Lynn and to let her try to talk to them; ensure that others understand that Lynn's intelligence is not impaired and to treat her as an adult.
- Ensure that any follow-up speech therapy is arranged, if required, when Lynn is ready for discharge from hospital.

Mobilising. Lynn's mobility is restricted due to her right-sided weakness and, initially, because of bed rest; she may have impairment of proprioception which will affect her mobility.

Nursing goal
- To assist Lynn with moving and changing her position; to provide support for paralysed/weak limbs and to prevent contractures and joint damage; to encourage a return to independence (a series of short-term goals is set to encourage Lynn to achieve realistic capabilities).

Nursing care
- Change Lynn's position at least 2 hourly whilst she is in bed — gradually encouraging her to do this herself (with assist-

ance, if necessary) — to aid lung ventilation and circulation, to reduce discomfort and to relieve pressure; record change of position during acute stage.
- Handle her gently, noting any pain or discomfort which should be alleviated by careful handling and positioning.
- Support her limbs and joints in a natural position, using aids such as pillows, foam pads or splints, if required, to prevent contractures, foot drop or wrist drop. Avoid over extension of joints when changing her position, to prevent damage — she may not be aware of this if sensation is impaired.
- Provide passive exercises to Lynn's affected limbs, putting all joints through their range of movements (this could be done when changing her position); this will prevent joint stiffness and muscle wasting and aid circulation — thus helping to prevent deep vein thrombosis and pulmonary embolism.
- Encourage Lynn actively to exercise her other limbs, and, when she is able, she is encouraged to use her unaffected side to exercise her affected limbs, e.g., by clasping her right hand in her left and raising her arms.
- Liaise with the physiotherapist to implement a programme of rehabilitation, including the use of any special aids or equipment. (Most physiotherapists use methods based on the 'Bobath technique' and the nurse should be familiar with this.)
- Ensure that Lynn's environment allows her maximum independence, e.g., whilst she is confined to bed, place locker and items she may require where she can reach them; when she begins to mobilise, allow plenty of space so that she does not trip or walk into furniture.
- Monitor her progress and provide continual encouragement and praise — even for small achievements — to help her to accept and to cope with her restricted mobility.

- Encourage Lynn to achieve as much independence as possible, within limitations of any residual neurological deficits.
- Educate her family/friends about the implications of her physical handicaps; encourage them to help Lynn to achieve maximum independence.
- Ensure that a home assessment is made, prior to Lynn's discharge from hospital, and that any aids or equipment, support, and outpatient physiotherapy are arranged, if required.

Eating and drinking. Initially, Lynn is unable to take food or fluids by mouth while unconscious; coughing and swallowing reflexes may be impaired; she may have difficulty in eating and drinking while lying in bed; her right-sided weakness will result in problems in feeding herself; she may experience nausea and vomiting due to the cerebral lesion.

Nursing goal
- To maintain adequate nutrition and hydration and to establish normal oral feeding as soon as possible.

Nursing care
- Pass a nasogastric tube and institute a regular feeding regime, in consultation with the dietician; ensure that the tube is in her stomach and that feeds are being absorbed; chart the amounts, type and time of feeds to ensure that she is receiving an adequate nutritious intake; report any difficulties to the nurse in charge or the doctor. (In some units fine-bore continuous feeding may be used.)
- Observe Lynn for any vomiting and prevent inhalation of fluids, so that her airway is not obstructed and a focus for infection in the lungs does not arise. Do not change her position immediately after giving feeds, as this may cause regurgitation with the risk of inhalation of fluid.
- Administer anti-emetic drugs, if prescribed by the doctor, and observe the effectiveness of these.
- Observe Lynn for the return of coughing and swallowing reflexes (if these were absent), so that normal oral feeding can

be introduced when she is conscious; fluids and food should be introduced gradually and the nasogastric tube removed when oral intake is sufficient.
- Observe for any diarrhoea, especially while tube feeding is in progress — modify feeds if this occurs.
- Assist Lynn to eat and drink, as required, but encourage her to feed herself; provide equipment such as a feeding cup and special utensils which will aid her independence; allow her sufficient time to cope with her disabilities.
- Protect Lynn's clothing and bed as necessary, but maintain her dignity.
- Find out which foods and drinks she likes and provide these if possible as she is likely to take them more readily.
- Give her small amounts at first, as her energy demands will be less due to her limited activity; diet can be supplemented by nourishing drinks if she is unable to take much solid food.
- Continue to record her fluid intake in order to ensure adequate hydration.
- Liaise with the dietitian to meet Lynn's changing nutritional needs as she becomes more active.
- Encourage her family/friends to assist her, at first, if present at meal times; this may help them to feel more useful if they can participate in some of her care. Explain the need for Lynn to become more independent as her condition improves.
- Provide reassurance and encouragement to Lynn, to help her to achieve independence in feeding; maintain her privacy if she is embarrassed about being assisted or about spillages but gradually help her to socialise with other patients at meal times.
- Make provision for any aids which she may require at home, by consulting with the occupational therapist.

Eliminating. Lynn is unable to control bladder and bowel function while unconscious and, therefore, is incontinent of urine and faeces; she may have problems in establishing full control when returning to consciousness. Constipation may occur owing to a change in environment and routine, lack of privacy, anxiety, limited mobility, a change in normal fluid and food intake, medications and impaired communication.

Nursing goal

- To keep Lynn clean and dry while incontinent; to anticipate her need to eliminate; to prevent constipation and impaction of faeces; to re-establish normal elimination patterns.

Nursing care

- Observe for any incontinence; wash and dry her skin and change clothing/linen as necessary.
- Observe her for signs of restlessness, which may indicate the desire to eliminate — provide a bedpan if required.
- When Lynn is conscious, establish communication and attend to her promptly when she expresses the desire to eliminate; this will help to relieve her anxiety and prevent soiling of clothing/bed linen.
- Provide assistance as required, maintaining her privacy.
- Institute bladder retraining, if necessary, e.g., by providing a bedpan 2 to 4 hourly, in order to prevent incontinence or retention of urine.
- Provide handwashing facilities for her, after using the bedpan, commode or toilet, and assist her as necessary.
- Monitor and record Lynn's urine output to ensure that her kidney function is normal.
- Collect and test specimens of urine, as required, to detect any abnormalities.
- Catheterise only as a last resort, i.e., if she has acute retention of urine or renal problems — in order to minimise the risk of urinary tract infection. Provide appropriate care if she is catheterised.
- Observe Lynn for incontinence of faeces, while she is unconscious, and keep her clean and dry.
- Note any diarrhoea, especially while she

is being tube fed, and modify diet if necessary.

- Observe for constipation and try to prevent this — encourage mobility as soon as possible; provide diet with adequate fluid and fibre content; administer suppositories, enema or suitable medication if required (according to the doctor's prescription).
- Reassure Lynn about regaining control of normal functions, and encourage gradual independence in attending to her own elimination needs.

Personal cleansing and dressing. Lynn is unable to maintain her own hygiene, or to dress/undress herself while unconscious; on her return to consciousness she will initially require help with cleansing and dressing due to her physical disabilities and limited mobility.

Nursing goal

- To keep Lynn clean and dry and to establish self-care as soon as possible; to keep the skin intact; to provide suitable clothing.

Nursing care

- Bed bath Lynn, as required, whilst she is unconscious and confined to bed; maintain her privacy and dignity throughout the procedure; keep her skin clean and supple, and prevent dryness by applying oil/moisturiser cream.
- Provide mouth care — oral toilet 4 to 6 hourly while unconscious — and keep her teeth clean; when conscious, and coughing/swallowing reflexes are present, she may require a mouthwash, particularly after meals.
- Trim her nails as necessary, preferably keeping them short so that there is less risk of injuring herself, and ensure that they are clean.
- Provide regular eye care, ensuring that her eyelids are closed while she is unconscious/asleep — eyepads may be required. Keep her eyes clean and free from infection.

- Ensure that her nostrils are clean, especially while the nasogastric tube is in place.
- Wash her hair, as required, in order to maintain a good body image and to keep it clean.
- If a menstrual period occurs while Lynn is in hospital, ensure that she has adequate sanitary protection and that the vulval region is kept clean.
- Assess Lynn's risk of developing pressure sores, e.g., using the 'Norton scale'; observe skin for signs of redness or soreness, particularly over bony prominences; change her position regularly and keep her skin clean and dry, using a barrier cream if she is incontinent; provide appropriate aids to help to relieve pressure; avoid friction to the skin when lifting or moving her, and avoid using patched or wrinkled bed linen; record changes of position on a chart. (Prevention of pressure sores is also mentioned briefly in the section relating to maintaining a safe environment.)
- When Lynn is conscious, allow her to take part in decisions about washing/bathing herself and encourage self-care, providing assistance as necessary.
- Carry out aseptic procedures if her skin is not intact, e.g., at site of intravenous infusion.
- Select suitable clothing for Lynn (in some units, unconscious patients are nursed without clothing, so that they can be observed more easily); when she is conscious, allow her to make decisions about her clothing; advise about clothes which will be easier to put on and take off, as she will have some difficulty due to her affected right side, e.g., front fastening clothes, zips rather than buttons, slip-on shoes. When she begins to mobilise, she may prefer to wear comfortable trousers while carrying out exercises; she should be advised to wear firm, supportive shoes with a flat heel, to aid walking.
- Encourage her to dress/undress herself, allowing plenty of time; explain how she may find it easier, e.g., to put her affected arm into a sleeve first. Liaise with the occupational therapist and physiotherapist who may be involved in helping Lynn with some of these tasks.

Controlling body temperature. Potential problems are alteration in normal body temperature, due to cerebral damage and changes in environment.

Nursing goal
- To maintain body temperature within normal limits and to provide an acceptable environmental temperature.

Nursing care
- Measure and record body temperature as often as required, e.g., hourly when she is first admitted and less frequently as her condition stabilises; use a suitable route for taking her temperature, e.g., axillary/rectal while unconscious, oral when conscious and able to cooperate.
- Provide appropriate measures to reduce Lynn's temperature if she becomes pyrexial, or to keep her warm if she has a low body temperature.
- Regulate the environmental temperature so that she is comfortable, e.g., provide a draught-free area, supply suitable clothing and bed linen.
- Report any abnormal changes in temperature, i.e., pyrexia, hyperpyrexia, subnormal temperature.

Sleeping. Lynn has a disturbance in the normal sleep/waking mechanism while she is unconscious, due to a depression of the reticular activating system in the central nervous system; on her return to consciousness, the change of environment and her normal routine, and potential discomfort, may interfere with normal rest and sleep patterns.

Nursing goal
- To differentiate between unconsciousness and normal sleep; to help Lynn to

return to full awareness; to minimise discomfort and disturbances.

Nursing care
- Monitor changes in her level of consciousness, allowing rest periods between provision of nursing care and observational techniques.
- Ensure that Lynn is comfortable and free of pain.
- Promote a suitable restful environment, with minimum noise; help to relieve any stress or anxiety.
- Facilitate normal routines as far as possible, with additional rest periods if required.
- Consult with the doctor if sedatives/hypnotics are required when Lynn's condition has stabilised.

Expressing sexuality. Lynn may be embarrassed about intimate procedures; lack of privacy due to hospitalisation; restrictions on normal sexual activities during hospitalisation and she may worry about the effects of her illness in the future; altered body image due to physical disabilities and problems with communication, which is likely to make her feel unattractive.

Nursing goal
- To reduce Lynn's anxieties, minimise embarrassment and maintain privacy; to encourage her to take a pride in her appearance and maintain a good self-image; to encourage her to resume normal sexual activities and role when she returns home.

Nursing care
- Ensure that any embarrassing/intimate procedures are carried out with minimum fuss and maximum privacy; allow Lynn to attend to her own needs when she is able to do so.
- Allow her to talk over any fears/anxieties that she has, remembering that she may have added difficulties due to her dysphasia; deal with her in a tactful and sympathetic way.
- Provide information to both Lynn and her

husband, if required, about resuming normal sexual activity and about contraception; the contraceptive pill, which Lynn was taking previously, will be contra-indicated.
- Assist Lynn, and encourage her, to maintain an attractive appearance and presentation, e.g., hair care, make-up, clothing, perfume, deodorant.
- Allow some privacy between Lynn and her husband, so that they can discuss the situation.
- Provide an opportunity for contact with her children, so that Lynn can maintain a relationship as a mother.

Working and playing. Lynn is in a different environment with changes in her normal routines and activities; she is separated from her family, friends and work; she has a potential problem of being unable to return to all of her previous activities, because of her physical disabilities and problems with communication; she may become bored while in hospital.

Nursing goal
- To prevent boredom, loneliness and isolation; to provide stimulation and encourage a return to independence; to help her to accept her limitations.

Nursing care
- Talk to Lynn and encourage her to communicate when she is conscious.
- Encourage contact with other patients and her visitors.
- Provide suitable diversional therapy, in which she has an interest and is capable of participating.
- Liaise with others who can help, e.g., occupational therapist, physiotherapist, and provide aids which will help Lynn to be more independent.
- Help Lynn to accept her limitations and to cope with frustrations which may arise from these; suggest new interests and hobbies if necessary; her previous interests, such as reading and cultivating plants should be encouraged; if she

regains some use of her right hand, she may be able to use an electric sewing machine, with care.

- Plan, with Lynn and her family, for long-term problems, e.g., the social worker can help with financial problems, if Lynn is unable to return to work.

Worshipping. Lynn is unable to communicate any specific spiritual needs while she is unconscious; there is a potential problem of inability to express these needs when she is conscious, due to communication problems; she may have difficulty in participating in normal religious practices (if any) due to her physical disabilities.

Nursing goal
- To determine her religious beliefs and needs (if any), and to help her to meet these and to participate in usual religious activities if desired; to respect her beliefs.

Nursing care
- Assess her normal practices (if any) by discussing with her husband; determine how important/significant these are in her normal life.
- Contact the relevant religious advisor/minister if required, to visit her and her husband, if this will reassure and comfort them.
- Provide opportunities for Lynn to participate in any usual religious activities, if necessary.
- Ensure that any special requirements relating to her religion (if any) are met, e.g., dietary restrictions.

Dying. There is a potential problem of death on Lynn's admission to hospital, owing to her critical condition and the possibility of an extension of her cerebral haemorrhage.

Nursing goal
- To prevent death, if possible; to institute resuscitative measures if respiratory/cardiac arrest occurs; to enable Lynn and her family to come to terms with the possibility of dying.

Nursing care
- Careful observation and monitoring of Lynn's condition, so that prompt action can be taken in the event of a deterioration in her condition.
- Have suction, oxygen and resuscitation equipment at hand, ready for emergency use if needed.
- Be familiar with resuscitation techniques and life support equipment, so that these can be used effectively if needed.
- Allow Lynn and others to express any anxieties/fears about death and listen to these; help them to cope with their anxieties/fears.
- Recognise the process of coming to terms with death and dying, and allow for changes in behaviour related to this.
- Provide information, explanations and emotional support.
- Alleviate any discomfort, pain, loneliness or feelings of isolation.
- Respect Lynn's and her family's wishes in relation to death and dying.
- Encourage a positive outlook on Lynn's recovery, as she may still have a fear of dying.

Promoting health. Lynn and her family may lack knowledge about her illness and its effects, and factors which predispose to stroke.

Nursing goal
- To help Lynn and her family to acquire relevant knowledge about the illness, and to cope with any residual disabilities; to be willing to provide education about other aspects of health and well- being.

Nursing care
- Establish what is already known about her condition, by discussing it.
- Listen to questions and comments and provide information.
- Ensure understanding of any information given.
- Set realistic goals for Lynn's rehabilitation.
- Adopt a positive approach to her recovery and the future.

- Encourage co-operation in any continuing treatment or therapy which is required.
- Advise about risk factors and encourage Lynn to avoid any she is able to in the future.

Evaluation of nursing care

As stated earlier in the text, it is important to evaluate Lynn's care and to reassess her needs, especially in relation to any changes in her condition. Evaluation will help the nurse to note the effectiveness of care provided, and to be aware of Lynn's progress. However, an evaluation is not included here, as it is not possible to assess the hypothetical situation. It is assumed that Lynn makes a good recovery and responds well to treatment and care.

Planning for discharge

As Lynn becomes more independent and she and her family are able to cope with residual problems, plans can be made for her discharge from hospital. She may be allowed home for short periods, e.g., a day or a weekend, to help her and her family to re-adjust in the home situation.

A discussion between all staff involved and Lynn and her family will be helpful. Decisions can be made about any support services and follow-up care which she may require. A home assessment may be carried out by the social worker, occupational therapist and physiotherapist (involving the community liaison nurse, if necessary) — i.e., a home visit with Lynn to assess her home environment and how she copes. This would enable Lynn to be provided with suitable aids and adaptations, if required, before she is discharged from hospital.

The nurses who have helped to care for Lynn — assessing her and her family's needs and priorities of care, implementing appropriate nursing care and evaluating the results — can be confident of maintaining a high standard. In meeting Lynn's needs as an individual, the reward is to see that she returns to her home and family and is able to resume a fulfilling role in society.

CONCLUSION

Caring for the patient with a stroke requires understanding and a great deal of time and dedication on the part of the nurse. Because of the high incidence of stroke, the majority of nurses, at some time in their career, are likely to be involved in the care of these patients. Whether or not the patient is in a specialised unit, the principles of nursing care remain the same. For those patients who survive, the nurse must adopt a positive approach in order to encourage the patient (and others involved) to achieve as much independence as possible. It is also important to remember, at all times, that the patient is an individual human being — psychological and sociological factors play a large part in recovery of physiological functions. The nurse who cares for the 'person', rather than the 'patient', is more likely to see a rewarding outcome.

BIBLIOGRAPHY

Amery A et al 1985 European working party on high blood pressure in the elderly: morbidity and mortality results. Lancet 1:1349
Bobath B 1970 Adult hemiplegia — evaluation and treatment. Heinemann, London
Brown A 1976 Physiological and psychological considerations in the management of stroke. Warren H Green, St Louis
Conway-Rutkowski B L 1982 In: Carini and Owens' Neurological and neurosurgical nursing, 8th edn. C V Mosby, St Louis
Hunt P, Sendell B 1983 The essentials of nursing — nursing the adult with a specific physiological disturbance. Macmillan, London
Marshall J 1976 The management of cerebrovascular disease, 3rd edn. Blackwell Scientific, Oxford
Myco F 1983 Nursing care of the hemiplegic stroke patient. Harper and Row, London
Purchese G, Allan D 1984 Neuromedical and neurosurgical nursing, 2nd edn. Baillière Tindall, London
Roper N, Logan W, Tierney A 1983 Using a model for nursing. Churchill Livingstone, Edinburgh
Roper N, Logan W, Tierney A 1985 The elements of nursing, 2nd edn. Churchill Livingstone, Edinburgh
World Health Organization 1971 Cerebrovascular diseases — prevention, treatment and rehabilitation. Technical Services Report No 469

11

Craniotomy — intra-operative and postoperative care

ANAESTHESIA

Neuroanaesthesia is a specialised area of anaesthetics. Pre-operatively the patient's intracranial pressure is, to a greater or lesser extent, elevated and any further increases caused by the anaesthetic process may rapidly lead to brain shift and damage. Anaesthesia should not raise intracranial pressure, should not cause impairment of cerebral oxygenation and should provide optimum conditions for the surgeon. It should enable the patient to be responsive as soon as possible following the operation so that postoperative deterioration can be differentiated from deficits directly related to the surgical technique. It is for this reason that no premedication is given.

Induction and intubation are associated with a marked rise in intracranial pressure and this can be minimised by the anaesthetist's choice of drugs. The patient is then given regular supplements of muscle relaxants to prevent him fighting against the ventilation. The nitrous oxide and oxygen used as carrying agents also raise the intracranial pressure and hyperventilation is used to compensate for this.

Control of blood pressure is important during the intra-operative period. It can be lowered to reduce the blood volume within the skull and induced arterial hypotension is often used during aneurysm surgery to reduce the risk of rupture and to ensure more readily controlled bleeding if rupture does occur.

163

Position

It is important to ensure minimal venous congestion particularly when easy access to the site of the operation requires the patient's neck to be rotated. The normal craniotomy position is supine with a slight head up tilt. A foot board elevates the feet slightly and removes the pressure from the back of the calves so reducing the risk of deep vein thrombosis. Foam pads are used to protect the peripheral nerves in the arms which are supported and immobilised.

A sitting position is assumed for posterior fossa surgery, the anterior aspect of the head being well supported. The advantages of this position include easy access to the site of the operation and correct spatial orientation of the surgeon which would be affected if the patient was positioned prone. Good venous drainage is assured. However there are also disadvantages, in particular hypotension and the risk of air embolus. Under normal circumstances the sitting and lying blood pressure of a particular patient varies slightly; under the effects of general anaesthesia there is no compensation and the difference is greater. Because the venous pressure is low and no blood escapes when the vein is cut it may not be obvious when there has been a cut and where there is a potential entry site for an air embolus. Additionally the veins traversing the skull are held open by the rigidity of the bone and so cannot collapse when they are emptied as do normal veins. There are several alternatives in the prevention of air emboli and these include bimanual neck compression, an inflatable neck collar and leg bandaging. Most commonly, however, an anti-gravity suit, inflated to a pressure of 60 mmHg, is used and the abdomen and the legs are compressed in order to force the blood upwards. There are cut out areas in the suit, for example, around the knees which protect the nerves and other than the uncommon complication of nerve entrapment there are no other known disadvantages. If an air embolus occurs, it passes via the superior vena cava to the right atrium of the heart where it causes the blood to be frothy. This can be detected by Doppler ultrasound and a detector is strapped to the patient's chest. However this does not indicate the extent of the embolus and the detector automatically cuts out when cautery is being used. As the air reaches the lungs the capillaries which are used in gaseous exchange are blocked and the excretion of carbon dioxide is reduced. The capnometer monitors end tidal carbon dioxide and so detects this change. A central venous pressure (CVP) line with its tip in the right atrium remains in situ throughout the procedure and arterial monitoring also takes place. If an air embolus occurs, the CVP increases and the arterial pressure falls. The early detection of an air embolus allows immediate aspiration of the frothy blood via the CVP line and can prevent the situation progressing to cardiac arrest.

The third common position is often used for the removal of an accoustic neuroma and is known as the park bench position. This involves the patient being positioned on his side so that there is easy access to the area for the surgeon.

SURGICAL TECHNIQUES

Various terms describe the ways in which the surgeon gains access to the brain across the skull.

Burr hole. This is a hole drilled through the cranium and is often sufficient for evacuation of a haematoma or biopsy of a tumour.

Craniotomy. This is the formation of a bone flap through which the surgeon gains access to a larger area of brain. A series of burr holes are made in a circular formation and all but one side are cut by means of a wire saw. The remaining side is broken, rather than sawn, in order to encourage more rapid healing when it is replaced.

Craniectomy. This is a hole made in the bone which is made larger by the chipping away of the bone. As a consequence this bone cannot be replaced when the operation is finished. A craniectomy is usually performed in the posterior fossa where the bone is particularly thick.

Transphenoidal approach. This approach

gains access to the pituitary gland. The incision is in the upper submucosa gum area and the approach traverses the sphenoidal sinus to reach the pituitary fossa from beneath.

A cranioplasty is another surgical technique whereby a synthetic replacement is used to restore the integrity of the cranium when an area of bone has been previously removed.

AIMS

The aim of the immediate postoperative care of each patient is threefold:

- a safe recovery from the general anaesthetic
- the maintenance of satisfactory neurological progress and the prevention or minimisation of any problems consequent to surgery
- the maximum degree of comfort within the postoperative limitations.

Of great importance are:

— a safe environment with emergency equipment
— knowledge of the patient's pre-operative neurological state
— knowledge of other pre-existing health problems and the patient's pre-operative emotional state
— an understanding of the nature of the operation, of specific postoperative regimes and potential complications.

The recovery area should be situated near to the operating theatre to facilitate the patient's rapid return if necessary and to allow easy access to surgeons and anaesthetists. Oxygen and suction must be available as must equipment to measure vital signs and to monitor both cardiac and respiratory function. There must be provision for arrest situations. Sufficient numbers of skilled nursing staff are necessary as observation and correct interpretation are essential components of the patient's care at this time.

An understanding of the patient's preoperative neurological state and other preexisting health problems enables the nurse to anticipate and prepare for situations that may arise during his recovery. The patient who has a history of generalised convulsions is more likely to experience post-operative fits (Mathew et al 1980), or the person with chronic obstructive airways disease to require a cylinder of compressed air if his respiratory condition necessitates the administration of bronchodilators via a nebuliser. If specific complications can be anticipated the nurse can ensure that all the equipment that may be required is readily available. With this knowledge of the patient the nurse can also distinguish between real and apparent problems. For example, the significance of a postoperative hemiparesis depends on whether it was a pre-operative feature of the patient's condition. An unknown preoperative 3rd nerve palsy can be temporarily misinterpreted as a sign of neurological deterioration. Knowledge of the nature of the operation and of the related postoperative complications are also essential so that all these factors can be considered together to gain a greater understanding of the postoperative needs of the patient. The nurse will then be able to provide appropriate care and respond properly to situations that arise throughout his recovery. If the management of the patient remains calm and efficient, the discomfort he experiences can often be reduced.

Throughout surgery and the recovery period the needs of the relatives also merit attention. Recovery staff may be in a position to accept responsibility for their care, or it may be that it is better that relatives remain the responsibility of the ward staff. However the time of surgery is a very anxious one for them as a result of total isolation from the patient and a complete lack of knowledge of his progress in theatre, and if relatives sometimes appear impatient and demanding this is often only a normal response.

RAISED INTRACRANIAL PRESSURE (ICP)

All postoperative patients have some degree of raised intracranial pressure and this is a fundamental consideration in recovery care. The nurse must be aware of factors that affect intracranial pressure so that she can prevent further, and possibly devastating, increases. The promotion of venous return from the head helps to reduce the blood 'compartment' of the intracranial contents and consequently ICP. This can be assisted by even slight head elevation as the veins are valveless and gravity aids their drainage. A curled up position slows the venous return by increasing intra-abdominal and intrathoracic pressure, and therefore raises ICP. Extreme flexion and extension or lateral rotation of the neck will also have this effect, again by prohibiting free drainage, and the ideal position for the head is forward-facing with the nose and the chin in alignment with the sternum and the symphysis pubis.

Cerebral vasodilation raises the ICP because of the increased volume of the blood vessels. This is commonly caused by a rise in the level of carbon dioxide (CO_2) in the blood and, as a consequence, the quality of the patient's respiration and the condition of his chest are of great importance and demand attention. The autoregulatory function of the cerebral vessels is reduced under the effects of general anaesthesia and a rise in blood pressure (BP), as associated with pain or fear, can lead to a rise in the pressure being transmitted to the vessels and so to an increase in cerebral oedema. Pain therefore must be controlled as rapidly as possible and the patient's discomfort minimised.

Each aspect of nursing intervention causes an increase in ICP, e.g., suction, and measurement of BP, and it is preferable to perform the required nursing activities over a period of time rather than to complete them as quickly as possible with the impression that the patient can then rest. Each of these factors is of importance in the control of ICP and the nurse can incorporate them as necessary into her care.

ADMISSION TO RECOVERY

The recovery staff receive the patient from theatre having already made a provisional plan

for his care. As quickly as possible priorities have to be confirmed or reidentified. The bed head, unless contraindicated, will be elevated to improve venous return, in some centres the degree of elevation being according to the specific instructions of the surgeon. Details of the operation that may influence the immediate care or progress should be given at this point but less critical information can wait until the patient has been assessed and the nurse is satisfied with his condition. The name of the patient and the specific operation performed are extremely important as are the identities of the surgeon and the anaesthetist so that later enquiries can be directed toward the appropriate individuals. The volume and nature of fluids infused are recorded as is the estimated blood loss. Drugs administered during the operation that may affect the patient's postoperative condition need to be recorded as do other details of the intra-operative period that may have a similar effect. An awareness of the surgeon's expectations for the patient's short-term recovery is often of value to the nurse and, later, his expectations of the longer term prognosis.

POSTOPERATIVE CARE

The immediate care of the patient includes assessment of respiratory and cardiovascular function and of neurological status, and confirmation and maintenance of intravenous (i.v.) access.

Respiratory function

Potential problems following anaesthesia

- Obstructed airway
- Inadequate respiration
- Lung congestion — due to anaesthesia and inactivity — leading to inadequate gaseous exchange and consequently a rise in ICP and an increased risk of chest infection.

Objectives

- To maintain a clear airway

- To maintain effective respiration
- To regain a normal breathing pattern with adequate gaseous exchange
- To have clear lung sounds.

Relevant information

1. *An obstructed airway is a threat to life.* Both complete and partial obstruction are instrumental in raising intracranial pressure by increasing the intrathoracic pressure and so reducing venous return from the head. Equally the presence of an artificial airway when the patient no longer tolerates it also raises ICP.

2. *The patient is artificially ventilated* throughout his operation and it may take some time before a satisfactory breathing pattern is re-established. If respiration is not adequate, neither is the oxygen intake or the elimination of carbon dioxide, and as the level of carbon dioxide in the blood ($PaCO_2$) increases so does the intracranial pressure.

3. At least 100 ml of secretions are produced each day and, under normal circumstances, these *ensure that the lung tissue is kept moist.* In theatre as the patient is immobile and has a constant tidal volume, pooling of the secretions occurs. This causes both a loss of secretions from the non dependent areas and a congestion of the dependent areas and if postanaesthetic respiration is shallow or if cilial activity is reduced then these areas of congestion remain. This not only increases the risk of postoperative chest infection but also reduces effective gaseous exchange. In turn this can lead to an increase in ICP particularly in those people who already have compromised respiratory function.

4. To prevent their collapse *alveoli need to be expanded hourly.*

5. Just as a rise in the $PaCO_2$ causes cerebral vasodilation, a reduction leads to vasoconstriction. If the patient hyperventilates the resultant vasoconstriction reduces the blood flow to the head and consequently the oxygen supply. Therefore *the blood level of oxygen must remain high* in order to maintain an adequate supply.

6. In the assessment of respiration *the colour of the patient* is an important factor. If pallor is present and is peripheral only, then it is generally of cardiovascular origin, often in the immediate postoperative period due to peripheral vasoconstriction as a result of hypothermia. If it is both central and peripheral the level of oxygen is low and it is generally of respiratory origin.

7. Those people who are *'at risk' include the elderly and the obese*, those with pre-existing respiratory problems and those who smoke. The pulmonary compliance in the elderly is reduced and more energy is required to inflate the lungs adequately. The obese also need more energy for adequate inflation which is further compromised by the weight of the abdominal contents on the diaphragm when the patient is lying down. Smoking paralyses the cilia and so reduces the mobility of the secretions which also tend to be more viscous. Those patients with respiratory disease generally have a reduced number of effective alveoli and often underlying infection.

Action

1. Prior to the patient's admission *ensure the availibility of equipment* that may be required for respiratory assistance. Check that it is functioning correctly.

2. *Maintain the patient's airway* until he no longer requires assistance. Because the patient is lying on his back he may require positional support as well as an artificial airway. Where this is so, the assistance of a second nurse is invaluable allowing further assessment and care of the patient to continue. As he begins to reject his artificial airway it is removed. Suction may be required.

3. *Remain with the patient* until his respirations are satisfactory and stable.

4. *Administer oxygen* at a rate of 4 l/min according to the regime of the unit, or according to the specific instructions given by the anaesthetist.

6. *Assess central and peripheral colour.*

7. If the patient is *hyperventilating* continue

the administration of oxygen to ensure an adequate supply to the cerebral tissue.

8. When the patient is awake *encourage hourly deep breathing*, with coughing if the lung sounds are not clear. Air and gaseous exchange is also improved by yawning, laughing, talking and moving in bed, all of which alter and increase the tidal volume. Those patients whose conscious level precludes active exercises or are 'high risk', or who have undergone lengthy surgery, require particular attention from the nurse and the physiotherapist.

9. Pay particular attention to those patients who have undergone *posterior fossa surgery*.

Cardiovascular function

Potential problems

- Cardiovascular instability or insufficiency
- Non-achievement of cardiovascular conditions most suitable for a good neurological recovery.

Objectives

For the patient to maintain:

- a stable BP at normal levels or as directed by the surgeon
- a heart rate within normal limits, usually 50–100 beats per minute, of satisfactory rhythm.

Relevant information

1. *Hypovolaemic shock* is characterised by tachycardia, a falling BP, shallow and rapid respirations and a cool pale skin. This is caused by general fluid loss particularly when large doses of diuretics, commonly mannitol, are given in theatre. Hypovolaemia may only become apparent when the patient's temperature starts to return to normal.

Haemorrhagic shock is characterised by a rapid and thready pulse, a low BP, and a cold, clammy skin. There is a greater likelihood of significant blood loss if the surgery involves vascular structures, e.g., a meningioma, or if

an aneurysm bleeds during surgery.

2. *The heart rate* may be affected when the operation has resulted in temporary damage to the vagus nerve which is the parasympathetic supply to the sino-atrial node. This may occur for example during the removal of an acoustic neuroma. Cardiac irregularities may also be apparent, again following posterior fossa surgery, if an air embolus occurred during the operation.

3. The patient may be given *hypotensive agents* in theatre by means of a controlled infusion and these can be gradually withdrawn postoperatively. Until the infusion has been discontinued arterial monitoring continues.

4. *Blood pressure* is a major consideration following intracranial surgery. A rise in BP increases the cerebral perfusion pressure and so increases both cerebral oedema and the risk of postoperative haemorrhage. However, following, surgery for intracranial aneurysm, the blood pressure is maintained at normal pre-operative levels even though these may be considered hypertensive. This assists in the maintenance of the microcirculation and the prevention of cerebral vasospasm which is a significant risk following this type of surgery. The surgeon may indicate limits of acceptability.

Action

1. Observe the *general appearance* of the patient.

2. Ascertain the estimated *blood/fluid loss* during surgery.

3. *Monitor and record the blood pressure and heart rate* at frequent and regular intervals. Reduce the frequency over several hours as the patient's condition allows but maintain hourly observations over the first postoperative night.

4. *Monitor cardiac function* if this is indicated.

5. *Record postoperative blood loss and urine output* (especially where intra-operative diuretics have been administered.)

6. The use of position, analgesia, antiemetics and appropriate nursing care help to reduce blood pressure, and position can be

used to increase it. *Report BP values that are outside normal or agreed limits.* On occasion the surgeon may commence an infusion of a hypertensive agent in order to achieve the required blood pressure levels.

Assessment of neurological status

Potential problem following surgery

- Neurological deterioration.

Objectives

- To monitor and record the patient's post-operative progress
- To detect deterioration as rapidly as possible
- To refer to medical staff appropriately.

Relevant information

1. *Observation and correct interpretation* are two of the most important requirements of the nurse in her care of the patient immediately following intracranial surgery.

2. *Early postoperative assessment* is essential in order to differentiate between problems consequent to the surgical procedure itself and subsequent deterioration.

3. In the immediate recovery period the post-surgical neurological state is clouded by the continuing effects of the general anaesthetic and the main consideration is that the patient *continues to show a steady improvement.* When he arrives from theatre the immediate neurological assessment is of his pupils and his level of consciousness. As he recovers from the anaesthetic all aspects of his general condition should improve at a similar rate and any aspect that fails to do so should receive particular attention as it may have a neurological rather than an anaesthetic cause. If his general recovery appears to be particularly slow the anaesthetist can be consulted with regard to the expected duration of the effects of anaesthesia and this will either reassure the nurse or help to confirm her suspicions that there may be a neurological basis for his lack of progress. The more experienced nurse may be able to distinguish between a slow recovery from anaesthesia and a neurological problem but if there is any doubt concerning the progress of the patient the surgical staff must be consulted. Once the effects of the general anaesthesia have diminished the patient's actual neurological state can be more easily assessed.

4. Pain causes a significant increase in intracranial pressure therefore *painful stimuli* should only be used when absolutely necessary.

5. As the patient recovers from surgery and anaesthesia *any reduction in his level of consciousness*, his degree of orientation or in any aspect of his neurological status is unacceptable and must be reported to the surgical staff and, if necessary, to the anaesthetic staff. The classic alteration in the vital signs indicative of raised intracranial pressure are late signs and the patient's deteriorating condition should be appreciated before these changes become apparent.

In some cases specific deficits are expected following the surgical procedure undertaken and the recovery nurse must be aware of them so that she can appreciate those which are unexpected. Again, quite commonly, the experienced nurse may be aware of a deterioration in the patient although there are no obvious or recordable reasons, and she is able to involve the medical staff at the earliest possible time.

6. The records may be in the form of a written account or they may involve the use of a coma scale, but they must *show clearly the patient's progress* and any departures from that which was expected or normal. Whereas the coma scale ensures that the most basic observations are recorded, more detail is often required in the recovery period when subtle changes are of such importance. The written account allows a more complete record but care must be taken to prevent ambiguity and a false representation of the patient's condition.

7. As the patient recovers from surgery and general anaesthesia any reduction in his level of consciousness, his degree of orientation or

in any aspect of his neurological status is unacceptable and must be reported to the surgical and, if necessary, the anaesthetic staff. Ideally there is a nurse to care for each particular patient and she must be aware of any factors that may influence his care, his progress or her interpretation of his condition. Throughout his recovery she must satisfy herself that she is fully aware of the patient's neurological state and progress. With an understanding of the patient's operation the nurse can apply her knowledge of the anatomy and physiology of the nervous system and can anticipate the most likely postoperative complications. An example of this is the special consideration given to the motor power of the legs following the removal of a parafalcine meningioma. The classical alteration in the vital signs indicative of raised intracranial pressure are later signs and the patient's deteriorating condition should be appreciated before these changes become apparent. Sometimes the surgeon may expect specific deficits or complications as a result of the particular operation he has undertaken and if the nurse is informed of these expectations she can more easily identify the unexpected changes. Quite commonly the more experienced nurse may be aware of a deterioration in the patient although there are no obvious or recordable reasons, and she is able to involve the medical staff at the earliest possible time.

Action

1. *Continuous observation and frequent assessment* of neurological status and vital signs. Initially the recordings are made every quarter hour the frequency being reduced to every half hour if the patient makes satisfactory progress over the first 2 hours. After a further 2 hours, if his progress continues, the frequency is again reduced and recordings are made hourly over the first postoperative night.

2. *Interpretation of observations* and appropriate action.

3. *Complete and accurate recording of progress.* Consider use of a standardised coma scale.

Intravenous access

Problem

● Need to have intravenous access.

Objective

● To maintain the i.v. route.

This enables emergency and other drugs to be given intravenously and have a rapid onset of action. It also allows administration of fluids to compensate for the lack of oral intake.

Action

1. Ensure that the i.v. infusion is patent as one of the priorities on admission of the patient to the recovery ward.

2. Ensure that the i.v. infusion progresses as prescribed and does not block or run through the giving set. This enables emergency drugs to be given at any time.

Once the most immediate assessment of the patient is complete and any required action has been taken, further considerations include the wound drain (if present), the patient's temperature and, as he regains consciousness, his pain and/or nausea. All of these are important and all have in common their direct or indirect relation to the amount of discomfort experienced by the patient as a consequence of surgery.

Wound drain

Patient's need

● To experience minimal discomfort and rapid wound healing.

Nursing objective

● To maintain an intact and functioning wound drainage system.

The drain is used following supratentorial surgery and serves to prevent the collection of blood under the skin. If it is allowed to remain the blood tracks down beneath the skin and results in gross peri-orbital oedema and discomfort for the patient. The wound site becomes 'boggy' and wound healing is delayed and the risk of infection increased. The proximal end of the system is positioned beneath the galea, the tough fibrous layer of the scalp, and the drain is sutured in position. It can be used for suction drainage or drainage by gravity according to the wishes of the surgeon. The presence of a drain also allows easy assessment of postoperative blood loss. Normally this slows and becomes minimal over the first few hours. If, immediately following the operation, the drainage by suction is extremely rapid and the fluid drained appears dilute it may be that cerebro-spinal fluid is also being removed. This is prevented by reducing the degree of suction or removing it entirely to leave a gravity drain. As well as minimising loss of CSF this again promotes wound healing, and the drainage system must be labelled to prevent it from being unknowingly revacuumed. If the vacuum in a suction drain cannot be maintained, then it is left in position as a gravity drain.

Action

1. Initially *check that the drain is patent* and draining and that the required degree of suction is present.
2. *Secure the drainage bottle.* The gravity drain must be lower than the level of the head and preferably suspended from the side of the bed to encourage the drainage of blood.
3. *Check the suction and patency and the amount* of drainage with each set of observations.
4. *Revacuum the drain if necessary* using asceptic technique.
5. *Ensure that the patient does not inadvertently remove the drain,* for example in the act of pulling at the head dressing.

Temperature

Patient's need

● To regain a normal temperature; to feel warm.

Objective

● To maintain the patient at a normal temperature.

Relevant information

1. *Patients are often cold immediately following surgery,* the temperature sometimes as low as 31°C per axilla. This is due to the muscle relaxants given in theatre which prevent the production of heat by muscular activity and, where the blood pressure has been lowered, this is also contributory.
2. *The patient may continue to lose heat* postoperatively if he is slow to recover.
3. *The patient needs to regain a normal temperature* in order to regain good peripheral perfusion and to accelerate the action of intramuscular analgesia (a reduced blood flow to a muscle slows the absorption).
4. *The patient may develop pyrexia* due to the presence of blood in the CSF or if the operation site was near to the hypothalamus. Pyrexia due to postoperative infection does not generally occur immediately following the operation.
5. *Every 1°C rise in temperature increases oxygen requirements* significantly by increasing the metabolic rate.

Action

1. *Have the electric heating pad warmed* and ready for use as soon as the patient arrives from theatre.
2. *Apply the heating pad* if the patient's temperature is below 36°C per axilla and ensure that it is covered to prevent heat loss to the atmosphere.
3. *Record the patient's temperature* quarter-to-half hourly initially.
4. *Remove the heating pad* when the

temperature reaches 36°C and is continuing to rise.

5. *If the temperature rises* above 37.5°C measures can be taken to reduce it.

6. *Be aware of the surgeon's upper limit of acceptability.*

Pain

Patient's need

● To have the pain reduced to tolerable levels.

Objective

● To minimise pain.

1. *Pain increases the blood pressure* and, with the associated restlessness, leads to a rise in intracranial pressure.

2. The patient experiencing severe pain is more likely to remove his head dressing and so dislodge his *subgaleal drain.*

3. The patient can often *distinguish between headache and pain* originating from the wound site.

4. Following transphenoidal surgery the patient is relatively free from pain at the *suture line.* The pain receptor fibres have been cut and the *suture line* will be healed before these regenerate and the pain perception returns.

5. There are *cultural differences* in the experience and expression of pain and discomfort and these must be incorporated into the care of the patient.

6. There are also *differences related to age* in the experience and expression of pain and discomfort, with younger people often having less experience of pain and so finding the experience more difficult.

7. *Codeine phosphate* is the analgesia of choice and is given intramuscularly either prior to the patient regaining consciousness or as he does so. Its administration while the patient is unconscious reduces the period of discomfort prior to the onset of action of the analgesic and it removes the additional discomfort of the injection itself. However,

very occasionally, the patient can be more than usually sensitive to the codeine and the value of its later administration is that his initial progress can be observed. Another possible advantage in some cases is the psychological benefit to the patient of his being aware of the analgesia having been administered.

8. If *the initial dose* of analgesia has a limited effect the anaesthetist may prescribe *a further dose* which often achieves a greater degree of pain control.

9. Occasionally *the head bandage* may be too tight and require reapplying.

10. Some patients will require *further surgery* and if the recovery period is made as comfortable as is possible then this may have a beneficial effect on the patient's feelings toward any future operations.

Action

1. Administer analgesia according to the prescribed regime in the attempt to achieve pain control. If this is not achieved, refer to the anaesthetist or the surgeon.

2. General and thoughtful nursing care.

Nausea and vomiting

Patient's need

● To have facilities for vomiting
● To experience minimal nausea and vomiting.

Objectives

● To provide for vomiting and to minimise the related discomfort
● To control nausea and vomiting.

Nausea and vomiting commonly occur following posterior fossa surgery due to the close proximity of the operation site to the vomiting centre situated on the floor of the fourth ventricle. It may be unresponsive to the prescribed anti-emetic and an alternative may be required although this may also have little effect.

Action

1. *Administer anti-emetic* as prescribed, routinely following posterior fossa surgery or where the patient is of Mediterranean origin as they often experience nausea postoperatively. Otherwise administer as necessary.

2. *Refer to the anaesthetist* if vomiting remains uncontrolled.

3. *Minimise the large scale movements of the patient* as these often exacerbate the patient's nausea.

4. Consideration must be given to the *possibility of depressed cough and gag reflexes* when giving mouth care to patients following posterior fossa surgery.

The catheterised patient

Potential problem

- Distress/discomfort related to urinary catheter.

Objective

- To enable the patient to tolerate the catheter until it is removed.

Relevant information

1. *A urinary catheter* is inserted in theatre if diuretics are to be used. The patient may not have been prepared for this situation pre-operatively.

2. In the recovery period women often tolerate a urinary catheter better than men who can become extremely restless. As a consequence these patients experience *a related increase in intracranial pressure.*

3. *If more than 5 ml water is inserted* into the balloon it is more likely to irritate the bladder wall. Irritation can be caused simply by its presence.

4. *If the catheter is not draining* it may be because of the patient's lack of understanding and his attempt by voluntary muscle contraction to prevent the embarrassment of wetting the sheets.

5. If inserted solely because of the administration of diuretics it can be *removed as soon as drainage returns to normal.* If possible it is retained until this time as, if removed while drainage remains rapid, the patient will become uncomfortable if he experiences postanaesthetic retention. If the patient has undergone suprasellar surgery the catheter may have to remain in situ in order to assess hourly urine output.

Action

1. *Explain as often as necessary* about the catheter and show the patient the drainage bag in order to reinforce your explanation. Explain that the irritation will subside. Indicate when the catheter will be removed.

2. Confirm that there is *only 5 ml water* in the balloon.

3. If the catheter is not draining and the cause may be *obstruction by muscle contraction,* encourage the patient consciously to relax his muscles and reassure him that the catheter is starting to function when it does so.

4. *If the patient is very restless* then the catheter may need to be removed despite any advantage attached to its presence.

Position

Knowledge of the use of position is essential to the nurse in her aim to ensure the optimal conditions for the patient's recovery. The degree of head elevation is also important. Following craniotomy for tumour the usual degree of head elevation is 20–30° as this encourages venous return and so reduces the volume of the blood 'compartment' of the intracranial contents. However patients having undergone infratentorial surgery are positioned at 60+° in order to maximise the venous return but also to minimise cerebral oedema which can lead to rapid deterioration when it occurs in the posterior fossa. Following surgery for intracranial aneurysm the degree of head elevation is reduced and in some neurosurgical centres the patients are nursed flat. This enables the slightly higher intracranial pressure to support the aneurysm and, where applied, the clip, and so helps to prevent rebleeding.

Those patients who have had a shunt system inserted also lie flat. If the head is elevated, the shunt is allowed to work to its full capacity and the intracranial pressure is rapidly lowered to normal levels. As these patients are accustomed to a high intracranial pressure this not only leads to a low pressure headache but also can result in the development of a subdural haematoma which requires the patient's return to theatre for its evacuation and for temporary tying off of the shunt. A more gradual reduction in pressure is achieved by the patient being allowed to sit up in stages over several days. Any patient who has had a haematoma evacuated also lies flat in order to prevent its re-accumulation and again is sat up over several days.

Adequate hydration

Patient's need

- To remain hydrated while unable to take fluids orally.

Objective

- To administer fluids intravenously and maintain hydration.

Relevant information

1. The patient will have taken *nil orally* for several hours and will only be able to recommence if his recovery is satisfactory over the first 2 hours. If his operation involved the posterior fossa then his gag and cough reflexes may be temporarily diminished and he will remain 'nil orally' until the following morning when these reflexes will be tested. If he has had a ventriculoperitoneal shunt inserted he may be required to wait until the presence of bowel sounds has been confirmed.
2. Following the *removal of a suprasellar tumour* the patient may develop diabetes insipidus and so require larger volumes of

replacement fluid prior to the administration of DDAVP.

3. In some neurosurgical centres the patients are dehydrated in the attempt *to reduce cerebral oedema*. Fluids are often restricted to 1000–1500 ml daily.

Action

1. Ensure that the intravenous *infusion progresses as prescribed*.
2. *Commence oral fluids* with consideration to normal regimes, and the patient's condition.

EXPECTED AND UNEXPECTED CHANGES FROM THE PRE–OPERATIVE NEUROLOGICAL STATUS

The nurse must be able to differentiate between expected and unexpected changes in the patient's condition. Some changes occur as a matter of course following the type of operation performed, others may be expected by the surgeon having performed the patient's operation and others may be simply due to the patient's deteriorating condition. In each case the nurse must understand the implications of the postoperative changes. She may be aware of the routine management of a particular situation, or of the surgeon's decision with regard to management, and be able to incorporate this knowledge into her care of the patient, but she must know when it is necessary to consult the surgeon. For her action to be appropriate she requires not only a sound understanding of neurosurgical nursing and knowledge of the patient's pre-operative neurological state, but also information regarding the intra-operative progress of the patient that will influence his care, his progress or her interpretation of his condition.

Routinely expected changes

One example of a routinely expected change is a unilateral facial weakness following the removal of an ipsilateral acoustic neuroma. This is due to damage, temporary or permanent, to the 7th cranial nerve which lies in close proximity to the 8th nerve. Because this damage is virtually unavoidable, assessment is primarily of the degree of weakness rather than of its presence. A tarsorrhaphy may have been performed in theatre in order to prevent corneal complications occurring as a result of the patient's inability to close his eye fully and eye care is given as necessary. If the patient is dysarthric as a result of the weakness he is given encouragement and time to express himself and communicate effectively with the nursing staff. His weakness may improve with time but there is no intervention that will accelerate this process and only basic nursing care is required.

Another expected occurrence is the development of diabetes insipidus following the removal of a pituitary or other suprasellar tumour. The onset is usually several hours postoperatively when the level of circulating antidiuretic hormone falls. Because the incidence of diabetes insipidus in these patients is so great they are often catheterised so that the hourly urine output can be measured. Their management is routine and generally involves a regime whereby if the patient passes more than a specified amount of urine within a specified period, for example 1000 ml in 4 hours, the nurse gives the pre-prescribed DDAVP (artificial ADH) keeping the doctor informed of the development. All these changes are a direct and often unavoidable result of the surgical procedure.

Expected changes in an individual patient

As well as those changes which are routinely associated with the operation, complications arising from the way this particular operation has gone may influence the patient's recovery. Ideally, the surgeon informs the recovery nurse of the possibilities and remains with the patient until the initial postoperative assessment is completed so that any queries that the nurse may have can be answered. Examples include any pupillary abnormalities caused by local nerve damage during the operation that, under normal circumstances, would lead the nurse to suspect a critical or deteriorating neurological condition. The pupil on the same side of the operation may be larger or it may be constricted so that the contralateral pupil appears dilated. During the period of unconsciousness immediately following surgery, the patient's pupils are the most important guide to his condition and the nurse must have any relevant information.

A second example is where the site of the operation is in close proximity to the optic chiasm or the optic nerve and the patient's vision may be affected. Again this disturbance may be permanent or temporary and again, once assessed, no intervention is required other than the care appropriate for any patient with a newly developed visual handicap of the nature experienced by the patient. A visual deficit which is not apparent immediately following the operation but which develops as a later consequence of surgery is considered differently. This may be due to cerebral oedema rather than to specific damage during the operation and the surgeon must be informed.

It may be considered that the patient may have a seizure, or that he will be expressively or receptively dysphasic or confused, or that he will have developed a limb weakness due to the area of the brain involved. The surgeon can explain his proposed management of these expected deficits. If, at any stage, an expected deficit becomes more profound, the surgeon must be informed. Where, particularly following a posterior fossa operation, the expected degree of cerebral oedema would be dangerous to the patient the intracranial pressure is often maintained at acceptable levels by the use of artificial ventilation. This prevents the occurrence of expected problems.

Without the knowledge of these expected changes in the patient's neurological state the nurse can still help the patient to recover adequately. However, with an understanding of his condition the nurse is in a better position to interpret her observations and to implement appropriate care to assist the patient's recovery. And when the nurse's understanding of the patient's condition is similar to that of the medical staff, both have a greater understanding of each other's actions and the recovery period is more satisfactory for all the staff involved.

Deterioration

Deterioration can present as a reduction in the level of consciousness or the degree of orientation, or the patient may have a localised, or more commonly, a generalised convulsion, or he may develop changes such as limb weaknesses, expressive or receptive dysphasia or develop respiratory problems. Changes can be extremely subtle or they can be easily apparent.

A reduction in the level of consciousness can be gradual or it can be rapid. In the early postoperative stages it can be easily identified due to the frequency of the required assessments. This serves to reinforce the need for constant observation of the patient even after his initial recovery and for the nurse to be aware of the patient's condition at all times.

As the patient recovers from general anaesthesia he may require some explanation in order to reorientate himself. However if his level of orientation subsequently decreases this is indicative of a deterioration in his condition. Care must be taken to differentiate between apparent confusion and expressive or receptive dysphasia, and the general manner of the patient is often of value to the nurse in this situation.

A generalised convulsion is often heralded by subtle changes in the patient. Those with a supratentorial lesion and who undergo supratentorial surgery are at risk of convulsive activity as the site of the operation and subsequent oedema can affect the motor cortex. Those who undergo infratentorial surgery are not at risk. Consequently those patients undergoing supratentorial surgery are usually prescribed prophylactic anticonvulsants whereas those undergoing infratentorial surgery are not. A history of pre-operative seizure activity also leads to an increased risk of postoperative convulsion as does extensive retraction during surgery or the site of the operation being in close proximity to the motor cortex. Examples of these 'high risk' operations include the removal of a meningioma, the clipping of an aneurysm and the intracranial removal of a pituitary tumour. The convulsion itself is often less violent than a usual generalised fit but it is similarly composed of tonic and clonic stages. In this critical postoperative period the exchange of oxygen and carbon dioxide is temporarily reduced, not only diminishing the supply of oxygen to the brain, but also increasing the level of carbon dioxide in the blood and consequently leading to a rise in intracranial pressure. The metabolic rate also increases with increased production of carbon dioxide thus raising the blood levels further. Once the intracranial pressure and the degree of cerebral oedema is increased the risk of the occurrence of further fits also rises and this cycle of deterioration must be controlled.

An intravenous infusion of chlormethiazole may be commenced at a rate sufficient to prevent further convulsive activity. The required dose, however, may render the patient unable to maintain his own airway and if this is probable then elective ventilation will be started. During this period anticonvulsants are given via the nasogastric route and the chlormethiazole is reduced and, like the ventilation, discontinued as therapeutic blood levels are achieved. The administration of oxygen is recommenced during the fit and is continued until the patient's neurological state returns to the pre-ictal level.

The respiratory centre is located in the brain stem and is affected by pressure, both indirectly as a result of transtentorial herniation of the supratentorial contents, and directly by oedema or haemorrhage in the posterior fossa. For those patients who have undergone infratentorial surgery respiratory changes may be the first signs of deterioration and the onset and subsequent decline can be rapid. Respiratory arrest may occur with little warning or the respiratory pattern may first become abnormal. In the latter case gaseous exchange is reduced as respiration becomes less effective and the level of carbon dioxide in the blood rises leading to an increase in intracranial pressure. As the pressure increases, the respiratory centre is further compromised and the patient's condition continues to deteriorate. The recovery nurse must observe the patient carefully and any signs of abnormal respiratory changes must be reported immediately.

Deterioration is most commonly caused by haemorrhage, by cerebral oedema or by cerebral vasospasm. A CT scan is usually performed to identify or confirm the cause of deterioration and treatment may involve medication to reduce intracranial pressure, to control convulsive activity or to alter the patient's blood pressure, and it may involve the patient's return to theatre and/or elective or emergency ventilation.

Common causes of deterioration

Haemorrhage

Hypotensive agents are often used in theatre to help to provide a blood-free field for the surgeon. When the bleeding points are being cauterised prior to closure the patient's blood pressure is returned to normal so that these points can be seen to withstand the normal conditions. If a haemorrhage does occur, several of these points are usually involved and the consequent deterioration may be rapid or gradual depending on the rate of bleeding, the extent and position of the haematoma and the underlying degree of raised intracranial pressure. Localised signs may be initially apparent or general deterioration may be immediate. If haemorrhage occurs following surgery for aneurysm it is often due to the rupture of that aneurysm, for example if the clip becomes displaced. Deterioration is extremely rapid and requires the patient's immediate return to theatre for evacuation of the haematoma. Haemorrhage following the removal of a tumour is managed differently. The patient is treated conservatively until a CT scan confirms the cause of his deterioration. If surgery is indicated then he will return to theatre. The risk of haemorrhage

in these patients is affected by the nature of the tumour removed. If the tumour is compact and total removal is possible, a space remains which allows a greater movement of the surrounding structures and therefore a greater risk of haemorrhage. The tumour that is infiltrative and surrounded by grossly oedematous tissue is often only partially removed and as the surrounding tissue quickly fills this space, the potential bleeding points are supported and the risk of haemorrhage is less high.

Oedema

A certain degree of oedema is inevitable following intracranial surgery particularly where there was a significant degree of pre–operative oedema and there was prolonged and extensive retraction during surgery. A CT scan discounts a haematoma and demonstrates the swollen brain tissue by showing the shrunken ventricles. Management is generally conservative although if this proves unsuccessful the patient can return to theatre for decompression, either by the removal of a bone flap or a partial lobectomy. However this is not often required.

Oedema following posterior fossa surgery causes a more rapid deterioration with the brain stem compressed and herniation of the cerebellar tonsils through the foramen magnum an immediate danger.

Cerebral vasospasm

Cerebral vasospasm leads to areas of ischaemic brain tissue and ultimately to areas of infarct. As a result, the consequences for the patient are extremely serious and the prevention of vasospasm, or its early recognition and reversal, is of paramount importance.

Vasospasm often occurs following spontaneous subarachnoid haemorrhage and again most commonly occurs in the postoperative period following surgery for aneurysm. There are a variety of methods used in the attempt to prevent it, one example being a regime whereby the patient has regular infusions of low molecular weight dextran over the first few postoperative days. However a major consideration in the nursing care of the patient is his blood pressure which, post-operatively, must be maintained at his normal pre-operative levels although they may be ordinarily considered hypertensive. Periods of relative hypotension can result in the collapse of areas of microcirculation and focal deficits then become apparent. Even at the patient's normal blood pressure, vasospasm can occur. The surgeon in either case may intervene and increase the blood pressure by starting a controlled infusion of a hypertensive agent, and a 'cut off' point may be apparent where the circulation is re-established or conversely lost. The other major complication following surgery for aneurysm is haemorrhage and these are easily distinguishable from each other. Haemorrhage results in extremely rapid deterioration whereas vasospasm, as already described, results in focal changes.

RELATIVES' VISITS

The 'family' involves not only the individual members but also the relationship between them. Within these relationships a support system develops which helps the family and its members to cope with and overcome, or adapt to, difficulties that arise. It is essential to maintain this system of support during the period of hospitalisation as it is this rather than external sources of support that is fundamental in the long-term. Attention to the needs of the whole family rather than to those solely of the patient is extremely important in the attempt to achieve this aim.

Molter (1979) and Daley (1984) showed that relatives of critically ill patients were not only able to identify their own needs but also rate them according to their importance. When 'need' was divided into different categories, the category concerned with being with the patient was of less significance than that for the relief of anxiety and that for information. (Bouman 1984, Daley 1984). However, the individual need 'to be with the family member' and to stay nearby at other times was rated very highly in several studies (Breu 1978, Molter 1979, Fuller & Foster 1982). To be allowed to visit at any time was considered important and there was a significant correlation between the family's perception of the patient's condition and the ranked importance of visiting frequently.

Visiting, however, is often restricted by both hospital visiting policies and the limited facilities available to the recovery unit. These restrictions must be thoughtfully implemented. The effect of visiting on the patient has to be closely observed but Fuller & Foster (1982) showed that although individual interactions could be either stress-producing or stress-reducing for the intensive care patient, family visits were no more or less stress-producing than were nurse/patient interactions.

The first postoperative visit is often an emotional time for relatives and their responses can be unpredictable and not always related to the apparent severity of the patient's condition.

Any remaining denial of the patient's situation is abruptly confronted and although many will appear brave in the presence of the patient they will need subsequent reassurance and explanation. Their confidence in the nursing and medical staff is extremely important at this stage and the staff must demonstrate and so confirm their skill and expertise. Repeated visiting helps to increase their confidence and serves to reduce the acute anxiety caused by the situation. Subsequent telephone contact is made easier and more helpful by each person's knowledge and understanding of the other.

Not all relatives want, or are able, to visit, and may, therefore, prefer to rely exclusively on telephone contact. Again this can be made more helpful and reassuring if the nurse not only gives an account of the patient's progress but also facilitates communication between the relative and the patient, e.g., by passing messages between them.

If the needs of the relatives, general as well as related to visiting, are known to the staff they are more easily and more successfully met. The ward staff are in a position to gain an understanding of each family's needs and they can pass this information on to the recovery staff. Of value is the finding that the ranking of needs did not correlate with demographic variables, i.e. age, sex, socio-economic class and education, or with the relationship to the patient (kin or significant other) or with the type of unit (Bouman 1984).

ONGOING CARE OF THE PATIENT WHO HAS HAD CRANIOTOMY

The time period covered by this section is that following transfer from recovery to the patient's discharge home.

THE AIMS OF CARE

1. Assess and evaluate the patient's neurological status in order to aid early recognition of raised intracranial pressure.
2. Control those factors known to increase ICP.
3. Aid rehabilitation, involving the prevention of complications and added disabilities, maintenance of intact skills and functions and a restorative period, allowing the whole person to adapt and make the best possible use of remaining abilities.

Wilson-Barnett (1981) cites a number of factors which influence recovery and thus the planning of care:

- previous health and risk factors
- the presence or absence of complications
- any past experience of illness and/or hospitalisation
- the individual's personality and understanding of his condition and necessary care
- the individual's expectations and doctor/nurses' expectations and advice
- age, sex and cultural background

- pre-morbid occupation and employer's attitude
- financial situation and other life events
- family and friends and the flexibility of roles within this group.

When the patient is transferred from the recovery area to the ward, information which is necessary to allow care to be planned, must be obtained:

— age, diagnosis and existing pre-operative signs and symptoms
— presence of pre-existing health problems
— details of surgery including duration, site and reasons
— any drugs administered such as mannitol
— type and volumes of intravenous fluid and blood administered
— intake and output record
— occurrence of problems during or following the operation
— respiratory and cardiovascular state
— vital and neurological signs
— state of head dressing and drain — presence, character and amount of drainage
— any test results, e.g. arterial blood gas, CT scan
— specific postoperative instructions to be followed, e.g. regarding elevation of the head
— involvement of the family — what they know.

The initial assessment of the patient should identify potential problems that may adversely affect recovery and establish the baseline with which future comparisons will be made. A visit to the recovery ward during the immediate postoperative period may assist in anticipating needs in the ward.

NEUROLOGICAL ASSESSMENT

Neurological assessment should be carried out and recorded immediately in the presence of the recovery nurse so that any queries may be answered. According to the patient's condition, the necessary frequency of observations can be determined. This will usually be not less than 2 hourly on the first post-operative day. The patient's best eye opening, motor and verbal responses are recorded according to the coma scale in use, level of consciousness being the most important indicator of neurological change. (Allan 1984) Early reporting of any change should allow appropriate treatment to be instituted. The patient should be asked to report any headache or nausea. In conversation, facial expression, asymmetry or abnormal movements should be noted. The quality of speech is assessed for signs of dysphasia and whether any difficulty is primarily in expression or understanding. Dysarthric speech, which is slow, slurred, hoarse or monotonous, may be a problem in the patient who has had posterior fossa surgery. Attention span, mood, behaviour and memory should also be evaluated. Reaction to illness and appropriateness of behaviour should be observed along with evidence of anxiety, excitement, depression or paranoid responses to questions.

Equality and reaction of pupils are assessed along with occular movement including presence of nystagmus.

Assessing motor function

Comparison of muscle strength must be made for symmetry with each side of the body. Both distal and proximal muscles of the limbs should be tested. The patient should be instructed to push against the observer's fixed resistance and this motor function graded. The patient should also be instructed to extend his arms with palms facing upwards, and keep this position for about 10 seconds, note any upward or downwards drift of the arms. Bilateral response to touch, pain and temperature can be estimated. Perception of position and evidence of inattention to one side of the body are noted.

If the patient's cerebellar function seems to be impaired, gait, balance and co-ordination are assessed. Any unsteadiness, lurching to one side or broadening of the gait will be particularly obvious if the patient is asked to walk heel-to-toe on a straight line.

Vision

Gross visual acuity may be estimated by asking the patient to count fingers. Any complaints of blurred vision or diplopia are reported. Visual field changes can be examined by confrontation. The patient is asked to face the nurse and cover one eye. The nurse positions her fingers to the side at eye level. The nurse's fingers are then moved into the main boundaries of the visual field, and the patient asked to state when the moving finger is seen. This exercise is repeated with the other eye. Visual field assessment is particularly important in the patient who has had pituitary surgery.

Lower cranial nerve assessment

If the patient has had surgery to the posterior fossa, the functions of the glossopharyngeal 9 and vagus 10 nerves, which control the gag and swallowing reflexes and articulation, must be assessed. The patient's ability to deal with his own secretions should be observed. If he is instructed to open his mouth and say 'ah', the soft palate and uvula should elevate in the midline. The gag reflex is elicited by asking the patient to stick out his tongue, the tip of a tongue depressor being used to gently stimulate the back of the pharynx. Any asymmetrical contractions of the palate, uvula and pharynx are also noted.

Cerebral oedema and raised intracranial pressure must subside before the permanence of neurological deficits can be predicted.

Potential neurological problems

Cerebral oedema

This may present as increased drowsiness and focal signs up to around 4 days after surgery and may follow an initial bright period following recovery from anaesthesia. Patients particularly at risk are those who have undergone prolonged surgery and brain retraction, those with large meningiomas which have caused significant brain compression, those with partially resected gliomas and those with cerebral contusions or abscess. Dexamethasone (usually 4 mg every 6 hours) is prescribed over the operative period to control cerebral oedema, probably by inhibiting CSF production. Prolonged use may exaggerate the normal physiological actions of corticosteroids and result in immunosuppression and side-effects such as diabetes mellitus, fluid and electrolyte imbalance, osteoporosis and mental disturbances such as paranoia, depression or euphoria. Dexamethasone should be administered with or after food along with an antacid to reduce the risk of gastrointestinal irritation. The dose is reduced gradually to allow recovery from adrenal cortex suppression.

Mannitol 20% (2 g/kg infused over 30 minutes) can be given to reduce cerebral oedema rapidly by removing fluid from the brain and thus reducing intracranial pressure. It is effective within 15 minutes of infusion although reduction of oedema may persist for several hours. Side-effects include pulmonary oedema, tachycardia, fluid and electrolyte imbalance and angina-like chest pain. Any crystals present in the solution should be dissolved by immersing the bag in warm water for around 15 minutes, shaking when cool enough to handle and cooling to body temperature before infusion.

Intracranial haemorrhage

There is increased risk of intracranial haemorrhage in those who have had surgery for meningioma or chronic subdural haematoma, where the brain is compressed, atrophied and non-expansive, and following shunting procedures. The risk is also present in those with vascular lesions, coagulation problems or extensive injury, where release of thromboplastin may lead to disseminated intravascular coagulation. Neurological deterioration due to haemorrhage is usually rapid.

Hydrocephalus

This may develop where a shunt becomes obstructed, is wrongly positioned, becomes detached or has a faulty valve. It may be a complication of subarachnoid haemorrhage or posterior fossa surgery due to impairment of CSF flow or absorption, e.g. when the outlets to the fourth ventricle are blocked. Meningitis or arachnoiditis may also cause hydrocephalus. This may present acutely with signs of raised intracranial pressure or develop insidiously with ataxia, confusion and incontinence.

Cerebral infarction

This may follow vascular surgery, e.g. for aneurysm, arteriovenous malformation. In patients with subarachnoid haemorrhage cerebral arterial vasospasm may lead to infarction. This tends to appear 4 to 11 days following the last haemorrhage regardless of when the surgery was performed. The development of spasm is insidious. Symptoms will vary depending on the area of altered blood flow. Focal deficits such as a hemiparesis or dysphasia may be transient or cumulative over hours or days resulting in ischaemia and infarction. The patient may recover from anaesthesia to his pre-operative state and subsequently deteriorate. Management aims to improve cerebral perfusion pressure and prevent infarction. Elevation of systemic blood pressure with drugs such as dopamine hydrochloride will necessitate close monitoring of blood pressure (quarter hourly or continuously) and side-effects such as tachycardia and hypovolaemia. Dopamine is usually infused via a large central vein as extravasation at a peripheral infusion site may cause necrosis. Rheomacrodex (dextran 40 intravenous infusion) may used to expand blood volume and increase flow to the ischaemic area.

Where the patient's condition is deteriorating the possibility of a metabolic cause such as hypoxia, fluid and electrolyte imbalance, hypoglycaemia or endocrine disturbance should be considered. If the problem is metabolic, confusion and disorientation usually precede loss of consciousness and motor signs. If motor signs appear, they are usually symmetrical. Pupillary reaction and occular movement are usually unchanged.

Respiration

Goals:

1. Regular respirations at a normal rate for the patient
2. Maintenance of optimal gaseous exchange to meet the brain's metabolic requirements; hypoxia and hypercapnia will cause cerebral vasodilation, increasing cerebral blood flow and thus intracranial pressure
3. Prevention of chest infection.

Identification of those particularly at risk:

— pre-existing problems, e.g. chronic obstructive airway disease
— age — decreased pulmonary compliance
— debilitation — underweight and undernourished
— obesity
— cigarette smoking — paralysis of cilia diminishes mobility of secretions
— depressed cough reflex — stagnation of secretions
— absent or depressed swallowing or gag reflex — risk of aspiration
— altered level of consciousness — depressed respiratory centres in medulla and pons
— dehydration — more tenacious secretions difficult to expectorate
— immobility — restricted ventilation increases stasis of secretions and promotes atelectasis
— lengthy operation.

Assess

- Airway and ventilation
- Temperature, cough, sputum
- Breathing pattern, chest pain.

Cerebral ischaemia is the most likely cause of restlessness and altered level of consciousness in the postoperative patient. Early

preventative care of those at risk should be instituted rather than waiting for signs of respiratory complications to develop. Changing the patient's position at least every 2 hours, sitting the patient up as soon as possible and giving encouragement and help to perform deep breathing exercises should allow maximum chest expansion and prevent pooling of secretions. Early activity will help to restore normal respiratory function. If a productive cough develops the patient should be assisted to expectorate avoiding strain which may increase intrathoracic pressure and thus intracranial pressure. Chest physiotherapy and suctioning may be necessary to remove excess secretions. Attention to comfort and relief of anxiety will assist the patient to co-operate with respiratory care. Oral intake must be withheld until presence of gag and cough reflexes is verified. A nasogastric tube may be inserted to aspirate stomach contents. If the patient's respiratory state is inadequate on clinical assessment, arterial blood gases should be evaluated. Physiotherapy, administration of humidified oxygen and if necessary, intermittent positive pressure ventilation should be employed to maintain the PaO_2 above 80 mmHg and the $PaCO_2$ below 45 mmHg. Once a sputum specimen has been obtained, a broad spectrum antibiotic will be prescribed until a specific sensitivity report is received.

Neurogenic pulmonary oedema may occur when there has been a sudden dramatic rise in intracranial pressure. The patient should be observed for signs of dyspnoea, restlessness, tachycardia, cold clammy skin which is grey or cyanosed in appearance and expectoration of mucus and possibly blood. Preventative care should minimise the length of stay in hospital.

Prevention of deep venous thrombosis and pulmonary embolus

Potential problem

Thrombosis may occur in the deep veins of calf muscles a week or more after surgery. Causes include compression of femoral and popliteal veins if the knees are kept flexed for long periods. Increased viscosity of blood postoperatively, particularly if hyperosmolar solutions have been administered to control intracranial pressure.

Venous stasis is caused by immobility.

The patient should be encouraged to move and change position as exercise will prevent venous stasis, and the muscle action will improve venous flow. Constriction of the leg veins should be avoided and the patient instructed not to cross his legs. Anti-embolism stockings will promote venous return. Systemic and skin temperature should be monitored and each calf observed for pain or tenderness though there may be no overt signs.

Fluid balance and nutrition

Goal

To ensure adequate hydration and nutrition to maintain body function, promote healing and combat infection, to maintain weight relevant to age, height and physique.

Patients at risk

Those with absent or impaired swallowing reflex following posterior fossa surgery. Those with nausea, vomiting, gastric irritation or diarrhoea. Patients with impaired conscious level, or who are unable to feed themselves independently. Those with a poor state of mouth and teeth or poor appetite. Those who are anxious or in pain. Patients whose eating and drinking habits changed in hospital or who developed diabetes insipidus as a result of surgery in the pituitary/hypothalamic region. Those with increased needs e.g. in hyperthermia or where administration of osmotic diuretics has led to a large diuresis. Patients who were administered high protein tube feeds without sufficient water for excretion of nitrogenous waste products of protein breakdown.

In the presence of risk factors, ability to maintain an adequate intake must be assessed. Patients must be alert with intact swallowing and gag reflexes before oral intake is introduced to avoid the risk of aspiration. The intravenous infusion is maintained until oral intake is sufficient or nasogastric tube feeds are established. Fluid balance and food intake are monitored. Diet should be well balanced. The patient is given assistance with a light diet on the first postoperative day to avoid fatigue. Supplementary nourishing fluids can be given and the family encouraged to bring in foods from home that may be more acceptable for the patient. Sufficient assistance and supervision should be given to ensure adequate intake and aids such as adaptive cutlery and non-slip mats provided if necessary to increase independence. The occupational therapist should be asked to assess the patient's needs and develop a rehabilitative programme. The patient must be in a comfortable position to aid digestion and anti-emetics or antacids administered if required. Those with a facial weakness should be advised to take food through the unaffected side of the mouth. Oral cleansing is carried out before and after meals to remove food debris.

The advice of the speech therapist should be sought to develop a feeding regime for the dysphagic patient. Small amounts of semi-solid food are easier to swallow than fluids.

In some units fluid intake is restricted for those with significantly increased intracranial pressure. This must be explained to the patient and the allowance divided up evenly over the day.

Diabetes insipidus

This develops when there is a decrease or absence of circulating antidiuretic hormone. ADH is produced in the hypothalamus and stored in the posterior pituitary gland. It acts on the kidney where it promotes water reabsorption. Diabetes insipidus may be transient where it is due to postoperative oedema, presenting within the first few days with a duration of several days to weeks. Patients with diabetes insipidus pre-operatively should not expect surgery to improve the disorder and it is often more severe postoperatively.

Excessive urinary loss of water occurs regardless of fluid intake. Output in excess of 200 ml an hour with a specific gravity of less than 1005 and weight loss indicate diabetes insipidus (1 litre of fluid weighs 1 kilogram).

In the alert patient thirst is an important symptom. Polyuria may occur postoperatively for reasons other than diabetes insipidus. Administration of large volumes of fluid during surgery is a common cause. The serum sodium in these patients will be low or normal and postoperative weight higher than pre-operative. When excess fluid is excreted, output, weight and serum sodium return to normal, usually within 24 hours of surgery. Hyperglycaemia also causes polyuria and may result from steroid therapy. The patient will be thirsty but the urinary specific gravity will be higher than in diabetes insipidus and glyco-suria will be present.

The patient with diabetes insipidus may not be able to compensate for a large output with large volumes of oral fluid, particularly if he is not fully alert. A urinary catheter may be necessary for accurate recording of output and the comfort of the patient. The specific gravity of each void should be recorded on all patients at risk and cumulative totals calculated. Treatment will consist of fluid and electrolyte replacement, thirst being a good indicator of needs in the fully conscious patient.

Frequency of urination and degree of thirst may interfere with other activities such as sleep and rest. If ADH replacement is necessary, desmopressin (DDAVP) is usually given intramuscularly at first. A typical regime may involve administration if the urinary output exceeds 1000 ml over 4 hours with a specific gravity of 1000. Administration will prevent diuresis but will not correct existing dehydration. If the patient is not receiving adequate cortisone replacement, diabetes insipidus will subside until levels are increased, as cortisone is necessary for water regulation. Patients with known diabetes insipidus must receive i.v. fluids when fasting for procedures.

If diabetes insipidus has not resolved prior to discharge from hospital, preparation for home management must be made. DDAVP can be administered intranasally once or twice a day. Fluid retention or pressor effects such as raised BP leading to the patient complaining of headache are rarely a problem. Often these patients will have other health problems to deal with such as cortisone and hormone replacement and poor vision. The patient's ability to learn and participate in his care must be assessed and family members included in any teaching sessions as they may have to assume responsibility for this. Time must be allowed for explanation, questions and demonstrations. Written instructions and diagrams for home reference should be included. The patient should understand that the severity of diabetes insipidus may change over time, that thirst is a protective mechanism which requires a response and that limiting fluid intake will not decrease urinary output.

If the patient is unsure whether to use DDAVP he should wait until thirst and urination increase. Patients who understand that DDAVP is a convenience for them may be less afraid. The district nurse should be asked to visit and assess ability to cope at home.

Inappropriate antidiuretic hormone

Inappropriate ADH secretion will cause fluid retention with an increase in urinary specific gravity and low serum sodium. It may follow head injury, hypothalamic or pituitary surgery or carcinoma of bronchus or lung. Fluid intake will be restricted and sodium supplements may be necessary. Hyponatraemia can cause headache, confusion, generalised weakness and fitting.

Hyperthermia

Problem

Cerebral metabolic demands and oxygen requirements are increased.

Identification of cause

Within 24–48 hours of surgery the cause may

be pulmonary atelectasis. It may be urinary tract infection, particularly if the patient has been catheterised, is dehydrated or immobile. Wound infection may become obvious 3–4 days after surgery. External ventricular drainage is a high risk of infection. Surgery in the region of the third ventricle or hypothalamus (near the temperature regulating centres of the brain) may be the cause if hyperthermia is unremitting. There may be CSF leakage leading to meningitis; subarachnoid haemorrhage; a transfusion reaction or phenytoin reaction in which case pyrexia is associated with erythematous rash or chest infection.

Investigations

Blood, urine, sputum, wound exudate or CSF culture.

Action

Measures should be taken to reduce temperature by approximately one degree an hour. Temperature is monitored via the axilla or rectum. Use of oral thermometers is contra-indicated due to risk of postoperative epilepsy. Minimal bed clothing, tepid sponging, fanning and administration of aspirin may be employed. Evaluation of fluid balance for increased needs should include assessment of loss through sweating.

Care of the wound

Goal

A well healed wound.

Potential problems

Wound infection caused by contamination during surgery, at dressing change or by the patient touching the incision. Meningitis caused by spread from wound infection, contamination at operation or through dural tear. Infection of bone flap or intracerebral abscess can occur. If the drain is not functioning blood will accumulate beneath the skin leading to peri-orbital oedema and discomfort for the patient.

Patients at risk

Elderly, debilitated patients or those who have undergone lengthy surgical procedures. Those with penetrating head injuries, compound skull fractures, external ventricular drains or CSF leaks. Those who have re-exploration of recent wounds, drainage of abscesses, removal of infected bone flaps.

Assessment of signs

— elevated temperature
— drainage from wound and presence of CSF (suggested by a haemoserous central patch with a clear or yellow outer ring)
— rhinorrhoea (clear drainage from the nose)
— inflammation and tenderness of the wound
— elevation of the bone flap
— symptoms of meningitis:
    restlessness and irritability
    headache and neck stiffness
    photophobia.

If the head dressing is dry, it is left in place until suture removal, usually between 2 and 5 days postoperatively for supratentorial wounds and 7 to 10 days after posterior fossa surgery. A wet head dressing will provide a medium for organisms to be transported and therefore should be changed in a strictly aseptic manner. The importance of not touching the incision should be stressed to the patient. Confused patients must be closely supervised. The bandage should be firm to discourage bleeding under the skin flap but may be changed if it is too tight with evidence of swelling for the comfort of the patient.

A specimen of any CSF drainage should be sent for culture and sensitivity and samples from external ventricular drains obtained each day for early identification of infection. Nasal suctioning is avoided in the patient with rhinorrhoea who should be instructed not to blow the nose.

The subgaleal drain should be well secured

to avoid traction and positioned below the level of the patient's head. Suction is maintained according to the instructions of the surgeon. Drains are usually removed 24–48 hours after surgery and the entry site observed for drainage.

Collection of fluid under the skin flap may necessitate aspiration and application of a pressure bandage though this carries further risk of infection. Surgical repair of a dural tear may be considered if CSF leakage does not abate. Removal of an infected bone flap is usually necessary.

Personal cleansing and dressing

The skin must be kept clean, odour free and intact. Risk factors such as incontinence or limb paralysis must be assessed to identify those vulnerable to pressure sore development. Position change, selection of type of mattress and skin care are then appropriately employed. Attention to the condition of hands and nails, scalp and remaining hair will help to improve self-image. The ability of the patient to carry out care independently should be assessed. Problems may include dyspraxia, where despite normal limb power the patient is unable to carry out a learned voluntary movement. The critical components of each activity to be learnt must be analysed. The physiotherapist and occupational therapist will help to develop a planned programme for the development of skills such as dressing.

Eyes

Eyes must be kept clean and well lubricated to prevent complications such as infection or corneal abrasion. Patients particularly at risk are the unconscious and those with periorbital oedema or those with facial weakness or loss of the corneal reflex following posterior fossa surgery.

The eyes are gently cleaned with sterile saline to remove crusting. Administration of drops such as hypromellose will counteract tear deficiency. The patient who is unable to close an eye due to facial (7th) nerve palsy will need a protective eye shield. If it appears that facial and trigeminal nerve damage is likely to be long-term, a lateral tarsorrhophy may be performed to keep the eye closed. Cold packs may be applied to relieve periorbital swelling.

Mouth

Oral hygiene must be maintained to keep the mouth clean, moist and odour free and to prevent discomfort and complications such as parotitis, ulceration or dental caries. Patients unable to take oral fluids because of bulbar palsy and those with a facial nerve palsy will require particular attention.

The teeth should be brushed regularly and mouthwashes given as necessary. Excess secretions and food debris should be removed particularly before and after meals. The patient should be assisted to be as independent as possible in his own care.

Mobilising

The head of the bed should be elevated to promote venous return unless a sudden reduction in intracranial pressure is contraindicated, e.g. following shunt insertion, evacuation of a subdural haematoma or clipping of aneurysm, when specific instructions from the surgeon regarding the length of time the patient is to lie flat must be followed. Neck and head rotation or flexion can impede venous return and should therefore be avoided. Activities where intra-abdominal or intrathoracic pressure are increased can raise intracranial pressure. Extreme hip flexion and actions such as pushing against the footboard of the bed with the feet should be avoided. The patient should be instructed not to strain when coughing, sneezing, blowing the nose, opening the bowels or repositioning. Rest periods should be provided between activities such as respiratory care and repositioning which are particularly associated with small increases in intracranial pressure (Snyder 1983).

While the patient is in bed, the limbs must

be kept in normal alignment using pillows and foam pads where necessary to maintain position. If a limb is paralysed, each joint should be put through its full range of normal movement at least every 2 hours to prevent musculoskeletal deformities such as contractures. The patient should be encouraged to move independently and participate in his own care to maintain muscle strength and tone. Changes of position and limb exercise will help to prevent skin breakdown and will promote circulation. If muscle tone is increased in a limb, frequent repositioning will be necessary.

The patient should be allowed out of bed for short periods as soon as possible from the second postoperative day. The nurse must be aware of physiotherapy programmes to be able to reinforce skills learnt by integrating them into all aspects of care. Goals must be realistic for the patient's motivation to be maintained. Only when balancing and sitting have been mastered can transfer activities from chair to bed and then from sitting to standing be commenced. The patient must be able to stand and balance safely before starting to walk.

Independence in bathing, toileting, grooming, hygiene, dressing and eating must be assessed. Deficits in perception, motor activity, communication, vision and intellectual function will all be barriers to relearning. The advice of the occupational therapist should be sought in assessing the need for adaptive devices to increase independence.

Eliminating

Goals

Normal bowel and bladder function, prevention of urinary tract infection.

Potential problems

— Incontinence due to diminished level of consciousness; loss of social control and judgement due to frontal lobe disturbance
— Retention of urine causing discomfort from distended bladder, restlessness, stasis of urine and increased risk of infection
— Incomplete upper motor neurone bladder causing diminished perception of bladder fullness, diminished ability to empty bladder; feeling of urgency to void
— Constipation due to inactivity, administration of analgesics such as codeine phosphate, lack of dietary fibre.

An indwelling urinary catheter may be inserted at the time of operation for accurate measurement of output if mannitol is administered or if it is anticipated that the patient will develop diabetes insipidus. Ensuring an adequate fluid intake and regular catheter hygiene will help prevent ascending infection. The catheter should be removed as soon as possible.

Adequate assistance and facilities for eliminating must be provided. Providing privacy and allowing the patient to get out of bed to use commode or toilet as soon as possible will help to relieve inhibition or discomfort.

Where sensation or control are diminished a bladder or bowel retraining programme may need to be initiated.

Regular administration of stool softeners and attention to dietary fibre and fluid intake should help to prevent constipation and are preferable to the use of enemas which may increase intra-abdominal pressure.

Fluid intake, urinary output and bowel function must be accurately recorded.

Pain

Pain will have undesirable consequences for the patient such as fatigue, discomfort, distress and restlessness, which will interfere with sleep and relaxation. Pain can stimulate the release of steroids from the adrenal cortex which affect protein, fat and carbohydrate metabolism. An increase in protein breakdown can delay wound healing. Where the immune response is depressed there will be an increased risk of infection (Boore 1979).

Headache is expected in the first 24–48

hours following surgery and usually originates from stretching or irritation of the scalp nerves or traction on the blood vessels of the dura. Facial expression, pallor, sweating or an increase in respiratory rate, pulse and blood pressure may indicate that the patient is in pain. The patient should be taught the importance of asking for analgesia before pain becomes severe. Analgesia which does not depress respiration or conscious level, such as codeine phosphate or paracetamol, should be administered on a regular basis to keep pain under control. If the patient decides that analgesia is necessary it will be more effective. Time and opportunity should be provided to discuss pain experienced or anticipated.

Individual needs are assessed. As anxiety increases, the awareness of pain increases. Reduction of uncertainty about future events, giving the patient information regarding his condition and recovery may reduce anxiety and pain experienced.

The bed should be comfortable and the head well supported, avoiding traction on the drain or overtight head dressings. Activities such as physiotherapy should be carried out when pain is being controlled successfully. Adjustment of light, noise and temperature may promote rest.

Epilepsy

Problem

Increase in cerebral metabolic demand; systemic hypertension which leads to increase in cerebral blood flow.

Patients at risk

Those who have undergone supratentorial surgery, particularly for meningioma, abscess, arteriovenous malformation, intracerebral haematoma, middle cerebral artery aneurysm.

The patient must be protected from physical injury and airway obstruction, avoiding placing anything in the mouth or restraining limbs. The nature of the fit should be recorded. This may be focal, e.g. muscular twitching of the face or hand caused by irritation of the responsible area of motor cortex. There may be a focal onset to a generalised convulsion. The eyes deviate away from a hemispheric lesion towards the side of motor involvement. The presence of post-ictal limb weakness or altered state of consciousness should be reported.

Because of the risk of postoperative fits, patients who are about to undergo supratentorial surgery are given prophylactic anticonvulsants such as phenytoin (300 mg daily). Even if a patient does not experience a fit, drug therapy may be continued for up to a year according to the surgeon's assessment of risk. Development of side-effects such as ataxia, tremor, confusion, gingival hypertrophy and tenderness and skin eruptions may dictate stopping administration or the substitution of a different anticonvulsant. Care of mouth and skin will have to be reassessed accordingly. Phenytoin should not be given intramuscularly as absorption is very unpredictable. As rapid intravenous administration depresses myocardial function, arryhthmias and cardiac arrest are possible.

If the patient is thought to be at risk of fits when discharged home, the family must be taught what to do should a fit occur. Social and occupational implications will have to be considered.

As a general guideline, the UK DVLC recommend that patients do not drive for a year following supratentorial surgery. Advice should be sought from the surgeon regarding individual risks. While safety must be of paramount importance, there may be social and occupational consequences if the patient is not allowed to drive.

Maintaining a safe environment

Neurological impairment will result in a diminished ability to provide for personal safety. Safety needs have to be assessed on an individual basis and the nurse must anticipate those which the patient is unable to maintain for himself. An inattention to one side of the body will necessitate teaching to improve perception, providing stimuli, encouraging handling of affected limbs and checking of the patient's position. Safety measures might include correct matching of chair to patient, leaving the bed in a low position, providing cot sides for the bed, or close supervision and attempts to orientate the confused patient.

The patient's ability to take prescribed drugs must be assessed. All patients should be protected from exposure to potential sources of infection.

Communicating

For those undergoing cranial surgery, the prospect of intellectual deficit, distressing for all, will be particularly so for those whose occupation or pleasures largely depend on thinking abilities. Perception of emotional needs is very subjective and such needs will be individual for each patient and family member. Family members whose loved one has undergone brain surgery may feel increased physical separation when there is neurological dysfunction. The patient may respond inappropriately or uncharacteristically or be unable to respond at all. This adds to the disruption of the family unit and decreases the ability of family members to assess progress for themselves. Increased effort is necessary for them to maintain or restore family unity and they must rely on communication with staff to understand the patient's progress. Nurses must aim to assist them to meet their personal needs. Family members need to feel confident in the abilities of the hospital staff. They need to feel that there is hope, that the staff accept them and care about their relative. They need regular information about the patient's condition and exactly what is being done and have questions answered honestly. They should know that they will be called at home if there are changes in their relative's condition (Mathis 1984).

For there to be communication, a relation-ship must be established between nurse, patient and family. Family members should be welcomed and allowed to feel that they play a vital role in the patient's recovery. Teaching and information must be given clearly and repeated as often as necessary. If the patient and/or family are asked to explain in their own words what they have been told, the nurse is able to assess what they have retained and understood. Diagrams and written material may be useful, particularly for the patient with memory impairment.

Communication between staff is particularly important. Ideally, the nurse should be present at discussions between surgeon, patient and family. Liaison between them and therapists and social workers is an important part of the nurse's role.

The patient's capacity for communication will depend upon his ability to speak, hear, see, read and write. Intelligence, vocabulary and native language, anxiety, mood and level of self-esteem may be influencing factors. The nurse should assess personal appearance, touching, eye contact, gesture, orientation and response to the environment and whether body and verbal language are congruent. Pain, discomfort and social embarrassment will also affect communication. A reassuring, unhurried and positive approach to the patient with speech problems may help prevent frustration leading to fear and depression. Simple sentences can be rephrased if not understood and picture boards may be useful. Those with receptive dysphasia may need gestural guidelines. Advice about individual approach should be sought from the speech therapist.

Attempts should be made to orientate the patient in time and place. Talking about family, friends and current affairs and passing on telephone messages may help reduce feelings of isolation.

Communicating is necessary for co-operation and motivation and lack of information will lead to fear and apprehension. Choice and input into decisions are often taken away from patients and their families in an acute ward and staff should be aware that they have rights.

Expressing sexuality

Potential problems

— Anxiety or embarrassment about intimate procedures.
— Disability or disfigurement , e.g. loss of hair, facial weakness, hemiparesis;
— Changes in function, e.g. impotence, amenorrhoea, as a result of pituitary disturbance.

Maximum privacy for patient and family should be maintained as far as possible. The nurse should try to minimise disruption to established relationships during hospitalisation. The patient's self-image may be enhanced by attention to grooming and preserving the dignity of those requiring assistance. The patient may choose to wear a wig, hat or headscarf. Communicating concern for and interest in the patient's body may help them begin to accept change in body image. Grieving behaviour should be recognised and the patient encouraged to express his feelings. Sexual needs are individual, covering a wide range of behaviour and attitudes and the subject must be handled with care and sensitivity. Help to understand changes in function should be given and any endocrinology follow-up explained. Information should be provided about resuming sexual activity after surgery. There are usually no restrictions after craniotomy, but the surgeon's advice should be sought as to any contra-indication to the continuing use of oral contraceptives. Helping the person to take part in his or her own care and encouraging independence will improve self-esteem. If the patient wants guidance about modification of activity, specialised written information or counselling they may be referred to the Association to Aid the Sexual and Personal Relationships of the Disabled (SPOD).

REFERENCES AND BIBLIOGRAPHY

Allan D 1984 Glasgow coma scale. Nursing Mirror 158(23):32

Arsenault L 1985 Selected post-operative complications of cranial surgery. Journal of Neurosurgical Nursing 17(3):155

Boore J 1979 Nursing surgical patients in acute pain. Nursing 1:37

Bouman C 1984 Self perceived needs of family members of critically ill patients. Heart and Lung 13(3):294

Breu C, Dracup K 1978 Helping the spouses of critically ill patients. American Journal of Nursing 78(1):51

Daley L 1984 The perceived immediate needs of families with relatives in the intensive care setting. Heart and Lung 13(3):231

Fuller B F, Foster G M 1982 The effects of family/friend visits versus staff interaction on stress/arousal of surgical intensive care patients. Heart and Lung 11(5):457

Hampe S O 1974 Needs of a grieving spouse in a hospital setting. Nursing Research 24(2):113

Hickey J 1986 The clinical practice of neurological and neurosurgical nursing, 2nd edn. Lippincott, Philadelphia

Howe P 1979 The respiratory effects of surgery. Nursing 1(7):324

Ingrar D 1975 cited by Zegeer L J 1982 Nursing care of the patient with brain oedema. Journal of Neurosurgical Nursing 14(5):268

Jones J 1982 Give and take. Nursing Mirror 154(7):xiii

Kaminiski D 1975 Air embolism during surgery in the sitting position:its prevention, detection and treatment. Journal of Neurosurgical Nursing 7(2):65

Lassen N A, Christensen M A 1976 as cited by Zegeer L J 1982 Nursing care of the patient with brain oedema. Journal of Neurosurgical Nursing 14(5):268

Lockstone C 1982 It's what the patient says it is. Nursing Mirror 154(7):ii

Mathew E et al 1980 Seizures following intracranial surgery: incidence in the first post-operative week. Canadian Journal of Neurological Sciences 7:285

Mathis M 1984 Personal needs of family members of critically ill patients with and without acute brain injury. Journal of Neurosurgical Nursing 16(1):36

Molter N C 1979 Needs of relatives of critically ill patients:a descriptive study. Heart and Lung 8(2):332

Smith J 1983 Nursing management of diabetes insipidus. Journal of Neurosurgical Nursing 13(6):313

Snyder M 1983 Relation of nursing activities to increases in intracranial pressure. Journal of Advanced Nursing 8(4):273

Stillwell S B 1984 Importance of visiting needs as perceived by family members of patients in the intensive care unit. Heart and Lung 13(3):238

Sutherland M 1982 Informed consent - the informed neurosurgical patient and family. Journal of Neurosurgical Nursing 14(3):195

Viahov D, Montgomery E, Tenney J H, Kahn-Eisenberg S 1984 Neurosurgical wound infections: methodologcal and clinical factors affecting calculation of infection rates. Journal of Neurosurgical Nursing 16(3):128

Watson C, Ross J, Ramsay M 1984 Identification of neurosurgical patients susceptible to pulmonary infection. Journal of Neurosurgical Nursing 16(3):123

Wilson-Barnett J 1981 Assessment of recovery with special reference to a study with post-operative cardiac patients. Journal of Advanced Nursing 6:435

Wilson-Barnett J, Fordham M 1985 Recovery from illness. John Wiley, Chichester.

12

Care of the patient with a spinal injury

Injury to the spinal column and/or cord is, for many patients, a devastating occurrence. It has been clearly demonstrated that good early nursing management of such a patient considerably improves the eventual outcome in terms of reducing neurological deficits.

MECHANISM OF INJURY

The principal mechanism of a spinal injury is the excessive movement in any direction of one or more of the following:

— extension
— flexion
— lateral flexion
— rotation
— vertical compression.

The common reasons for harmful excessive movements in an industrialised society are accidents at work, sporting accidents and road traffic accidents. A knowledge of the mechanics of an injury is necessary in order to understand the type of injury sustained and whether the injury is stable or unstable.

A spinal injury is classed as unstable when the posterior ligament complex (supraspinous and interspinous ligaments, ligamentum flavum and facetal joint capsules) is no longer intact. A stable injury is one which implies that the ligaments are intact thus preventing further cord damage and dislocation. Joint dislocation occurs when the articular surfaces are no longer in contact and subluxation is described as a partial dislocation.

IMMEDIATE MANAGEMENT FOLLOWING INJURY

Following an injury all patients who suffer loss of consciousness, facial injuries, pain around the spinal column or altered sensation or power to any limb should be suspected as having sustained a spinal injury. The spinal injury must be treated as unstable until proven otherwise. Incorrect handling could mean the difference between complete recovery and quadriplegia.

Further spinal cord damage must be prevented during removal of the patient from the scene of the accident and transport to hospital. The head, shoulders and pelvis must be moved as one. A minimum of four people, one of whom should be an experienced first aider, if possible, are required to lift the patient onto a stretcher. The experienced first aider should maintain the patient's head in a neutral position, along with a slight degree of traction when a cervical spine injury is suspected. All large and hard objects should be removed from the patient's pockets to reduce the risk of pressure sore development (see Fig. 12.10).

On arrival at hospital the patient should be placed on an emergency room trolley. Care is maintained to prevent movement of the spinal column. In a suspected cervical spine injury sandbags may be placed on either side of the patient's head. No pillow or similar object should be placed under the patient's head unless specially asked for by the medical practitioner.

This helps to maintain the spinal column in good alignment.

Removal of clothing must be carried out by nursing staff experienced in the handling of a patient with a suspected spinal injury. If conscious, the patient will be extremely anxious and therefore constant reassurance is required. This reassurance should also be extended to relatives and/or friends who may be in attendance at the hospital.

INVESTIGATION

On admission a full neurological examination is made by an experienced practitioner which is repeated at regular intervals during the first 48 hours.

Radiological examination

Radiographs

Antero–posterior and lateral radiographs are the common initial views requested. In a suspected cervical spine injury, views of the odontoid process and C7–T1 junction may also be requested. The former view is taken through the patient's open mouth; the latter requires traction on the upper limbs to achieve good visual appearance of the stated area.

Flexion and extension and/or oblique views of the cervical spine may also be requested, but this is usually following the initial investigative radiographs, as subjecting the new patient to this type of X-ray could increase his distress.

Computerised axial tomography (CT)

When available this procedure is useful in confirming subluxation of a joint, and also allows the medical practitioner to note the position of posterior bony fragments in burst fractures of the vertebral column. At present, CT scan is not used as an initial diagnostic aid.

CERVICAL SPINAL INJURY

This type of injury can be associated with trauma to the head and therefore can be easily overlooked, while priority is given to the head injury.

Whiplash injury

This is a common injury following a road traffic accident. On impact the head is violently thrown backwards, and then immediately catapulted forward as the person's trunk hits the back of the seat.

Whiplash injury is a form of extension injury to the cervical spine and surrounding tissues. Often there is no radiological evidence of bony injury, but an injury to the spinal cord can occur. This could be due to pressure from the damaged ligament flavum or the cervical laminae of the cord.

The patient will complain of pain in the neck region and movements of the head and neck will be limited. If momentary pressure on the spinal cord has taken place, he may also complain of paraesthesia of the limbs. In extreme cases quadriplegia may occur. If no damage to the spinal cord has occurred the patient will be fitted with a cervical collar made of a mouldable synthetic material to be worn for a 10–12 week period. The collar will assist pain relief but analgesia will also be required.

Wedge compression fracture of a vertebral body (Fig. 12.1)

This occurs when a severe flexion force, such as a heavy blow across the shoulders or neck, causes crushing of the cancellous bone of one or more vertebral bodies. The posterior ligaments remain intact therefore the fracture is stable.

The patient will present with a history of trauma followed by pain and immobility of the neck.

As the fracture is stable the treatment consists of support by a cervical collar for 2–3 months and analgesia for pain.

Burst fracture of a vertebral body (Fig. 12.2)

A vertical compression force transmitted along the line of the vertebral bodies while the cervical spine is straight will result in a burst fracture. The bodies of one or more vertebrae are burst open because the compressed intervertebral disc is driven forcibly into the vertebral body. Occasionally posterior fragments of the vertebral body may be driven backwards, damaging the spinal cord.

The patient will have a history of a fall from a height, in the erect postion, e.g. a fall off a ladder or a severe blow on the top of the head.

Pain and stiffness of the neck will be experienced. If a bony fragment has travelled backwards a neurological deficit will be apparent.

Provided there is no neurological deficit, external support by a well fitted cervical collar

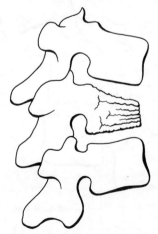

Fig. 12.1 Wedge compression fracture.

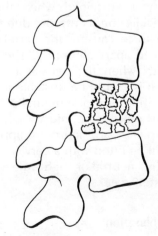

Fig. 12.2 Burst fracture.

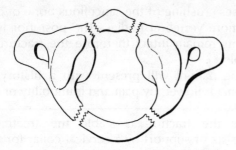

Fig. 12.3 Fracture of the arch of the atlas (viewed from above).

to relieve pain will suffice. Analgesia will be required for a temporary period following the injury.

Fracture of the atlas (Fig. 12.3)

This is sustained when a vertical force acting through the skull causes the occipital condyles to be forced onto the anterior and posterior arches of the atlas, causing the arches to fracture. Lateral displacement of the fragments occurs and the spinal cord is seldom injured.

The patient will give a history of a weight falling onto the head, followed by pain in the neck. Again, a cervical collar is worn for about 10–12 weeks to relieve pain and analgesia is provided.

Extension subluxation

This injury is sustained when the anterior longitudinal ligaments rupture due to a severe extension force causing the vertebral bodies to be forced apart anteriorly. The spine will only sublux when the neck is in extension, therefore it is said to be unstable in extension but stable in flexion or a neutral position. The spinal cord can escape injury.

If no spinal cord injury is apparent, the patient will be fitted with a cervical collar with the neck in a neutral or slightly flexed position for at least 10 weeks.

Flexion subluxation

This occurs more commonly in the lower part of the cervical column. There is a forward

displacement of one vertebra on another due to rupture of the posterior ligaments. The patient will have severe pain in the neck and be unwilling to move it. If osteoarthritic changes are present in the spine, the spinal canal may be narrowed and damage to the spinal cord by osteophytes could occur.

The subluxation is reduced by extending the cervical spine and the neck is held in extension by a well fitted collar for 10 weeks. Flexion and extension subluxation can recur following acute treatment. If this complication arises, surgical spinal fusion may be required.

Dislocation and fracture dislocation (Fig. 12.4)

This is a very unstable injury and is due to a flexion or flexion-rotation force to the spine. The articular surfaces of the vertebrae are forced out of contact causing an overriding of the articular processes. The articular processes become locked in the dislocated position. Spinal cord involvement, when it occurs, will be variable. If complete transection of the spinal cord occurs above the level of C4 this will result in death.

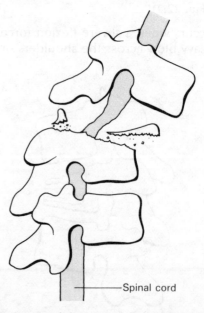

Fig. 12.4 Fracture dislocation of the vertebral column showing transection of the spinal cord. The fracture is of the vertebral body.

The patient presenting with this injury may give a history of diving into the shallow end of a swimming pool. Pain will be severe and the patient will be very unwilling to move his neck.

The extreme instability of this injury demands careful handling of the patient to prevent further displacement, which could cause or aggravate spinal cord involvement. Skull traction will be applied under local anaesthesia and the weights gradually increased (Fig. 12.5). Regular radiological examination of the spine will be performed until the over-riding articular processes have disengaged. It is important that close observation of the patient's neurological state is recorded during the period of heavy traction, as further damage to the spinal cord could occur. The articular processes are then reduced by gradual extension of the cervical spine with the use of a small firm pillow placed between the patient's shoulder blades. Once reduction

has occurred the traction is reduced thus allowing the articular surfaces to return to their pre-injured state. The patient can then be managed by a variety of methods such as:

1. *If cord involvement is absent* a Minerva plaster jacket can be applied 2–3 weeks following reduction of the dislocation. Once the plaster jacket is dry, the patient can be mobilised and may be allowed home (Fig. 12.6).

2. *Traction* is maintained for 6–10 weeks followed by the fitting of a well moulded cervical collar.

3. *A halo-thoracic or pelvic traction system* may be used. This consists of a metal ring (halo) around the head into which metal pins are attached. These pins are inserted at regular intervals around the patient's skull. Metal struts leave the halo on either side and pass down the side of the face to the shoulders. These struts are then attached to a moulded thoracic jacket or pins which have been inserted into the iliac crests. The jacket can be made of plaster or a mouldable synthetic material. The main disadvantage of this system is the weight and unwieldy nature of the apparatus.

4. *Surgical spinal fusion.* If the articular processes cannot be disengaged, open reduction followed by a spinal fusion is necessary.

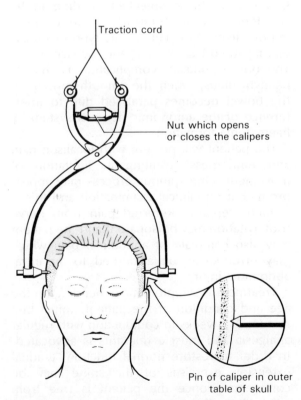

Fig. 12.5   Skull traction using cone calipers.

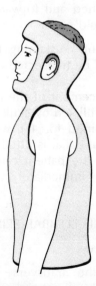

Fig. 12.6   Minerva weight.

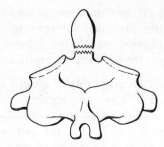

Fig. 12.7 Fracture of the odontoid process-posterior view of axis.

Fusion will also be used if the initial reduction is complicated by gradual displacement of the articular processes or fresh neurological signs develop. Early operative treatment by spinal fusion, following reduction of the dislocation is being utilised more frequently.

Fracture dislocation of the atlanto-axial joint

This injury can occur in two ways:

1. *Direct violence* to the neck causing a fracture of the odontoid process (Fig. 12.7). The odontoid process along with the atlas may be displaced in an anterior or posterior direction.

2. In *chronic inflammatory disease* such as rheumatoid arthritis the transverse ligament becomes softened and forward displacement of the atlas could occur.

In some patients sustaining this injury, the spinal cord will be transected which will result in death.

When displacement of the joint is present, reduction is achieved by skull traction, which is then maintained for 4–6 weeks, following which a cervical collar is fitted. If no displacement is noted the patient can be fitted with a cervical collar immediately.

THORACIC AND LUMBAR SPINE INJURY

Transverse process

Fractures to the transverse processes are caused mainly by direct violence such as a fall or a blow to the spine. They occur most often in the lumbar region. The patient will complain of localised pain and tenderness at the site of injury.

The main aims of treatment are to avoid adhesion formation and to disperse any haematoma. The fracture itself does not require any treatment. The aims are achieved through early mobilisation and adequate analgesia. The main potential complication involves the renal system, due to the proximity of the kidneys to the site of injury. The patient is admitted to hospital for 24–48 hours to observe urinary output and monitor for haematuria.

Wedge compression fractures of the vertebral body

These are sustained when a vertical compression force is directed onto the spinal column when the spine is held in a position of flexion, e.g. a fall from a height landing on the feet or buttocks or a heavy object and landing on the shoulders. The nurse must be aware of other injuries likely to occur in this type of injury, e.g. fractured base of skull and the calcaneum. The only significant complication is that of paralytic ileus, when the smooth muscle of the bowel becomes paralysed due to interference of the autonomic nervous system by haematoma formation.

The patient will present with localised pain and tenderness resulting in limitation of movement. One spinous process may appear prominent on clinical examination and this is termed stepping. Referred pain from nerve root irritation may be apparent and the patient may also complain of abdominal pain which may erroneously be attributed to an intra-abdominal injury.

Treatment is symptomatic depending on the age and condition of the patient. Initial bed rest for 1–3 weeks in conjunction with regular analgesia and muscle relaxants is advocated. In order to restore normal function, gradual extension exercises of the spine may be commenced once the patient is free from pain. Normally support for the spine is not

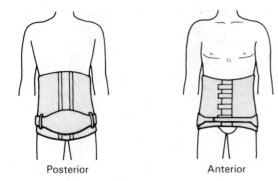

Posterior   Anterior

Fig. 12.8 Lumbosacral support.

needed but in cases of persistant pain a corset may be necessary (Fig. 12.8).

Burst fractures of the vertebral body (Fig. 12.2)

Burst fractures of the lumbar and thoracic spine are similar to wedge compression fractures except that the spine is held straight when the vertical compression force is applied. The vertebral body erupts into numerous fragments which are scattered in all directions; those displaced posteriorly may damage the spinal cord or cauda equina. Although the posterior ligament is intact these fractures can be classified as either stable or unstable depending on the position of the posterior fragments.

The patient will present with localised pain and tenderness on examination with limitation of movement and extensive bruising. If there is any cord involvement there may be loss of power and sensation of the lower limbs.

If the injury is stable, the treatment is as that for a wedge compression fracture. If unstable, the treatment is as that for a fracture dislocation, which is discussed later

FRACTURES OF THE SACRUM

This is a very uncommon injury and is usually stable. When unstable, some displacement may occur causing damage to the cauda equina or sacral plexus. The cause is by a direct blow or fall and the patient presents with pain, local tenderness and bruising. Analgesia is prescribed to relieve pain.

Fractures of the coccyx are even rarer. The presentation is similar to that for a sacral fracture and treatment is the same.

FRACTURE DISLOCATION OF THE SPINE

The most common site for this injury is at the thoraco-lumbar junction, between thoracic 12 and lumbar 1. A violent force causing flexion and rotation of the spine is responsible for this type of injury. The posterior ligament is almost always divided and the cord is usually damaged. This is a serious and unstable injury. At the thoraco-lumbar junction, the lower segments of the cord and cauda equina lie together, therefore injury could be partly cord and partly nerve root.

The signs and symptoms depend upon the degree of injury. If the patient has no cord involvement, these will be as previously outlined for wedge compression fractures. If the cord has been damaged, there will be varying degrees of motor and sensory loss, ranging from paraesthesia in the lower limbs to complete paraplegia with flaccid paralysis. 'Spinal shock' is the term given to complete suppression of autonomic function in the segments below the lesion. This results in a flaccid paralysis and can last from 48 hours to a few weeks. Bladder, bowel and visceral reflexes are also suppressed and overdistension of the bladder and bowel must be avoided. The only evidence to demonstrate that a lesion is incomplete is preservation or early return of voluntary motor power and sensation below the lesion.

Return of reflex activity without voluntary motor power improvement is diagnostic of complete transection of the cord and paralysis at this stage is normally spastic in nature. Continued neurological examination of the patient is important in the first 48 hours following injury in order to ascertain if the lesion is complete. Treatment, in terms of surgical intervention, can vary. If there is a chance of improvement, spinal decompression and internal fixation will be performed as soon as possible. If there is no cord involvement, conservative measures are employed. The patient is nursed flat with a pillow inserted at the lumbar region to maintain the neutral lordosis position. Confirmation of the reduction would be by X-ray examination. This process of healing can take 6–8 weeks.

NURSING MANAGEMENT

Ideally, a patient sustaining a transection of the spinal cord, with a neurological deficit, will be managed in a specialist spinal injuries unit. Nursing and paramedical staff within such units are experienced in the rehabilitation of such patients. Following admission and initial treatment of the injured patient, the nurse will receive the patient with either a cervical collar in position or skull traction in situ (or about to be set up) (Fig. 12.5, 12.9).

Nursing care of the patient experiencing different problems will now be discussed. Although each is dealt with separately for clarity, in practice the care often overlaps in many instances.

NURSING CARE OF THE PATIENT IN A CERVICAL COLLAR

The patient is unlikely to be fitted with the definitive collar immediately but will have a temporary collar in position. This collar is usually made from high density foam, Sorbo rubber or a similar material which is then covered with an absorbent material and secured with Velcro straps or a similar fastening (Fig. 12.9A). This form of collar can be used as a permanent collar when the patient does not require such rigid immobilisation or may be used as a night collar for sleeping. When a more rigid collar is required (Fig. 12.9B) this will be moulded 24–48 hours after the injury, by which time the patient will be more comfortable. This type of collar will be individually moulded by an experienced orthotist using one of the many synthetic

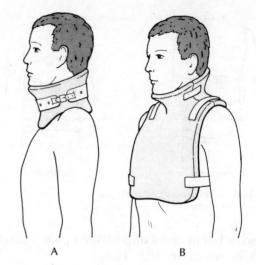

Fig. 12.9 Cervical collars.

materials which are available, e.g. Plastazote, Neofract, polythene or orthoplast.

Patient problems

Communicating

Pain following cervical spine injury can be severe and adequate analgesia must be administered, including, possibly, use of narcotics. Muscular spasm may also be a contributing factor and anti-spasmodic drugs, e.g. diazepam, are frequently prescribed in small regular doses. Some patients may realise the serious nature of their injury and correct information must be given at all times. The nurse must be approachable at all times to allow easy communicating to develop between the patient, relatives and herself. Patients who have sustained some neurological deficit must be helped to voice their fears and apprehensions regarding their recovery and rehabilitation.

Breathing

The more rigid cervical collar which extends down anteriorly and posteriorly over the rib cage may cause limited respiratory movements if fastened too tightly. Potential breathing problems could develop if the patient is unable to mobilise due to another injury.

Eating and drinking

Due to slight swelling around the neck and the presence of the cervical collar, difficulty in swallowing may be experienced by the patient. Mastication is restricted as the collar limits the range of normal mandibular movements. Introducing the patient to a softer diet is usually of benefit. As extension of the neck is reduced Flexi straws and spouted feeding cups may allow the act of drinking to be made easier for the patient.

Personal cleansing and dressing

The cervical collar is removed for a short time each day to allow personal hygiene to be carried out and the patient should be instructed in this before discharge. The skin should be inspected at regular intervals for signs of pressure or irritation. The common pressure points are the occiput, the chin and mandible region, the clavicular region and over the sternum. Skin irritation can be induced by some of the synthetic materials used to make the collar. Some patients have found it beneficial to wear a 'polo neck' of stockinette between the skin and the collar. The stockinette is cut to a length which will allow sufficient to be folded over the top and bottom of the collar. In male patients who do not have a beard, the skin must be kept in a clean shaven state as short beard growth will act as a skin irritant. Patients may find it more comfortable to inspect and wash the skin under the collar when lying in bed.

Regular mouth care should be instituted as the limited mandibular movements may cause food deposits to build up on the teeth and oral mucosa.

Due to the friction of the occiput against the collar the patient's hair can become very tangled and matted, if not brushed or combed at regular intervals during the day. Hair washing should be left until the patient feels comfortable and confident to tolerate this

procedure. As some collars are made of plastic type materials which are water resistant, the collar could be kept in position if the patient wished and the collar would require to be dried thoroughly before re-application. All clothing around the neck should be worn outside the collar otherwise the collar will not provide the support required.

Patients who have neurological complications such as paraesthesia or reduced muscle power to the upper limbs will require nursing intervention in some or all aspects of this activity of living. Intervention by a physiotherapist and occupational therapist will also be required to aid the patient's independence.

Mobilising

The patient is mobilised out of bed as soon as his condition permits. When a patient's neck is encased in a collar all neck movements are reduced therefore the head and trunk are moved as one. If a neurological deficit has occurred, active and passive limb movements will be instituted by the physiotherapist and the patient will be instructed to perform these activities at regular times throughout the day. Physiotherapy will continue following discharge of the patient with a neurological deficit and on all patients after removal of the collar.

Expressing sexuality

Some patients may feel that the presence of the collar is an erosion of their normal body image. Reassurance by staff and relatives will alleviate this apprehension. Some patients may welcome the suggestion of individualising their collar with the addition of a scarf or cravat.

Working and playing

The occupational therapist may be asked to help the patient in this activity of living. The nurse will use her educational skills to help the patient adapt to the temporary or permanent changes to his working and social environment. If a patient has a manual job he should refrain from work until the medical practitioner states he is fit to return. This may prove to be financially difficult for the patient and referral to a medical social worker may be necessary. A patient who has a sedentary job may be allowed to return to work while still wearing his cervical collar provided he has the approval of the medical staff.

Sleeping

Altered sleeping patterns are extremely common in the first few days following injury. This can be due to the presence of the collar or the discomfort felt by the patient. Patients who have been fitted with a rigid collar may be given a soft collar to wear at night. Night sedation should only be used as a last resort.

Patient in skull traction (Fig. 12.5)

Skull traction is a form of skeletal traction used to correct the alignment of an injured cervical spine. The insertion of the pins of the skull calipers into the outer table of the skull can allow 15–18 kg to be applied to create a strong traction. The skull calipers (ice tong, Blackburn or similar) are introduced into the skull slightly above and behind the patient's ears. All caliper designs have pin guards incorporated to prevent penetration of the inner table of the skull which could lead to cerebral complications. Following insertion of the calipers under a local anaesthetic, the pin sites will be covered with a pin-hole dressing. The patient will then have the traction weight applied and be transferred onto a bed. The patient will be nursed on a selected specialist bed:

— ordinary hospital bed with cervical traction extension unit
— cardiac bed with cervical traction extension unit
— wedge turning frame (Stryker frame)
— Egerton Stoke-Mandeville turning bed
— circo-electric bed.

Pillows are not usually placed under the patient's head unless a non-neutral position is desired. A neck roll should be utilised as this will give support to the natural curve of the cervical spine. The neck roll is made from absorbent material which is rolled into a sausage shape approximately 15–18 cm in length and 8–10 cm in diameter. Due to the appearance of the skull calipers the nurse should explain the nature of the apparatus to the patient and relatives.

NURSING CARE OF THE PATIENT WITH SKULL TRACTION IN A WEDGE TURNING FRAME (STRYKER FRAME)

Maintaining a safe environment

The patient will be dependent on the nurse for this activity of living. He must lie recumbent on a Stryker frame to maintain the traction on the cervical spine. The patient may fear that he will fall out of the narrow frame or that the skull calipers may fall out of the skull.

The patient with minimal or no neurological deficit may be nursed on a cardiac bed. As this bed is similar to an ordinary bed the fears already outlined will be alleviated. In view of the potential problem of pin tract infection, the dressings over the pin sites should be changed at regular intervals, e.g. every 2nd or 3rd day unless any sign of infection is noted.

Communicating

As the patient is unable to move his head and trunk, eye to eye contact should be initiated prior to verbal communication. Relatives and friends should also be told this. As a result of the patient's anxiety, information given to him may not be fully comprehended. The nurse may need to reinforce the reasons for the treatment used and also the extent of the injury. The appearance of the skull calipers and the bed or frame could make the patient feel stigmatised by staff, relatives or friends who are not familiar with the equipment or find it difficult to accept the patient's appearance.

Breathing

When a neurological deficit has been sustained following injury there is a potential problem of breathing difficulties due to the possible interference of the nerve supply to the muscles of respiration. At regular intervals the nurse must observe the rate, rhythm and depth of the patient's respirations along with recordings of vital capacity. Some patients may require the support of artificial ventilation. Breathing difficulties can occur due to the development of a chest infection, as a result of the patient's position and immobility. When being nursed on a Stryker frame patients may find it easier to expectorate while lying prone.

Regular blood pressure recordings should be commenced on admission. Hypotension, in the absence of other injury, is suggestive of spinal shock (see p. 197).

Eating and drinking

Paralytic ileus is a common problem following spinal injury. The pins of the skull calipers are inserted through the temporal muscle of the skull therefore full mandibular movements may cause discomfort to the patient. The patient's diet may require alteration to reduce this problem.

Eliminating

The patient with no neurological deficits may be at risk of urinary retention, urinary tract infections and constipation. The nurse must use all her previous knowledge to reduce the development of any of these problems. Where it is necessary to use a urethral catheter it is preferred that a catheter size of 12 or 14 FG with a 5 ml balloon be used. This greatly reduces trauma to the urethra, urethral sphincters and bladder mucosa.

In the patient with a neurological deficit, eliminating constitutes major problems. Re-education of the patient is required and further elaboration on this can be found in the section on paraplegia.

Personal cleansing and dressing

Infection of the oral mucosa and dental caries can be a problem. If the patient is on a Stryker frame mouth hygiene is best carried out with the patient lying prone. Clothing will need to be able to be opened and fastened down the centre, back and across both shoulders. Studs of Velcro are very suitable for this purpose as they are smooth and cause little pressure on the patient's skin. The majority of relatives are usually willing to adapt some of the patient's own clothing in this manner.

Hair washing with water, if permitted, can be performed when the patient is nursed on a Stryker frame. Alternatively, the use of dry shampoos can be of benefit.

Controlling body temperature

Patients with spinal shock can present with a hyperpyrexia. The nurse will help the patient maintain his body temperature within the normal range.

Mobilising

Due to the complete immobility of the patient who has become quadriplegic or suffered some neurological deficit, problems of muscle wasting and joint stiffness will arise. Intervention by the physiotherapist will be required but the nurse will assist in maintaining a constant regular programme. Placing the limbs in a neutral position (or as near as possible) will lessen the problem of foot drop and joint contractures. Hand splints may be used to prevent joint contractures of the smaller, more delicate joints in the wrists and fingers.

Deep vein thrombosis and pulmonary embolism are also potential problems which will be alleviated with the use of anti-embolism stockings and passive physiotherapy.

Working and playing

Potential problems of boredom can be alleviated by ensuring access to radio, television and newspapers. When the patient is nursed on a Stryker frame he will require a mirror attachment to increase his range of vision. The floor and ceiling of a ward are not the best form of visual entertainment. Prism glasses are of benefit to allow the patient to read while lying supine. The occupational therapist can also be involved in providing activities. Computers are now also being utilised to provide another interest.

The social worker may need to give the patient advice on assistance with financial and/or social problems.

The patient who has a neurological deficit will require a great deal of support from all staff and relatives. It is better to concentrate on what the patient is able to do for himself rather than what they are not able to do.

Expressing sexuality

Patients will have potential problems with feelings of erosion of their body image due to the skull calipers and the position they have to adopt. Self-esteem will be reduced as the patient is dependent on the nursing staff for his personal appearance. Care appropriate to the patient's gender and use of cosmetics, perfume or after shave will be of benefit.

Patients with a neurological deficit may have anxieties about their future sex life and this is discussed in the section on paraplegia.

Sleeping

The abnormal position, bed and apparatus in use with the patient may produce altered sleeping patterns. Night is commonly a time when the patient's anxieties are more pronounced. The nurse should allow the patient to voice all fears, anxieties and ask any questions.

As sleeping patterns will be disturbed as a result of the turning regime, rest periods should be incorporated throughout the 24 hours of each day. Night sedation should only be given as a last resort.

Dying

Patients who have a neurological deficit may have fears of dying which may or may not be expressed. Some patients fear sleep as they think that they may stop breathing while asleep. Other patients may wish to be dead as they cannot face up to the future with the disability they have. It is only with constant support and reassurance that these fears and anxieties can be dealt with.

NURSING CARE OF THE PATIENT WITH A THORACIC OR LUMBAR SPINE INJURY

Communicating

Regular analgesia is needed and initially intramuscular preparations may be required but these can quickly be substituted for oral preparations. A muscle relaxant, e.g. diazepam, may also be given as a regular prescription, in conjunction with analgesic drugs to ease the muscle spasm related to bony injuries.

Eating and drinking

The first few days following injury may present a problem for the patient regarding eating and drinking. The most comfortable position is likely to be one of recumbency, therefore the patient may require assistance at meal times. Continuous close observation for early signs of a developing paralytic ileus, should be made.

Eliminating

Confinement to bed makes eliminating difficult. The nurse should afford the patient privacy in order to reduce his embarrassment. Constipation, due to decreased mobility, should always be prevented. An adequate fluid intake of 2–3 litres daily to decrease the incidence of urinary tract infection is necessary.

Mobilising

Mobilisation is severely restricted following injury, due to pain at the fracture site. Assistance will be needed with movement and lifting in the first few days.

Physiotherapists will assist with passive and active exercises during the period of bed-rest. Following this, the patient will commence gradual mobilisation which will vary in duration from patient to patient. Constant reassurance is required until full mobility is achieved.

NURSING CARE OF THE PATIENT WITH A FRACTURE DISLOCATION OF THE THORACO-LUMBAR JUNCTION

The patient without any neurological deficit will be nursed for 6–8 weeks on a wedge turning frame. The frame should be turned 4 hourly to check the patient's pressure areas. Those patients with normal power and sensation will know when there is excessive pressure on their skin and will ask to be turned more often. The psychological and nursing care of this patient will follow a similar pattern to the one for traumatic paraplegia (see below). These patients should be able to void urine without difficulty but may be prone to constipation.

When there is X-ray evidence of bony healing the patient will be transferred to an ordinary bed to be nursed flat with one pillow. Mobilisation commences slowly. The patient may feel dizzy when sitting upright for the first time and may suffer from supine hypotension. Once the patient starts to mobilise he is supplied with a rigid spinal support to be worn at all times. Ideally, it should be worn over a tee shirt or stockinette vest in order to protect the skin. The physiotherapist will assess what aids the patient needs for mobilising and by the time he is discharged he should be independently mobile. The spinal support should be worn for a further 4–6 weeks and the patient will be reviewed every 2 weeks. Once the spinal support has been removed, physiotherapy is continued to achieve full mobility of the spine.

CARE OF THE PATIENT WITH TRAUMATIC PARAPLEGIA

Maintaining a safe environment

The traumatically paraplegic patient requires constant reassurance from the moment he arrives in the ward. It is essential for the nurse to gain the patient's confidence. Care must be taken when transferring the patient from the trolley to the turning frame, as pain and discomfort are common. The transfer is super-

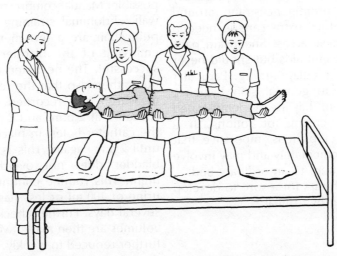

Fig. 12.10 Positioning of lifters when lifting a patient with a suspected cervical spine injury. Note also position of pillows when using an ordinary hospital bed or an Egerton Stoke Mandeville turning bed.

vised by the most senior nurse and at least four lifters are needed (Fig. 12.10).

Once the transfer is complete the nurse should spend some time with the patient explaining what is happening and how the turning frame operates and its purpose. It is at this stage that the patient will start to ask questions. These must be answered truthfully and in language that the patient understands. The nurse's role is to help the patient and his relatives to accept his condition and to come to terms with his paraplegia.

Personal cleansing and dressing

Prevention of pressure sores is of prime importance and all paraplegic patients should be nursed in a wedge turning frame or a similar device. This enables the patient's position to be changed without undue discomfort. A generalised, decreased resistance to infection and compromised circulation combine to increase the risk of pressure sore formation in the paraplegic patient. The patient's position is altered every 2 hours, day and night. While the patient is still on bedrest, the nurse is responsible for ensuring that he is turned. However, once the patient is in his wheelchair he has to accept responsibility for relieving his own pressure areas.

Pressure sores, when they develop, usually occur over bony prominences and around moist areas, therefore extra care is needed when observing these areas. Sheepskin pads and blankets are useful aids but should never be substituted for regular turning. Particular attention is given to general skin hygiene; although no benefit has been demostrated from the use of creams or lotions. If a pressure sore develops it is imperative that this is dealt with immediately and may involve transferring the patient to an ordinary bed.

It can take only hours for a sore to develop but it can take months to heal.

Eliminating

Any spinal cord lesion has the ability to impair the nervous supply to the bladder and/or bowel. As the pressure within the expanding bladder increases, the sphincter will be forced open and urine will be allowed to escape. Once the pressure falls, the sphincter closes again thus retaining a large volume within the bladder. This stagnated residual urine is a medium for infection.

On admission, an indwelling catheter is inserted and left on continuous drainage until there is evidence that the period of spinal shock has passed and that reflex action has returned. This will be obvious when the flaccid paralysis has become spastic and there are definite reflexes present. An attempt is now made to 'bladder train' the patient. A programme might include the following regime: the catheter is removed from the bladder at 2 a.m. and in the case of a male patient an external sheath is placed over the glans penis and a catheter bag is attached. For female patients, it is necessary to offer them a bedpan every 2 hours instead. If this is unsuccessful and the patient is being incontinent, the frequency of giving bedpans must be increased.

At 8 a.m. the patient is asked to empty his bladder. This can be achieved in many ways. A certain amount of urine will be passed spontaneously due to reflex action, but it is in the patient's interest to have as small a residual as possible. Manual compression of the abdominal wall, abdominal straining and pulling of the pubic hair are a few methods of aiding the emptying of the bladder which have been successful. The next step is to pass an in and out catheter so that the residual urine can be measured and recorded. This procedure is repeated at 2 p.m. and 8 p.m., at which time the catheter is left in place and not removed until 2 a.m. again. This is to ensure that the bladder does not overdistend during the night. This routine continues until a residual urine of 100 ml or less has been obtained for several days. Further checks on residual urine volumes are then made twice weekly and then further reduced to weekly. This can be discontinued once it is evident that the patient's residual urine remains low. The patient should be encouraged to maintain a good fluid intake and to drink 3–4 litres daily.

Urine samples are sent to the bacteriology laboratory each week for culture. It is not always possible to avoid urinary infections and urinary antiseptics and antibiotics may be needed. Once discharged, an intravenous pyelogram is performed every 6 months as a diagnostic aid to highlight impending urinary complications.

During the period of bladder training, additional problems with skin care can arise. When applying an external sheath, adhesive tape is needed and this can excoriate the skin. In female patients, skin breakdown can be caused by a poorly placed or roughly removed bedpan. The patient should not be allowed to remain on the bedpan for a prolonged period of time.

Some advocate surgical intervention with ileal conduit being the procedure of choice. There is no restriction in diet and fluid inake following this and the patient may feel more socially acceptable.

Efforts should be made to establish a 'normal' bowel pattern as soon as possible. Initially, an aperient would be given in the evening followed by 2 suppositories after breakfast the following morning. This regime continues with aperients on alternate evenings and suppositories every other day. It may take weeks for the patient's bowels to function 'normally'. Diet must also be considered and adequate roughage should be included. Each patient will settle to his own pattern and should aim to empty his bowels just after breakfast. This will make him more socially acceptable and avoid accidents.

Communicating

Some paraplegic patients may complain of pain below the level of their lesion. They find it difficult to explain this as they know they have no sensation of pain in that area. This can be severe and is thought to be under psychological control. Treatment should be aimed at allaying anxiety and prescribing mild sedatives.

Eating and drinking

Initially, the patient will need to be assisted with meals but as he settles into the routine of the turning frame he will establish the most comfortable position to eat in. This is usually prone, as the patient can see what is on his plate and will find it easier for swallowing and digestion.

There are many accessories for the turning frame, the most important being a mirror which enables the patient to see around the room.

Mobilising

Physiotherapy commences as soon as the patient is admitted. During the acute phase, when the patient is on bed-rest, deep breathing exercises will be taught to help prevent chest infections. Passive exercises to all limbs will be carried out several times daily to avoid muscle contraction. More time will be spent by the physiotherapist in exercising and developing the muscles of the arms. The paraplegic patient will need to depend on his arms for lifting himself from his chair into his bed or car.

Spasm is a convulsive, involuntary muscular contraction which occurs after spinal shock. Spasm occurs as a result of loss of influence from the higher centres on the affected segment of the cord. When the muscle spasm is severe, shortening of the muscles and ligaments occurs resulting in contractures. All care must be taken to prevent such deformities and this begins with gentle passive exercises to the paralysed limbs from the time of admission.

Spasm in the paralysed patient is uncontrollable and often exaggerated. Irritations to the body can cause spasm so these must be avoided, e.g. pressure on the skin, infection, constipation, anxiety and ill fitting clothes. It would appear that this is the body's way of compensating for the sensory loss. In some instances the spasm may be excessive and difficult for the patient to cope with. There are various treatments prescribed which may be of help. Certain drugs can be used to depress activity in the reflex arc. Tendons, muscles and nerves can be surgically divided in order to prevent spasm.

Working and playing

It is not easy for a paraplegic patient to balance in the sitting position after 8 weeks lying flat, so a lot of effort must go into his rehabilitation. This is the time when the physiotherapist, occupational therapist and social worker are more involved. The patient must learn to transfer from bed to chair, from chair to toilet, into the bath and also in and out of his car. All these procedures are new to him and will take time to master. Once the patient is established in his wheelchair, the importance of weight relief must be impressed upon him. This entails the patient lifting himself clear of the chair every 30–60 minutes. A mirror may be used by the patient so that he can perform self-examination of his pressure areas.

Many patients benefit from competing with each other in the gymnasium and there are now many sports in which they can participate.

It is now that the patient may attempt to walk with calipers. The success of this depends on the level of the lesion and the determination of the patient. It must be remembered that not all patients will be able to master calipers. The patient will require a lot of emotional support from his family and friends.

The occupational therapist will play an important role in the rehabilitation programme. She must teach him to dress himself and to care for himself.

In the early stages when the patient is still on bed-rest, the social worker should be involved in his care in order to commence work on any alterations which may be required in his home. There are many adjustments which may have to be made to the patient's home and in some instances, re-housing may be necessary. Prior to discharge some home visits will be made to ensure that any potential problems are dealt with. The social worker will also make the patient aware of any financial assistance he may be entitled to and of facilities available in the community for the disabled. Some are able to return to their previous employment, for others, the disablement resettlement officer is available to discuss future alternative options.

Expressing sexuality

This is a very serious problem which is often neglected. At some point in the patient's rehabilitation programme he may approach the subject of his future sex life. Some patients may never raise the subject so it is the place of the nurse who is experienced in dealing with paraplegic patients to broach the subject. It is usually found that the patient is more worried about not being able to satisfy his partner sexually, rather than about his own sexual pleasure and it is this that can lead to misunderstandings.

Preparation of the body for sexual intercourse is controlled by the forebrain which can be stimulated by smell, sight, touch, fantasy or just by closeness of a member of the opposite sex. Impulses are then sent, via the spinal cord, to the genital area where erection of the penis or clitoris occurs — 'psychogenic erection'. Complete transection of the spinal cord at any level will obviously prevent psychogenic erection. Once the spinal shock has passed, erection may be made possible by reflex action, from stimulation of the penis. The erection can only be sustained for as long as the stimulation occurs. If the spinal lesion is at the sacral level or if the sacral nerve fibres are damaged then even reflex erection is impossible.

Ejaculation is nearly always inhibited in paraplegic patients as ejaculation is controlled by nerve tissue at the level of the lumbar spine. Due to the changes in body temperature around the testicles the production of sperm deteriorates. Artificial insemination can be attempted but, due to the low sperm count, is often unsuccessful.

Once female paraplegic patients have recommenced a normal menstrual cycle there is no change in their fertility from the pre-injury phase. There is no reason why they should not bear children but extra care in pregnancy should be taken to avoid urinary tract infections and pressure sores. There are no greater risks involved in labour or delivery of the child. Forceps delivery may be indicated due to the patient's inability to bear down in the second stage. Advice on contraception should be given to all females on discharge.

Loss of sensation below the level of the spinal lesion will greatly impair sexual sensation and orgasm. Pleasure is often attained by the fact that their partner has been satisfied. In some, touching of the body above the level of the lesion may cause erotic sensations.

BIBLIOGRAPHY

Adam J C 1972 Outline of fractures. Churchill Livingstone, Edinburgh
Crockard H A 1981 Spinal injuries. In: Odling-Smee W, Crockard A (eds) Trauma care. Academic Press, London
Mills, J O M 1981 The use of X-rays in trauma In: Odling-Smee W, Crockard A (eds) Trauma care. Academic Press, London
Shepherd A M, Blannin J P, Smart M E 1980 In: Mandestam D (ed) Incontinence and its management. Croom Helm, London

SUGGESTED READING

Betts-Symonds G W 1984 Fracture: care and management for students. Macmillan, London
Guttman L 1973 Spinal cord injuries: comprehensive management and research. Blackwell, London
Fallon B 1975 So you're paralysed. Spinal Injuries Association, London
Spinal Injuries Association 1980 People with spinal injuries: treatment and care. SIA, London
Stewart W F R 1979 The sexual side of handicap. Woodhead-Faulkner, Cambridge

13

Spinal surgery — pre-operative and postoperative care

In relation to intracranial surgery, spinal surgery is sometimes seen as 'minor' or 'routine'. For the hospital staff it may not have the same glamour or excitement, and the nursing care can appear to reach an acceptable standard with less specific knowledge and skills. Even the patient and his family may view this type of surgery differently from intracranial surgery with its attendant risks and potential consequences. However, just as the vast majority of 'intracranial' patients and their families display different ways of coping and coming to terms with the diagnosis and the need for surgery, patients due to undergo spinal surgery and their relatives also display a wide variety of feelings. As an example, those patients whose surgery is being carried out for a spinal tumour may respond in a way similar to those whose surgery is to the brain. Both are faced with a serious situation which threatens their normal pattern of living and calls for long-term adjustment. Alternatively, families of patients undergoing surgery for prolapsed lumbar disc may have high expectations and consider the operation to be routine, hoping for an end to their period of adjustment and a return to their normal way of life. Although the physical care of these patients may itself be very similar, unless these profound differences are acknowledged while planning their care, many of their needs may be neglected.

As with intracranial, and indeed any other surgery, the preparation begins as soon as the patient is admitted to the ward. Again it is directed at the whole family unit and can be divided into three stages: the initial general care, the more specific period of preparation and the day of surgery. It takes account of his physical needs, his psychological needs and his spiritual, cultural and family needs. Although there are many facets to his care it is solely the preparatory care that is covered in this chapter. As many aspects have already been considered in some detail in Chapter 6 they will only be mentioned briefly here. However they are as relevant to patients undergoing spinal surgery as they are to patients undergoing intracranial surgery.

COMMON SPINAL SURGICAL PROCEDURES

Laminectomy

This involves the removal of a half or a whole lamina sometimes including the spinous process. This may be performed at more than one level and more commonly in the lumbar and cervical regions. A cervical laminectomy is used in preference to an anterior approach when there is extensive disease and where several levels are involved but is contra-indicated if there is any degree of instability, as this would be increased postoperatively.

Fenestration

This procedure can be used in cases of prolapsed lumbar disc when there is little sign of other degenerative changes, for example in a younger patient. An opening is formed in the ligamentum flavum and the disc fragments can then be removed.

Anterior cervical approach

The techniques that can be performed using an anterior cervical approach result in the fusion of the affected levels of vertebrae and so not only decompress the spinal cord but also reduce the subsequent radicular pain. The disc alone can be removed and then fusion occurs; bony if a bone graft is used,

otherwise fibrous in nature. The posterior osteophytes can be removed with the disc although this also involves the removal of part of the bodies of the adjoining vertebrae. A larger bone graft is used in this procedure, the Cloward's procedure, and again bony fusion occurs. This procedure is not usually performed when more than two levels are involved.

Costotransversectomy

This has replaced the laminectomy as the treatment of choice for anteriorly placed lesions in the thoracic spine. With the spinal cord already displaced backwards by the position of the lesion, posterior decompression, as produced by laminectomy, has shown to have the attendant risk of leaving the patient paraplegic. The more successful costo-transversectomy involves a lateral approach which prevents further backward displacement. Access is gained to the lesion by the excision of the transverse process of the vertebra and a part of the adjoining rib.

GENERAL PRE-OPERATIVE CARE

General pre-operative care consists of the development of a trusting and confident relationship between the family and the hospital staff so that the patient feels as safe as possible during his stay and so that anxiety about the forthcoming operation can be used positively to encourage a good postoperative recovery. This relationship develops, not automatically, but as the staff demonstrate that they are competent, kind and approachable, and that they are reasonable and flexible in their approach to care.

In each case the nurse must understand what the medical staff expect the patient to gain from surgery, not only so she can appreciate any discrepancies between that and the patient's own perceptions, but also so that her nursing care and the information and advice she gives is appropriate. This understanding is fundamental in determining the philosophy or general aim behind the care of the patient and without it the care can only be superficial.

'Spinal' patients can be classified in two ways and, although each patient is obviously individual, these may be helpful in planning the nursing direction. Firstly they can be divided into those who have a life-threatening condition and those who do not. This obviously leads to profound differences in response and expectations and is the most basic consideration in their care. At the same time they can be divided according to the expectations of surgery. The first category includes those patients for whom surgery may bring to an end a period of personal and family adjustment, or at least reduce the degree of adjustment required. The second includes those patients for whom surgery may reduce the need for further adjustment although the existing level will probably remain, and the third, those for whom the period of adjustment is indefinite and the degree likely to increase. So whereas all brain pathology is considered to be extremely serious and the variation is generally in people's methods of coping, the perceived implications of spinal pathology and surgery are a great deal more diverse.

Chronic pain and progressive disability are common features in the presentation of spinal pathology and a practical understanding of these and their effects on personal and family life is important in the attempt to understand the patient's feelings towards surgery. Chronic pain has been described as 'a situation rather than an event' (Twycross 1979). It becomes the dominating feature of the patient's existence and disrupts many aspects of his life. The related feelings of anxiety, depression and irritability alter the patient's outlook and often lead to tension within his family and other relationships. The disability consequent to his pain or other neurological dysfunction may force him to relinquish some of his normal responsibilities within his family and his employment. There is a commonly assumed association between a 'bad back' and the shirking of responsibilities and if the patient has been confronted by this attitude or has sensed this feeling in others his emotional state will be further affected. Many of the people with a longstanding history of back pain have already undergone a variety of conservative treatments and they have found no lasting relief. Now they face surgery, often considered the last resort, but once more with no guarantee of success.

Pain affects every aspect of a person's general condition and his nursing care can be extremely demanding. It is important that the nurse accepts each patient's pain as he describes it and understands its consequences in relation to his behaviour and his pre-operative preparation. If he always knows exactly the time of his next dose of analgesia surely this is the normal response of a person experiencing pain. If he is impatient with the strict regime then surely this is also understandable. His general manner may demonstrate a lack of tolerance. His concentration and memory for new information may be affected and difficult explanations may receive impatient responses. His appetite may be poor, his normal sleeping pattern may be altered and his general wellbeing affected. If, through conversation with both the patient and his family, a greater understanding of his premorbid personality and outlook, and the effect of his condition on himself and his family can be gained, this can provide a good basis for individualised and appropriate care.

Progressive disability affects the patient and his family in a variety of ways depending not only on the nature, extent and rate of progression of the disability but again on the long-term implications of the patient's condition. The disability may be relatively minor and restrict the patient only slightly in his daily activities. Alternatively he may be obviously disabled, for example, reliant on a wheelchair for his mobility. This can affect not only his ability to maintain his independence safely, but also have a great influence on the lifestyle of his family. As well as practical and emotional difficulties directly related to the patient's condition, the stigma that is still attached to physical handicap within our society can also affect the patient's relationships outside of the family and his own family self-image. There may be financial consequences of the patient's disability and there may be a change in the whole system of roles and responsibilities within the family, in itself of very great concern to them. Whatever the degree of disability, the patient and his family's ability to cope with it is important. An understanding of this and of their expectations of his prognosis will assist in the nurse's understanding of their feelings towards surgery and will provide a sound foundation on which to base the patient's care.

The control of anxiety is another important factor in pre-operative care. The degree of anxiety displayed by the patient is not necessarily related to the severity of his condition and prognosis; it is individual and has many component factors. However, patients who display a moderate degree of anxiety at this time have been shown to make a better postoperative recovery than those who display either high or low levels (Janis 1981), so the moderation of anxiety is the aim of care. The patient and his family must be convinced of both the credibility of the staff and of a genuine concern for their wellbeing. Being so they will place more value on the teaching, advice and information offered and feel more able to discuss their feelings. Both, but in particular the patient, need realistic explanation and description of what surgery involves so that the related discomfort may not be totally unexpected. The major stressors that are causing the anxiety response for example, the diagnosis, the operation and the uncertainty of the patient's prognosis, cannot be removed. However many of the attendant stressors can be reduced if they are identified, and studies have described many common examples encompassing all aspects of care. Hayward (1981) found that 70% of patients were concerned about one or more aspects of general anaesthesia, the older ones remembering frightening experiences of gas anaesthetics. 60% were unhappy about the depersonalisation, loneliness and acute anxiety produced by the ritual nature of the preparations immediately prior to surgery and 35%

were surprised by the severity of postoperative pain. General uncertainties about the roles of 'patient', 'relative' or 'visitor' are anxiety-producing as is the apparent isolation of the family from the patient, and a lack of understanding of his condition. To identify factors that are producing anxiety in individual patients or families, they must feel able to express their feelings. 'Accepting' rather than 'comforting' responses are helpful as in the example where the patient expresses his concern over the forthcoming operation. The 'accepting' response 'Is there anything you would like me to do/explain?' may help to identify his needs rather than the 'comforting' but dismissive 'I'm sure it'll be all right'. With thoughtful nursing care the moderation of anxiety becomes a more realistic goal; with only superficial nursing care it remains extremely difficult, if not impossible, to achieve.

The care of the family is extremely important. It should be remembered that they have experienced the effects of the patient's condition for as long as he has and they will influence his progress when he returns home. Some families require very little care other than courtesy and simple explanations, but others, perhaps where the patient's conditions has more serious long-term consequences, need a great deal more time and support. Families are usually able to identify their own needs and if they feel able to express those needs to the nursing staff and believe that the nursing staff can help them, the staff are in a position to respond to them. This confident and helpful environment, then, is one which is essential for the individual care of each family.

Physical preparation

Eating and drinking

The patient's nutritional health is important as this affects his ability to tolerate the period of catabolism consequent to surgery. This may last several days and, while the value of a high calorie-high protein diet during this period has not been agreed (Behrends 1982, Mogh-issi & Boore 1983), the value of a good pre-operative nutritional state has been accepted (Behrends 1982, Stotts 1982). The patient in poor nutritional health is more likely to experi-ence a delay in wound healing and has an increased risk of wound and other infections. Because of the relatively meagre blood supply to the centre of the back, wound infections are slow to resolve even in the healthy person. In the less well nourished person, resolution and subsequent healing take even longer. The patient with bladder dysfunction who has a degree of retention already has an increased risk of urinary tract infection. If he requires a urinary catheter postoperatively, even for a limited time, this is a further risk and if his nutritional state is poor the risk is even greater.

Signs and symptoms that may influence the patient's nutritional state include any motor or sensory dysfunction that prevents preparation and consumption of an adequate diet. The psychological consequences of the patient's condition may lead to a reduction in appetite or in the nutritional content of the food selected. Once in the hospital the situation may continue, as the patient who requires help at mealtimes may prefer to eat less rather than to monopolise the time of the busy nurse. He may be finding difficulty in coming to terms with being dependent, or feel embarrassed at needing help, and so may attempt to limit the duration of time that he is so obviously exhibi-ting and being faced with his disabilities. He may simply be in pain and benefit from the thoughtful administration of analgesia half an hour prior to some, if not all, of his meals. However factors unrelated to the patient's neurological pathology may also lead to poor nutritional health and the nutritional status and dietary intake of all the patients should receive attention.

Sleeping

A balance of sleep, rest and activity is essential to the wellbeing of the patient as it is to all people (Bruya 1981). Each of these can be

difficult to ensure within the constraints of the hospital and of the patient's situation and a balance of all three almost always remains an ideal rather than a reality. Appreciation of this problem, however, and of the mental and physical discomfort that results from an imbalance may help in the more sympathetic care of the patient and consequently in his preparation for surgery. For many patients this may not be a problem only associated with hospital admission, but a longstanding situ-ation resulting from their symptoms, their anxiety and their chronic pain.

Maintaining a safe environment

The comfort, safety and wellbeing of the patient are extremely important aspects of his preparatory care as they are measures by which he and his relatives assess the quality of care. Bouman (1984) found that this was the greatest emotional need of the family and obvious attention to these aspects helps to convey concern for the patient and helps to develop their trust and confidence in the staff prior to the operation and the more acute nursing care that it entails.

SPECIFIC PRE-OPERATIVE PREPARATION

When the investigations are complete and surgical intervention is confirmed as the appropriate course of action, the more specific preparation can begin. Some patients, for example those with a herniated lumbar disc, have been admitted with a view to surgery and have already accepted the need for it, although they may remain extremely anxious. Others, for example with a spinal cord tumour, may have been admitted 'for investi-gations' and they may be less well prepared for the idea of surgery. Their families may need more time to come to terms with the diagnosis and its immediate implications, and the starting of this more active stage of preparation requires sensitive timing. The surgical staff may now have more definite expectations of surgery, for example they may consider that a significant improvement is possible, or alternatively, that surgery will be essentially diagnostic and performed so that the patient's prognosis may be better understood. The nursing staff must be aware of these developments so that their care remains appropriate, and obviously the patients and their relatives also need up-to-date information from the surgical staff.

This stage still involves the giving of information, support and advice, but now also concerns more detailed aspects of pre- and postoperative routines. Teaching of respiratory and limb exercises by the physiotherapist is important and these can be reinforced by the nursing staff. A theatre or recovery nurse may visit the patient to explain those aspects of his surgical experience in greater depth and to identify the more individual priorities of his care in the theatre/recovery area. The relationship between the ward staff and the family has ideally developed so that anxieties can be expressed and discussed. Misconceptions can be corrected and again, realistic expectations can be reinforced.

To a certain extent the physical care of all patients undergoing surgery is similar and explanations can be given to each patient to the extent that he finds satisfactory. Similarly the physical care of the 'spinal' patient depends on the site of the operation and again the relevant explanations can be given. However patients should also be given more detailed explanations of what they can expect following their operation and how they can help to achieve a more comfortable and successful recovery.

The patient with a prolapsed lumbar disc should be made aware that his immediate postoperative condition does not necessarily reflect the degree of success of the operation. Although he may experience an immediate improvement he may equally experience pain similar to or greater than his pre-operative level. An initial reduction in pain can be followed by its return, but again this is often due to nerve root irritation and oedema and only subsides as the inflammation resolves. He may experience muscle spasms in the low back, thighs or abdomen and again these resolve over the first few days and do not indicate a lack of success. The true results of the operation will become evident over a longer period of time, although sciatica is more reliably relieved than back pain and neurological deficits are variable in their recovery. The knowledge that surgery cannot guarantee the relief of symptoms may concern some of the patients or their families, and they can often be reassured that surgery rarely causes a deterioration and that the stability and strength of the back will remain unaffected as none of the weightbearing structures are removed.

A patient about to undergo anterior cervical dissectomy and fusion (Cloward's procedure) needs to understand the importance of limiting the movement of the neck in the immediate postoperative period. A haemorrhage in this area can rapidly obstruct the airway and be fatal, and the possible dislodging of the bone graft may have disastrous consequences for the spinal cord. Without alarming the patient this understanding is essential. The pain following a Cloward's procedure is often severe with the pain of the surgical procedure, of incision and retraction, combining with the discomfort following intubation and the pressure of the cervical collar. All this centres on the patient's neck and can be very frightening. He should understand pre-operatively that the pain may be severe but that with analgesia it will be controlled as quickly as possible. He may be accustomed to wearing a cervical collar but if unused to the feeling he can experiment with those supplied by the physiotherapist for postoperative use. If a bone graft is to be taken, the nurse can ensure that the patient is aware of the planned donor site so that he has a greater understanding of his pain as he regains consciousness and will experience less fear. Because of the age group of many of the people requiring this type of surgery, pre-existing respiratory problems such as chronic bronchitis are quite common. These patients may be extremely anxious, particularly with regard to the anaesthetic, and they can be reassured that both the anaesthetist and the recovery nurse will be aware of their condition and that measures will be taken to prevent or minimise any related problems. They are often also concerned about the necessity to lie flat postoperatively and again they can be reassured that if they find this position does adversely affect their breathing then the bed head can be elevated if the cervical collar is in position.

The patient undergoing surgery for tumour must be aware that he may have to wait several days for final confirmation of the nature of the tumour but that the doctor will explain the extent to which he was able to remove the tumour and so decompress the spinal cord as soon as possible after the operation.

If it is considered that the patient may have difficulties with micturition in the postoperative period he may be catheterised in theatre in order to prevent further discomfort. It can be explained pre-operatively that this is a possibility so that he may more easily understand any initial discomfort or irritation in this area and be aware that this feeling is only temporary.

These are three common examples but all patients should have a sufficient understanding of what they can expect, that is, an understanding that they themselves find sufficient. All patients must be aware that postoperative pain and discomfort are inevitable and that although the analgesia given will control its severity it often cannot remove the pain entirely. However they also need to understand that they will be helped through this period by the medical and nursing staff and all will be done to minimise their discomfort.

To assist in the achievement of a smooth and uncomplicated recovery from surgery, both respiratory and limb exercises are taught at this stage. This is usually the responsibility of the physiotherapist but the nurse also plays an active and valuable part in their reinforcement. Respiratory exercises are important especially as mobility is often restricted postoperatively by the pain of surgery, by the regime of the surgeon or by the patient's neurological deficits. Those having cervical surgery, particularly from an anterior approach, must in particular be taught the value of frequent deep breathing as in the immediate postoperative period breathing may be painful and, as a result, shallow, and coughing may also cause pain. Limb exercises may be passive or active depending on the degree of dysfunction. The movement of joints that are immobilised by muscle weakness or pain soon becomes restricted and all joints should be moved through their full range of mobility twice daily to avoid this loss of flexibility. The post-anaesthetic risk of venous thrombosis could also be mentioned when explaining to the patient the reasons for these exercises. Passive straight leg raising should be avoided in patients with a prolapsed lumbar disc as it leads to the stretching of inflamed nerve roots and so severe pain. Active straight leg raising may be used as part of the initial assessment of limb function but again should not be included in the limb exercises, or indeed used as part of the routine assessment of the patient due to the severe pain it can cause.

THE DAY OF SURGERY

The priority of care on the day of surgery is the safety of the patient throughout and following his operation. The reduction of discomfort before and after surgery is also a major concern.

Ideally the general preparation has been completed so that the minimum of new information needs to be given at this time, and the patient can feel that he retains some degree of control over his situation. Reinforcement of previously taught information is of value and he should be reminded not to expect immediate freedom from pain. The physical preparation is often made easier by the use of a checklist (see Fig. 6.1) which helps to ensure the safety of the patient but it is important that the nurse tries to reduce the inflexibility and depersonalisation associated with its use. The degree of anxiety displayed by each patient is individual, not necessarily related to the degree of difficulty of the operation he is about to undergo, and care must be taken to reduce any last minute doubts and to confirm his trust and confidence in the medical and nursing staff.

When the patient has been taken to theatre the nursing records are forwarded to the recovery ward so that the staff responsible for his immediate postoperative care can identify their priorities for him. Any specific details that may influence his care, for example the duration and extent of pre-operative pain, can also be communicated verbally.

The time of the operation is often the most anxious period for members of the patient's family. If they wish to remain in the hospital they can be advised where to stay so that they can be informed when the operation is over. If they do not wish to, they can be advised when to telephone. Whereas the care of the patient by the ward staff is temporarily halted during the operation, the care of his family has no such interruption.

IMMEDIATE POSTOPERATIVE CARE

Just as in the care of the craniotomy patient there are three main aims of the recovery period: firstly, a safe recovery from general anaesthesia; secondly, the maintenance of satisfactory progress and the prevention or minimisation of problems consequent to surgery; and thirdly, the maximum degree of comfort within the postoperative limitations.

A safe environment with the presence of emergency equipment is essential, as is the nurse's knowledge of the patient's pre-operative neurological state in relation to his motor and sensory function, her knowledge of other pre-existing health problems and his emotional state, and her understanding of the nature of the operation, of specific postoperative regimes and potential complications.

The patient is admitted from theatre in a supine position. Respiratory and cardiovascular considerations are of immediate concern not only in connection with the

general anaesthetic but also following cervical and thoracic procedures when local damage may have occurred. The maintenance of intravenous access is of vital importance throughout this acute period so that the rapid onset of drug action can be ensured in an emergency situation and so that the intra-operative fluid loss can be replaced.

Information concerning the patient's progress in theatre is of importance and the theatre staff must ensure that all the relevant details are given.

The timing of the patient's return to the ward varies according to the policy of each unit. In some centres all 'spinal' patients return when their recovery is seen to be progressing satisfactorily. In others, because of their supine position and the careful observation that this necessitates, patients remain in the recovery unit until their recovery is more established. Those having undergone cervical surgery, in particular the Cloward's procedure, may remain for several hours to allow close supervision.

Assessment and general nursing care

Assessment is of the motor and sensory function below the level of the lesion (and surgery). The pre-operative level of neurological functioning should be known to the nurse and the main concern is that the patient regains this level as the effects of general anaesthesia diminish. The accurate recording of each assessment is important and if the patient does not regain his pre-operative status the medical staff must be informed.

Motor assessment can be performed almost immediately after the patient's admission to the recovery unit with the patient soon responding to request and touch. If he is moving his limbs spontaneously then observation alone may be sufficient for this initial assessment. As the patient recovers from the effects of the anaesthetic agents and the muscle relaxants, he becomes more able to demonstrate his increasing power. In the case of the 'lumbar' patient comparison between the power of the legs and that of the arms (the unaffected limbs), as well as the consideration of his general state can help the nurse to distinguish between weakness of anaesthetic origin and that with a neurological cause.

Subtle sensory function is more easily ascertained when the patient is sufficiently alert to respond to the questioning involved. Paraesthesia may be described in areas of previous numbness and the patient can be reassured that this is an improvement. Sciatic pain may or may not be reduced and, if necessary, the patient can be reminded that remaining pain does not indicate a failed operation.

Although painful stimuli will demonstrate both sensory and motor function very early in the recovery process this causes unnecessary pain and it is not used in the normal nursing assessment of the 'spinal' patient. The use of other actions that may also cause pain, for example straight leg raising in the lumbar patient, must also be limited, particularly before pain control is achieved.

Position is important in the postoperative care of the 'spinal' patient and the commonly accepted regime is one whereby the patient remains flat, initially on his back for 2 hours. There are, however, certain compromises that can be made to increase the patient's comfort and which are acceptable to the surgeon. Pain control increases the patient's comfort and also enables him to keep his back reasonably still.

Physiotherapy is carried out or supervised by both the physiotherapist and the nursing staff. The patients are reminded of previously taught respiratory and limb exercises. Whereas these exercises may have appeared straightforward pre-operatively they may now prove painful and difficult and the nurse can provide the help and encouragement that the patient requires. Where the limited muscle power of the patient prevents active limb exercises the nurse can perform passive movements to span the range of mobility.

Nursing care following lumbar surgery

Although there is a common assumption that the patient with low back pain gains relief by lying flat on his back on a hard surface this is not necessarily so. It cannot be assumed that this position will promote comfort in the postoperative period and as the commonly accepted management regime is one whereby the patient remains on his back for the first 2 hours, a degree of flexibility is required. However this position reduces strain on the wound site and and allows easier and more accurate assessment of neurological function and so is advantageous to both patient and staff in the majority of cases. Many patients can be helped to tolerate this position by the use of analgesia and those patients with remaining sciatic pain often appreciate the periodic reduction in the traction on the sciatic nerve by the positioning of pillows beneath the knees for short periods. The main concerns are that he lies flat, with his lumbar spine straight, and that he lies reasonably still. If he cannot tolerate lying supine then the nurse must enable him to find a position which meets both his immediate need for a reasonable degree of comfort and his longer term needs for an uncomplicated recovery and a successful result to surgery. Good positioning is essential with adequate support by pillows and this is usually acceptable to the surgeon. If the patient is obese then a lateral position may be of value in reducing the pressure of the abdominal contents on the diaphragm and it may be assumed solely for this reason. Breathing becomes easier for the patient and the tidal volume increases so reducing the risk of postoperative chest infection.

In the assessment of these patients the motor power of the arms does not need to be included. However this is often of value in interpreting apparent weakness in the legs as the patient recovers from the general anaesthetic. Under normal circumstances all limbs regain their motor power at a similar rate and any difference, particularly an increasing one, may indicate a neurological cause for the dysfunction. If all limbs remain equally weak the cause may be anaesthetic. Straight leg raising should not be used as part of the routine assessment of motor function. This not only causes stress to the wound site but can also be extremely painful for the patient due to the contraction of the lumbar muscles. Bladder function requires careful attention following a lumbar laminectomy. Where there is cauda equina compression there is often bladder involvement pre-operatively with urine retention being a major feature. These patients may be catheterised but otherwise both they and others who have experienced bladder problems, often in association with sciatic pain, need particular care.

Patients who have a long history of back pain may view surgery as a last resort after having undergone a variety of conservative measures, all proving unsuccessful. Although they will have been told pre-operatively not to expect immediate relief from pain and other symptoms they may retain this hope and be extremely disappointed when they regain consciousness and experience not only the discomfort that occurs as a consequence of surgery but again their usual pain. The post-operative experience is variable however and some patients will find their symptoms improved, commonly their sciatica rather than their back pain. This sciatic pain can subsequently return, or it can be increased, or the patient may complain of muscle spasms in the abdomen, low back or thighs. All these are not unusual changes and the patient must be reassured that they do not reflect the degree of success of the operation and that this will be apparent over the following days and weeks.

Nursing care following thoracic surgery

Following surgery on the thoracic spine the patient is nursed flat and helped to turn every 2 hours or as required for his comfort. Because of the curvature of the spine, and the convex nature of the thoracic spine in particular, a dressing in this area may prove more uncomfortable than one in the concave lumbar and cervical regions. The patient then may prefer to be in a lateral rather than a supine position. On occasion a wound drain may be inserted and this also limits the patient's choice of position.

Although respiratory function is carefully monitored following any period of ventilation, after thoracic surgery this is particularly important. The patient's colour and the rate, depth and ease of breathing together with the symmetry of chest expansion and audible signs all assist in the assessment of the patient's condition. If, during costotransversectomy, the pleura has been inadvertently cut the surgeon may insert a chest drain. Alternatively he may suture the cut while the lungs are inflated and order a chest X-ray to be performed in the recovery unit.

Nursing care following cervical surgery

Following cervical surgery, position is again important with the patient lying supine on a flat bed for the first 2 hours postoperatively. Elderly patients, however, make up a significant proportion of the people requiring cervical surgery and although the majority tolerate this position well, those with pre-existing respiratory problems often experience great difficulty. In these cases elevation of the bed head can be used, often in conjunction with bronchodilators, to help improve respiratory efficiency and comfort. Again an understanding of the principles involved in the care of these patients is important and allows the flexibility required for a successful recovery.

The mobility of the neck is restricted by the use of a soft foam collar which not only reduces rotational movement but also flexion and extension. It may be applied immediately following surgery or later before the patient is first turned or raised from the flat position. It should be used if head elevation is used for respiratory reasons. Many of the patients whose surgery involved an anterior approach find breathing uncomfortable and may complain of difficulty. This type of surgery can be extremely uncomfortable with the pain of the surgical procedure and retraction combining with the discomfort of intubation, the postoperative swelling of soft tissues and the presence of the wound drain and the collar, and all of this pain centres on the neck. The nurse must be able to distinguish between those respiratory problems which are related to the discomfort and those with other causes and must act appropriately. Analgesia is required as a priority when pain is a causative factor and reassurances and kindness can be of great value in the period before its control is achieved. As breathing tends to be shallow in many of these patients and, as a consequence, the risk of postoperative chest infection is increased, respiratory care is essential.

In the patients who have undergone anterior cervical dissectomy and fusion (Cloward's procedure) the nursing care and observation must take account of the additional risks involved. The consequences of haematoma formation can be extremely serious with the airway being in imminent danger. For this reason the insertion of a wound drain is a standard procedure. This is usually a suction drain but even on the occasion that this cannot be maintained it remains in situ acting as an outlet for blood and so continuing to protect the airway. Wound closure may be achieved by clips or sutures and it is important that the nurse knows which of these have been used. In this way she can ensure that the equipment required to remove them in the event of rapid haematoma formation when, for any reason, the drain proves ineffective, is easily available. A tape measure to help to detect a suspected haematoma or to measure its development is also necessary.

A further risk attached to this procedure is the dislodgement of the bone graft used to assist fusion of the vertebrae. This can obviously have disastrous consequences for the spinal cord and so for the patient, and as reduced movement of the neck is particularly important, rapid pain control is essential. However, unless an artificial graft has been used, these patients have the additional discomfort related to the donor site. Because of the retraction involved in this type of surgery the vagus nerve can be temporarily affected and cardiac arrhythmias are not uncommon. If these become apparent or they are expected, then cardiac monitoring is indicated.

Relatives

Most patients have relatives who are greatly concerned for their safety and their rapid return to optimal health. Each telephone enquiry is from a person to whom the patient is important. As the relatives or close friends rarely meet the recovery staff their confidence in them is based, to a certain extent, on these telephone conversations. If the nurse's manner is friendly, warm and competent the relatives will be reassured. A description of how the patient has progressed together with a positive reassuring comment, all given in easily understandable terms, is of value as is an estimated time for the patient's return to the ward. If the patient's stay in recovery is to be of any duration then a visit by a close relative may be beneficial to the patient and his family, particularly if they have spent the period of surgery waiting in the hospital. If so, this is usually possible to arrange.

CONTINUING CARE

Factors related to length of hospital stay

Most of these factors cannot be changed by nursing practice but identification of patients who are more likely to have longer stays will assist in the planning of care and discharge from hospital, recognising that these patients may need more attention from the outset. A study by Sutcliffe & Vincent (1985) found that patients with certain characteristics tended to stay longer in hospital following laminectomy:

— patients over the age of 40
— black patients
— those unemployed prior to admission
— those living alone
— following cervical surgery
— those with other medical diagnosis, e.g. diabetes, hypertension
— those with extensive pathology or who had

undergone extensive or 'partial' procedures — those who needed greater use of analgesia — where early activity was not possible.

Respiration

Postoperative care aims to promote normal respiratory fuction and prevent complications such as atelectasis or chest infection.

Pain will increase the tendency to shallow breathing and reluctance to move. The patient who is immobile and confined to bed will be at greater risk of respiratory problems. Tracheal oedema or development of a haematoma following Cloward's procedure may result in difficulty with coughing and managing secretions, or tracheal compression. Spinal cord oedema or haemorrhage, paralysis of intercostal muscles or involvement of the phrenic nerve (C4) will cause respiratory dysfunction.

The rate, rhythm and depth of respirations should be assessed regularly, particularly following cervical surgery. Anterior neck wounds must be inspected frequently for signs of swelling. Observation of diaphragmatic breathing without use of the abdominal muscles, shallow respirations with increased respiratory effort, asymmetrical chest movement, inability to cough, restlessness or confusion should be immediately reported. Suction and humidified oxygen therapy are employed as required. Any purulent sputum should be sent for culture and body temperature monitored. Turning the patient every 2 hours, encouraging deep breathing (at least 10 deep breaths an hour) and early activity will all promote adequate gaseous exchange and avoid pooling of secretions. Control of pain will allow the patient to breathe deeply and participate in physiotherapy.

Neurological assessment

Aim
- To monitor postoperative improvement and to recognise the development of problems such as nerve root compression or alterations in spinal cord perfusion due to oedema, haemorrhage or infarction.

Where the patient has undergone cervical surgery, assessment concentrates on arm strength and sensation. Following lumbar surgery, greater attention is given to the legs and feet. Observation of increasing motor and/or sensory deficit, swelling along the suture line, or increased pain proximal to the suture line, should be reported immediately. The spontaneous movement, muscle strength and tone and coordination of each limb should be assessed. Activities such as straight leg raising may be limited by pain.

Each limb is graded accordingly:

5 Full range of motion against gravity and resistance
4 Full range of movement against gravity with limited movement against resistance
3 Movement against gravity but not against resistance
2 Range of movement but unable to elevate limbs against gravity
1 Slight contraction observed
0 No movement.

Bilateral response to touch can be estimated by asking the patient to identify changes in sensation. A wisp of cotton wool can be used to touch gently various parts of the body, avoiding areas of excessive hair. Position sense can be assessed by moving the index finger or big toe at the last joint and asking the patient to close his eyes and identify upward or downward movement. Sensory changes such as paraesthesiae and change in nature or site of pain should be reported.

Care of the wound

The dressing should be observed for signs of haemorrhage or CSF leakage. It is important to note from the operative report if the dura was opened. If there is a risk of CSF leakage, contamination may lead to meningitis and prophylactic antibiotics may be prescribed. Swelling along the suture line may indicate the formation of a haematoma or the accumulation of CSF. Inflammation, severe incisional pain and pyrexia indicate infection of the wound.

Thoracic wounds are most prone to rupture and the patient should not be pulled by the arms. Contamination of the dressing may occur if the patient is incontinent or when a bedpan is used, therefore the wound must be cleaned and a dry sterile dressing applied should it become wet. The contrast media used in myelography or contamination of the wound may cause inflammation of the arachnoid, leading to the formation of scar tissue and adhesions and severe chronic pain. Surgical removal of adhesions is often unhelpful though there may be some response to steroid therapy. Osteitis of the vertebral body is rare but occasionally patients develop a chronic disc space infection which causes long-term pain.

Adequate nutrition and fluid intake will help to promote wound healing. Sutures may usually be removed on the 5th postoperative day following a Cloward's procedure and 7 to 10 days after a laminectomy. Once healed the wound site can be gently washed and the patient instructed to use clean tissues for thoroughly drying the area.

Pain

Aim
- Freedom from pain allowing the patient to participate in his own care and physiotherapy.

Pain may be due to postoperative incisional discomfort, oedema, muscle spasm or a result of nerve root irritation at surgery. The surgeon's expectations of postoperative pain should be ascertained so that expected pain can be distinguished from that arising from complications. If uncontrolled, pain will lead to restlessness, fatigue, tension and irritability, reluctance to move, cough or take deep breaths and may inhibit micturition.

Assessing pain
Note site, intensity and pattern — compare with any pre-operative pain

- Patient's appearance — frowning, grimacing, pallor, sweating
- Resistance to position change and movement
- Stooping posture when walking
- In the patient who has suffered chronic pain — whether there are secondary gains in maintaining pain behaviour, e.g. avoidance of home or work responsibilities; manipulative, controlling behaviour; if pain behaviour is reinforced by family; signs of depression or anger
- Response to analgesia.

If pain is constant or very intense, the patient will be unable to relax or be distracted from it. Motivation will be different in the patient who knows that pain will lessen in a few days from the patient who feels that it will be a lifelong experience.

Muscle spasm tends to present on the 3rd or 4th postoperative day. Possible reasons include nerve irritation at the time of surgery, overactivity of the patient or recovery of previously compressed nerves. The pain may be very discouraging for the patient and he can be assured that spasm should abate in a few days. Frequent change of position and adequate rest periods may help.

Pain and spasm may be relieved by supporting the body in alignment and turning the patient with care and adequate personnel to give the necessary assistance. All actions should be explained before proceeding so that the patient is not surprised by sudden movements. For the patient who has had cervical surgery, collars are applied with the neck slightly flexed for maximum relief of pain. The cervical collar should reduce the range of motion of the neck and diminish nerve root irritation.

Analgesia

Initially the patient may need narcotics such as Omnopon (10–20 mg 4 hourly) for adequate pain control. This should be given before pain becomes severe and 20 to 30 minutes before physiotherapy or getting out of bed. Anti-emetics are given to counteract any nausea. Administration of narcotics may also cause respiratory depression and cough suppression and contribute to ·urinary retention and constipation. Radicular pain may be treated with a short course of dexamethasone. Diazepam can be used as a muscle relaxant but may cause drowsiness and long-term use is associated with dependence. Spinal cord tumours may involve the corticospinal tract and spasticity is often a problem in patients who have had surgery for tumours.

Spasticity will interfere with movement and positioning and may be extremely painful for the patient. It may cause contractures and increase the risk of pressure sore development as the skin is irritated by friction and pressure. Spasticity may be interpreted as a return of voluntary movement by the patient. It may also contribute to inadequate bladder or bowel emptying.

Beneficial effects of maintaining muscle mass and tone and preventing muscle atrophy and establishment of bladder emptying by stimulation of trigger points, may be gained by a degree of spasticity. A relaxed, calm atmosphere with adequate time allowed for positioning and transfer activities can help to control spasticity. Touch should be gentle, yet firm and steady. Extremes of temperature should be avoided and clothing should not be tight. Nail care is important for affected patients as ingrown, infected toenails will contribute to stimuli which increase spasticity. Constipation, urinary tract infection or a distended bladder must be avoided. Range of motion exercises should be carried out in a slow, smooth manner, supporting joints and explaining each move beforehand. Drugs such as diazepam, dantrolene sodium and baclofen are widely used in the management of spasticity. Dantrolene may cause drowsiness vertigo and liver dysfunction. The side-effects of baclofen include gastrointestinal disturbance, headache and fatigue.

If surgery was successful in relieving pain the patient may feel elated but if pre-operative pain persists he is likely to experience anger or depression.

Recurrence of pain

Pain may recur after surgery if the diagnosis was wrong. For example conditions which may present with similar signs to a herniated nucleus pulposus include spondylosis, spinal cord stenosis, spinal cord tumour and arthritic disease, where a simple dissectomy will not relieve symptoms. The operation may have been performed at the wrong level or an adequate decompression of an affected nerve root may have proved impossible. Damage may be caused during surgery, if a nerve root is actually cut resulting in a painless deterioration in the patient's neurological signs. Pain may be caused by a new disc prolapse at the same level as the original operation or at a different level. The patient who has extensive degenerative changes will not benefit from a disc removal alone and may require an extensive decompression and possible spinal fusion. Arachnoid cyst formation, sterile abscess, meningitis, instabilty of the involved spinal level due to extensive surgical procedure may all cause persistent postoperative back pain. Formation of new bone impinging on spinous process following a spinal fusion may cause nerve root compression. Patients who are claiming compensation following back injury have a higher incidence of postoperative complications and report poorer subjective results.

Operative treatment may be followed if the patient appears to have pathology correctable by surgery but conservative methods of treatment are frequently used for recurrent pain. Bed-rest with firm support for the back, use of analgesia and antispasmodic drugs, instruction in body mechanics and back care, and physiotherapy, including hot or cold applications and gentle massage in the acute phase may be employed. An active exercise programme may improve the patient's range of movement and feeling of wellbeing. Patients suffering from inflammation in and around nerve roots may benefit from epidural block, which may need to be repeated, and the use of anti-inflammatory drugs. Transcutaneous nerve stimulating techniques and acupuncture are also used for relief of chronic pain.

Pain is both a psychological and a physical experience. It can be enhanced or modified at the cortical level, in the spinal cord or in the periphery. It is a subjective experience and the nurse must accept that it is whatever the patient says it is and that the discomfort cannot be managed without assistance.

Patients who have suffered chronic pain for months or years may exhibit manipulative behaviour and the risk of a breakdown in communication between nurse and patient, where the nurse becomes exasperated by what may appear to be many inconsequential demands, must be recognised. Staff may feel uncomfortable with the patient who does not get a good result from surgery.

Chronic pain may lead to dependent, passive behaviour, inability to cope, low self-esteem, fatigue and irritability. There is a tendency to make the pain experience the centre of life which does not occur in the patient with acute pain, who may be overtly anxious but is able to utilise coping mechanisms more successfully.

The patient's use of drugs — analgesia, tranquillisers and night sedation — should be understood and may influence their needs postoperatively, particularly where there is evidence of misuse or dependence.

Interests other than the patient's symptoms and healthy behaviour such as exercise and participation in physiotherapy should be reinforced. Administration of analgesia on a time, rather than pain dependent, basis may avoid rewarding the patient for having pain while still providing pain relief. The multidisciplinary team needs to work closely together to help improve the patient's resources to live a more productive life. Assistance from social or psychiatric services or a minister of religion may be appropriate. Physical, social or psychological problems, which may influence recovery, must be considered on an individual basis and a careful nursing history and plan of care are essential to dealing with them. Thorough evaluation of the patient's problems

should aim to restore confidence and give them hope.

Positioning and activity

Following a lumbar laminectomy immediate care involves log rolling the patient from side to side at least 2 hourly and checking body alignment regularly. The head of the bed should not be elevated more than 20 degrees. Knees and hips should be flexed and the top leg supported with a pillow along its entire length to decrease pressure on nerve roots.

Following cervical surgery, the head of the bed can be gradually elevated. The head and neck should be kept in a neutral position and the patient instructed to avoid pulling with the arms when sitting up, which might increase stress on the operative site.

Full range of motion exercises with each limb will maintain muscle tone, promote circulation and venous return, preventing venous stasis and deep venous thrombosis.

Unless contra-indicated, the patient should get out of bed for a short period on the first postoperative day which will help relieve any spasm and increase independence. Bed-rest will usually be for a longer period when the patient has had a spinal fusion to allow healing and permanent fusion to occur. When three or more vertebrae have been involved in the surgery or there is risk of CSF leakage through a dural tear, bed-rest will also be longer. Following an anterior cervical fusion the patient may be up on the first postoperative day, wearing a hard collar, after a lateral cervical X-ray to check the position of the graft.

Analgesia should be administered 30 minutes beforehand and the patient reassured that he will not do any damage to his surgery. He should be instructed to bend his knees and edge to the side of the bed and roll onto his side, placing the upper hand in front of the abdomen and pressing down firmly against the mattress. In one movement he should rise to a sitting position using the elbow of the other arm as a lever. The bed should be at a height that allows the patient's feet to touch the ground with the knees slightly flexed. This procedure is reversed when the patient gets back into bed. Once standing, tension may be relieved by concentrating on deep breathing. The degree of activity is dictated by the patient's level of discomfort and sitting is contra-indicated for the patient who has had lumbar surgery for the first week. The nurse and physiotherapist should assist the patient in getting out of bed on the first couple of days to encourage correct use of body mechanics and assess any gait problems. The patient should be encouraged to carry out grooming and hygiene with the exception of washing legs and back.

Application of a soft or hard cervical collar will reduce the range of motion of the neck and head, decreasing nerve root irritation and discomfort for the patient who has had cervical surgery. The collar should be worn with the neck slightly flexed to allow opening of the intervertebral foramen. Lying in a prone position should be avoided, as the head and neck are rotated which may be painful. Before discharge from hospital, patients should be advised that riding in a car may be uncomfortable due to vibration. Those who drive should use rear view mirrors when reversing to avoiding turning the head to look. Working areas should be arranged so that prolonged periods of flexion, extension or rotation of the cervical spine are minimised. The physiotherapist should instruct the patient in range of motion exercises to be carried out at home. Limitation of movement will be greater when there has been a cervical fusion. Exercise aims to increase the strength and mobility of muscles and supporting structures and may include:

— bending the neck and head forward trying to touch the chest with the chin
— bending the head and neck backwards
— trying to touch the left shoulder with the left ear without moving the shoulder, repeating on the right side
— making clockwise and anticlockwise circles with the head and neck

— turning head and neck to the left and then to the right.

The goals of exercise for the patient who has had lumbar surgery are to strengthen the low back muscles, to stretch muscles and tendons which may have been shortened before the operation, to keep the spine in alignment and to develop the attitude that proper care will prevent future injury. The nurse should work with the physiotherapist to learn the patient's individual treatment plan. For the first 2 weeks prolonged standing or sitting is avoided and time should be allowed for sufficient rest to prevent fatigue and loss of motivation. Chairs should be firm and provide good support for the back, allowing the knees to be as high as, or slightly above, the level of the hips. The patient should be instructed to sit always with the back straight and thighs supported on the chair. When lying on the back, knees should be flexed or the legs elevated, to help relieve spasm.

The patient may shower once sutures are removed and the wound is well healed. The ability of the patient to use the bath without slipping and risking injury to the back should be assessed by the occupational therapist who may advise on provision of aids such as non-slip mats or handrails. Provision of a shower at home is desirable if possible. If the patient has loss of pain and temperature sensation, safety measures must be taught. The temperature of water, radiators, etc. should be checked with an unaffected limb.

Prior to discharge from hospital, patients should be provided with a written guide to exercise and back care. Advice may include:

— resting for approximately 20 minutes each day either on a firm bed or on the floor
— standing with the back straight and weight evenly distributed between both feet, and not in one position for too long.

Rules for lifting

• Weight of the object should be tested
• Stand close to the weight to be lifted

- Stand with feet apart and toes pointing in the direction the weight is to be carried
- Bend knees and hips, keeping the back straight
- Grip the weight firmly with the palms of the hands
- Keep the chin tucked in and lift by straightening hips and knees using thigh and buttock muscles
- When carrying shopping either hold the bag into the chest or carry two equally weighted bags
- Avoid lifting whenever possible.

Working surfaces should be at a height that does not necessitate slouching forward and working position should be changed regularly to relieve stress on the back. The patient should receive advice to increase conscientiousness about the posture used in daily activities. Strenuous and competitive sports are not allowed until the patient is reassessed by the surgeon at the first outpatient appointment around 6 weeks after surgery and may be contra-indicated after that. The patient can usually resume sexual activity as soon as he or she feels comfortable enough to do so. Once the patient begins to drive again the car seat should be moved so that the knees are slightly higher than the hips. Driving is not usually advised for the first 3 weeks and may be uncomfortable for prolonged periods. Sudden jerking movements can cause muscle strain. Patients should be advised against wearing high-heeled shoes.

Pain should be a guideline for all activity and is a sign for the patient that he has done too much or done it incorrectly. As many patients feel stiff first thing in the morning a gentle exercise routine may be beneficial before getting out of bed. The patient should understand that taking care of his back will help prevent future strain and injury.

Personal cleansing

The condition of the skin should be assessed every 2 hours while the patient remains in bed, with particular attention paid to bony prominences. Colour, moisture, texture, temperature and elasticity are checked. The skin should be clean, well lubricated and free from moisture and bed linen smooth and unwrinkled. Patients particularly at risk of skin breakdown are those with paralysis and/or sensory loss, those who are incontinent, elderly or in a poor nutritional state. Position change, adequate fluid and dietary intake and exercise will promote skin integrity. If a prolonged period of bed-rest is unavoidable, use of sheepskin or special mattresses can be made to relieve skin from continuous pressure. Patients with sensory loss should be taught to examine their skin systematically and regularly for signs of pressure, and the importance of frequent position change.

Eliminating

The pre-operative state of the patient's urinary tract should be documented. As soon as possible the patient should be allowed out of bed to void. General anaesthesia, oedema at the site of the operation and pain will increase any difficulty.

Potential problems

— alteration in bladder tone
— distension of bladder
— overflow with retention
— stress incontinence
— decrease in urinary output
— frequency of micturition
— restlessness.

A fluid intake of 2.5–3 litres over 24 hours should be encouraged unless contra-indicated by the patient's cardiovascular state. Intake and output should be measured and accurately recorded. If the patient's bladder becomes uncomfortably distended, catheterisation may be unavoidable and measures to maintain the hygiene and patency of the catheter must be taken to avoid urinary tract infection. If it is suspected that the patient is not completely emptying his bladder a catheter may be passed to measure any residual urine. If the urine is offensive or cloudy, a specimen should be obtained for culture and sensitivity. Early activity and adequate pain control will help reduce the risk of voiding problems.

Lesions of the conus region of the spinal cord and of the cauda equina will destroy reflex bladder activity. Cord compression or transection will allow reflex or automatic bladder function as reflex pathways below the lesion are intact.

Neurogenic bladder

Where there has been upper motor neurone damage above the 2nd, 3rd and 4th sacral level (e.g. due to tumour), the bladder abruptly empties when the stretch receptors in the bladder reach their threshold. The patient has no sensation of fullness so voiding is involuntary. There may be inadequate emptying of the bladder due to spasticity of the external sphincter and detrusor muscle.

The patient may experience sweating, restlessness and abdominal discomfort and learn to relate these symptoms to a full bladder. Voiding may be triggered by stroking the inner thigh or abdomen, pulling the pubic hair or digital stimulation of the anus or doing push ups on the toilet. Once the urinary catheter has been removed and the patient has voided, the residual urine should be checked, and if this is more than 100 ml the catheter reinserted. If the male patient experiences dribbling, an external drainage device may be worn at night.

Flaccid atonic bladder due to lower motor neurone damage

Bladder evacuation may be assisted by pressure over the suprapubic area, or straining and contracting the abdominal muscles to increase pressure on the bladder. Intermittent self-catheterisation may be taught as a clean technique.

The key to success in dealing with a damaged bladder is the psychological adjustment of the patient. Loss of control over voiding can generate anxiety which may be related to childhood control difficulties and toilet training. The patient's self-image can be seriously affected and lack of activity and boredom will add to concentration on the loss of function. Providing information in an honest, unselfconscious manner can help avoid feelings of embarrassment or guilt. A planned programme with realistic goals which avoids unnecessary setbacks will help to promote a positive approach. Encouraging the patient to express his emotions will help adjustment to a new body image. Family members may experience similar depression, anger and helplessness and early involvement with the patient's care and treatment, providing information and expressing expectations can help them to adjust.

Bowel function

A high fibre diet, stool softeners and adequate fluid intake will help to promote normal bowel function. Constipation will exacerbate back pain by increasing pressure on the spine. Straining will increase pain and CSF pressure. Bowel sounds and function should be assessed and recorded daily. Most patients with a spinal cord lesion are able to retain bowel control. The patient should be in a comfortable position with feet flat on the floor before attempting to pass stool. If the abdominal muscles are weak, exerting pressure on the abdomen with the hands may be helpful. Normal routine for the individual should be followed as far as possible.

Paralytic ileus

Paralytic ileus is a possible problem in those with lesions at or above T6 level. The patient may exhibit abdominal distension, anorexia, vomiting, altered respirations or absence of bowel sounds. Diaphraghmatic movement may be altered and the patient may be at risk of aspiration. The patient should be given nothing orally and stomach contents should be removed via a nasogastric tube.

Radiotherapy

Where surgical treatment has been performed for spinal cord tumour, radiotherapy may be indicated. Extradural or intradural extramedullary tumours (neuromas and meningiomas) may be completely excised. Spinal cord tolerance to irradiation is less than that of the brain. Corticosteroid therapy is usually continued for the period of radiotherapy to help protect the cord. The patient's prognosis will vary greatly depending on the type of tumour and the neurological deficits it has caused. For the patient with a metastatic tumour, death is inevitable and the nurse should listen carefully to the patient and his family and assess their need for information and support.

Psychosocial considerations

Spinal surgery is associated for many people with fear of paralysis. The impact of spinal cord damage may involve fear of physical helplessness and loss of control of bodily functions. Grieving for physical losses is a normal response involving a process of shock and denial, leading to developing awareness of loss and finally, to resolution, when the patient is able to adapt to the change. Nurses have to develop support for patients and their families by facilitating this process and providing hope, counselling and education. They should foster open communication between the patient and his family and the multidisciplinary team, making appropriate referrals for specialised advice and care, e.g. sexual counselling for the patient with impaired function.

REFERENCES AND BIBLIOGRAPHY

Behrends E A 1982 Nutrition in neuroscience. Journal of Neurosurgical Nursing 14(1):44
Bouman C 1984 Self perceived needs of family members of critically ill patients. Heart and Lung 13(3):294
Bruya M 1981 Planned periods of rest in the intensive care unit: nursing care activities and intracranial pressure. Journal of Neurosurgical Nursing 13(4):184
Devoti A L 1983 Lumbar laminectomy: diagnosis to discharge. Journal of Neurosurgical Nursing 15(3):140
Hayward J 1981 Information — A prescription against pain. Royal College of Nursing, London
Hayward R 1980 Essentials of neurosurgery. Blackwell, London
Hickey J V 1986 The clinical practice of neurological and neurosurgical nursing, 2nd edn. J B Lippincott, Philadelphia
Janis I L as cited by Hayward J 1981 Information — a prescription against pain. Royal College of Nursing, London
Moghissi K, Boore J 1983 Parenteral and enteral nutrition for nurses. Heinemann, London
Novoty R W 1984 Psychosocial implications of a neurogenic bladder. Rehabilitation Nursing July/August:35
Robb D A, Dunscher S B 1981 Cervical spondylosis. Journal of Neurosurgical Nursing 13(2):72
Sharp B 1981 Nursing care of the patient with recurrent back pain after dissectomy. Journal of Neurosurgical Nursing 13(2):77
Stotts N 1982 Nutritional assessment before surgery. American Association of Operating Room Nurses Journal 35(2):207
Sutcliffe S A 1978 Comprehensive nursing care: the patient with a ruptured lumbar disc. Journal of Neurosurgical Nursing 10(3):86
Sutcliffe S A, Vincent P 1985 Factors related to length of stay of laminectomy patients. Journal of Neurosurgical Nursing 17(3):175
Twycross R as cited by Hunt J M 1979 Protracted pain and nursing care. Nursing 1(2):56

14

Care of the patient with back pain

BACK PAIN

In Britain 45–50% of the population is affected at some stage by back pain. Backache is one of the most common causes of morbidity and disability, and is a known threat to health, especially in the middle years of life. Backache is responsible for a high number of lost working days in Britain and the annual cost is approximately £1000 million.

Presentation may be:

1. Mechanical
2. Non-mechanical
     — related to possible spinal pathology
     — related to nerve roots.

Most backache is mechanical and results from minor trauma or degenerative changes. Specific physical activities such as bending, coughing or sudden movement make the pain worse, whereas others, such as lying in the appropriate position or applying heat, reduce the pain. This pain may vary with time, due to related physical activity in response to re-injury or treatment.

Non-mechanical backache is not relieved by rest or position and it may be worse at night when there are no other distractions. Recognition of this backache should make one suspect spinal pathology.

NERVE ROOT PAIN

It is important to distinguish between referred

leg pain and root pain. Leg pain is not necessarily due to nerve root involvement. Percutaneous needle stimulation of the ligaments, muscles, small facet joints or discs in the back can produce dull, ill-localised pain, which spreads to the buttocks, groin or posterior aspects of the thigh, but rarely radiates below the knees. This type of referred pain should simply be regarded as spread of backache. When the needle hits the nerve root, sharp, well-localised pain and paraesthesia are produced, which usually radiates to the foot. Apparently the distinction between referred and root pain is quite clear in 90% of patients.

As already stated, it has to be established that it is the nerve root that is being compressed and this can be demonstrated by manoeuvres which stretch or press on an irritable nerve to produce radiating root pain. Straight leg raising limited by reproduction of radiating leg pain is a critical sign. This may also be demonstrated by the straight leg raising of the asymptomatic leg, reproducing cross over pain in the symptomatic leg. Direct pressure also demonstrates radiating root pain and paraesthesia.

Compression of the nerve leads to muscle wasting, motor weakness, sensory disturbance or depressed tendon reflexes.

Prolapsed intervertebral disc often occurs following an injury, but it is believed that degenerative changes within the disc may be an important predisposing factor. Congenital weakness of a part of the annulus fibrosus is thought to be the cause in younger patients. The most common sites for prolapse are between lumbar 5 and sacral 1 or lumbar 4 and lumbar 5.

Part of the gelatinous nucleus pulposus protrudes through a weakened part of the annulus fibrosus which is normally posterolateral. When a small bulge protrudes through onto the sensitive longitudinal posterior ligament it causes back pain. If the protrusion is large, the disc herniates through the longitudinal ligament and may press on the nerve causing sciatic pain (see Fig. 14.1).

Treatment may comprise:

- conservative management
- chemonucleolysis — chymopapain injection
- surgical excision.

Conservative management

This type of approach is the most common. Management includes rest and support for the lumbar spine, which may be achieved by strict bed rest for a minimum of 6 weeks with the possible addition of traction. Alternatively, the patient may wear a lumbosacral support.

Chemonucleolysis

Chymopapain is a protein enzyme extracted from a South American plant. The preoperative investigations for chymopapain injection include:

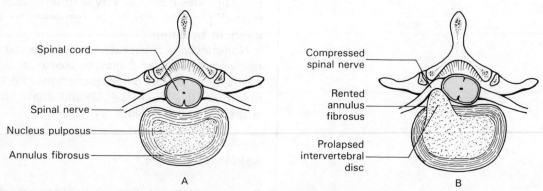

A   B

Fig. 14.1   (A) Position and structure of the intervertebral disc (B) Prolapsed intervertebral disc.

— plain radiographs of the lumbrosacral spine; antero-posterior and lateral views are obtained
— myelography.

Injection of chymopapain is usually performed under local anaesthesia. A rare complication of chymopapain is adverse patient reaction resulting in anaphylactic shock, the patient is fasted and an intravenous infusion commenced. This permits efficient and effective management should a reaction occur.

The patient lies in the lateral position on the theatre table and using an image intensifier X-ray control, a needle is introduced into the appropriate disc space. The chymopapain is injected into the nucleus polposus of the disc which is dissolved instantly.

On the patient's return to the ward, the colour, sensation and movement to both lower limbs are particularly noted along with routine postoperative observations. In addition observation of urinary function is noted.

It must be understood that although the patient has not had extensive surgery, adequate analgesia must be given, e.g. pethidine 50 mg i.m. This is because increased back pain is felt after this procedure due to chemical irritation within the disc, which in turn causes spasm in the surrounding muscles. After the nucleus pulposus has been dissolved, the annulus fibrosus of the disc shrinks and therefore no longer presses on the nerve root. The paraesthesia the patient experiences diminishes very quickly, but the leg pain may continue for some time.

An anti-inflammatory agent and a mild analgesic are prescribed for the patient, and the patient is seen in 6 weeks at the outpatient clinic. Up to 90% of patients do not suffer any further sciatica.

The patient may be discharged the following day provided that mobility is adequate and there is no elevation in temperature.

Surgery

Surgery may be indicated when the sciatic pain is so severe as to prevent the patient from sleeping and carrying out other activities of living or where the herniation is so large as to threaten the function of the spinal cord, e.g. to produce loss of sphincter control.

A range of surgical procedures is available, depending upon the initial diagnosis:

1. Hemilaminectomy — excision of part of the posterior arch of the vertebral lamina
2. Foraminotomy — surgical removal of part of the intervertebral foramen
3. Lumbar microdiscectomy — removal of disc material using an operating microscope.

The pre-operative investigations include:

— plain radiographs of the lumbosacral spine
— myelography
— other standard pre-operative investigations, e.g. ECG, blood screen.

Postoperatively colour, sensation and movement of both lower limbs and bladder function are recorded along with routine postoperative observations.

It is not unusual for the patient to experience retention of urine postoperatively but this is normally due to abdominal pain, muscle spasm and the supine position which the patient may adopt. The lateral and prone positions can be used if the patient chooses these, and finds them comfortable. It is important that when the patient is changing his position the nursing staff should assist to prevent the patient from twisting his spine. Adequate analgesia must be given regularly to control the pain.

On the first postoperative day the patient is normally on bed-rest but if the pain is well controlled it can be suggested that he sits at the edge of the bed, stands and perhaps takes a few steps with the assistance of two nurses. Normally the patient does not mobilise fully until the next day. No walking aids are used as they may encourage bad posture and are psychologically detrimental. If the patient had a lumbosacral support pre-operatively he may want to wear it after surgery if he feels it is beneficial. Gradually the patient increases his mobility over the next few days. Lifting, bending and twisting movements are discouraged while in hospital.

The wound dressing is inspected on the 5th day and if it is dry and clean, an airstrip is applied. If there is no elevation in temperature, the patient can be discharged after a week, returning on the 10th day for removal of sutures. Analgesia is provided on discharge. The patient is seen at the outpatient clinic 6 weeks postoperatively and is expected to return to work after 3–6 months, depending on the nature of his employment.

SPONDYLOLISTHESIS

Spondylolisthesis is a term applied to spontaneous forward displacement of a lumbar vertebral body upon the segment next below it. The patient presents with back pain and in many cases sufferers are below the age of 20 years. The operation carried out for this condition is spinal fusion although, in some cases, decompression of the nerve root is performed.

Lumbar posterior spinal fusion

Pre-operative investigations include:

— full haematology
— cross-matching of 2 units of blood
— full biochemistry profile
— ESR
— plain radiographs of the lumbosacral spine
— ECG.

The operation procedure involves the insertion of a wedge-shaped bone graft obtained from the iliac crest, between the affected vertebrae. The object of fusion is to stabilise that section of the vertebral column, which will mean some loss of mobility in that region.

Recently a stainless steel graft has been introduced. This is internally fixed to the neighbouring vertebrae for added and instantaneous stability.

On return to the ward the patient is nursed flat or on his side with a pillow placed alongside the operated area. Vital signs are recorded quarter-hourly and gradually decreased to 4-hourly as his condition stabilises.

Observation of the wound for staining is performed and a note made of any discharge. As before, observation of colour, sensation and movement of both legs are noted frequently. A check should be made that the patient voids urine postoperatively. Difficulties in micturition could be indicative of a postoperative complication.

On the first postoperative day the patient remains on bed-rest but is encouraged to move freely in bed. The patient should be taught how to mobilise in bed without twisting his spine. On the next day the patient is encouraged to sit up in bed and progress to standing beside the bed. Gradually mobility is increased from standing to taking a few steps and sitting in a chair. In most cases patients find it uncomfortable to sit in a chair and prefer to lie in bed. If the patient has worn a lumbosacral support, he can now wear it if he feels it is beneficial. Most patients feel more secure if they do. The wound drain is removed 36 hours following surgery. Prophylactic antibiotics are given over this period but if the patient's temperature is normal, the antibiotics are discontinued.

The wound dressing is removed on the 5th day and the wound is then covered with an airstrip, if the site is clean and dry. Sutures are removed on the 10th day and if the wound is healed and dry, and the patient is apyrexial and has attained assisted mobility, he can be discharged. A return to employment is usually achieved in 3–6 months.

Anterior spinal fusion of the thoracic lumbar spine

This procedure is normally performed in the treatment of tuberculosis or tumour of the thoracic spine.

The patient with tuberculosis is usually elderly and has had a tubercular infection at a younger age. Anterior collapse of the affected vertebrae leads to an angular kyphosis (posterior curvature of the spine) and a degree of cord compression. Degenerative changes in the spine also cause instability and pain.

The patient with a tumour may present with back pain and radiating leg pain. Bony destruction of the affected vertebrae will be seen on X-ray. Sensory and motor weakness with a degree of bladder and bowel dysfunction is also evident.

Spinal tumours are described according to their anatomical location. Extradural tumours are found in the extradural space and often are secondary deposits from a distant carcinoma. These may account for up to 40% of all spinal tumours. Intradural, extramedullary tumours lie in the subarachnoid space, often consisting of a benign neurofibroma or meningioma.

Intramedullary tumours occur within the spinal cord itself and are therefore the most difficult to treat. They are often malignant although on this occasion the malignancy occurs within the nervous tissue itself.

A needle biopsy is normally carried out for diagnostic purposes before any fusion is considered. This is carried out under local anaesthesia with an image intensifier, using a lateral approach.

Prophylactic antibiotics and steroids are commenced before surgery. The affected vertebral bodies are removed. To fuse this area a selected portion of fibula from both lower limbs is removed and split. This is inserted in position in the spine with intact vertebrae above and below the graft. Bone struts are also taken from the iliac crest and are placed into position alongside the fibula. Access to the vertebral bodies is through the diaphragm, via a thoracotomy.

Postoperatively the patient is nursed in a turning frame, e.g. Stryker frame. It is important that the patient becomes accustomed to the working and function of this bed pre-operatively. For elaboration of the care of the patient on the Stryker frame, see Chapter 12.

On return to the ward the patient is nursed supine. An intravenous infusion, chest drain, central venous line, urinary catheter and as many as three wound drains may be in situ.

Vital signs are checked quarter-hourly and gradually decreased to 4-hourly as the patient's condition stabilises. Urinary output is observed hourly and gradually decreased to 4-hourly when output is satisfactory; the catheter is normally removed on the 4th or 5th day. Bowel sounds should be listened for. Colour, sensation and movement of both legs are charted frequently. If there is any change or alteration in these observations this must be reported immediately. The chest drain is normally kept in place for 5 days by which time there is little drainage and the lung is well epanded. The nursing care appropriate to the management of the chest drain should be implemented. Observation of wound staining can only be done by inspecting the posterior mattress. If staining is excessive the patient must be turned for inspection of wound.

It is not until 24–36 hours after surgery that the patient is turned prone, adopting the safety measures outlined as before. Skin care is crucial. If the patient has a kyphosis it is sometimes covered by the wound dressing. To help relieve pressure here while the patient is lying supine, foam can be used. This is done by applying 2.5 cm (1 in) sheets of foam cut into the appropriate size to cover the kyphosis and a 5 cm (2 in) surrounding area. The middle portion of the foam is cut out so that the kyphosis can protrude and the surrounding foam relieves the pressure over the skin. It cannot be stressed enough how important the observation and prevention of pressure area damage are to the patient. Other pressure areas at risk are the heels and sacrum.

Sutures are removed 10 to 12 days postoperatively. The patient has to remain on the Stryker frame for 6 weeks, during which time he may return to theatre for further surgery to fuse the posterior facet joints at the previously grafted anterior area. The normal pre-operative work-up is carried out to a lesser degree but it is important that the patient is in the right psychological state and that he is fit for surgery.

At the end of the 6-week period, when the graft is stable and callus formation is demonstrated on X-ray, the patient can be transferred to an ordinary bed. Here he can mobilise freely for a few days. A plaster jacket may be required for added spinal support. Supportive walking frames are necessary at first because the patient feels very dizzy and weak.

Anti-tuberculosis therapy or radiotherapy is given to the patient as necessary. When the patient is confident, fit and mobile, he can be discharged.

BIBLIOGRAPHY

Adams J C 1981 Outline of orthopaedics, 9th edn. Churchill Livingstone, Edinburgh
Schott G D 1975 Spinal tumours — 1 Classification. Nursing Times 71(52):2055
Schott G D 1976 Spinal tumours — 2 Symptoms and signs. Nursing Times 72(1):21
Schott G D 1976 Spinal tumours — 3 Investigations, treatment and prognosis. Nursing Times 72(2):57
Waddel G 1982 An approach to backache. British Journal of Hospital Medicine 28(3):187

15

Care of the child with hydrocephalus and spina bifida

This chapter will deal with hydrocephalus and spina bifida in relation to the infant only and the reader is directed towards the section on hydrocephalus in the adult in Chapter 5 and to the physiology of the CSF pathways in Chapter 1.

HYDROCEPHALUS

This is a disorder characterised by an imbalance between the production and absorption of CSF, and the incidence varies between 2–8 per 1000 live births in the UK. It seldom occurs alone and one of the many commonly associated problems that can arise is that of spina bifida.

As in the adult, there are two types of hydrocephalus:

1. *Communicating*: in this type some of the CSF is able to pass out of the ventricles into the subarachnoid space. This occurs when the obstruction is beyond the tentorial opening.

2. *Non-communicating*: this is due to an obstruction somewhere in the ventricular system, more commonly at one of the outlets of the 4th ventricle.

These types are sometimes referred to as internal or expansive and external hydrocephalus which occurs when fluid accumulates in the subdural space. The latter is now termed subdural hygroma and is discussed on page 122.

Causes

Malformation

Aqueduct stenosis. This is a congenital condition where the tissues surrounding the aqueduct undergo cell proliferation thereby reducing or stopping the flow of CSF along this narrow channel. This may be a primary malformation or in association with spina bifida.

Arnold-Chiari malformation. This is a condition in which the medulla is elongated and misplaced through the foramen magnum. This will produce an obstruction to CSF flow through the basal cisterns and this too is associated with spina bifida.

Dandy-Walker syndrome. A large cyst may develop at the exit of the foramen of the 4th ventricle. This may follow inflammation or a primary malformation where the foramen is covered with a thin membrane and may also include cerebral hypoplasia. It is possible that the cyst development may produce a 'ball-cock' effect causing intermittent blockage as it develops.

Infection

Exudate may, in the post-infective period, block the flow of CSF at any point within the system. This may follow meningitis, *Haemophilus influenzae* and tuberculosis infection.

Birth injury

Adhesions following haemorrhage as the result of a birth injury may block the CSF flow. This can appear at any point along the pathways.

Neoplasm

Tumour formation, particularly of the posterior fossa, can compress the CSF pathways leading to the development of hydrocephalus.

Failure of absorption of CSF may be caused by meningeal irritation together with blockage of the basal cisterns. Increased venous pressure may also impair reabsorption of CSF as in a subdural hygroma or arteriovenous malformation. The causes of overproduction of CSF are not generally known and are rare.

Symptoms

The child with hydrocephalus will present with an increase in the vault of the skull resulting in a prominent forehead, stretched skin, which gives it a shiny appearance, and prominent scalp veins caused by stretching and engorgement. The child may have 'sunset eyes', a phenomenon that arises because the eyebrows and lids are drawn upwards to expose the sclera above the iris; and makes it difficult for the child to gaze upwards.

Other signs which may be present are those of raised intracranial pressure, i.e. restlessness and irritability due to headache and, vomiting. Raised intracranial pressure is not always immediately apparent in all cases as the flexibility of the newborn skull does accommodate some increase, but this mechanism is soon overridden. An increase in the size of the head, as shown when measuring the occipital-frontal circumference, in combination with delayed closure of the fontanelles, would also be indicative of the development of hydrocephalus.

Additionally, the child may display widespread sutures, bulging fontanelles, lethargy, seizure activity and in later development, may have difficulty holding his head upright. A distinct high pitched cry is also evident. Alterations in the vital signs are in keeping with those found in raised intracranial pressure, i.e. bradycardia, raised blood pressure and slow irregular respirations.

Diagnosis will be confirmed with CT scanning, which will demonstrate enlarged ventricles and possibly the original pathology which has led to the development of hydrocephalus. If access to CT scanning is not possible diagnosis may be based on skull X-ray, i.e. wide sutures, bulging fontanelles, possibly bone erosion, caused by deficient ossification which gives rise to flat bones (cranio-lacunia) or thin areas which indent on pressure. Percussion of the skull will produce a 'cracked pot' sound (MacEwen's sign). Papilloedema will also be present.

Treatment

Treatment in most instances is by the insertion of a shunt which will divert the excess CSF from the ventricles into either the atrium or the peritoneum for dispersal. Some sources advocate the use of the diuretic, isosorbide, in mild cases or following surgery on a child with a meningocele, where hydrocephalus is not immediately apparent. This may delay or avoid the need for surgery.

Modern shunting systems are available in a variety of forms. Most incorporate a device to allow testing or manual pumping of the shunt and valves which are set at low, medium or high pressure to prevent reflux and to control the rate at which CSF is drained. A burr hole is created in the temporal parietal region and a measured length of silastic tubing is passed into the lateral ventricle. A valve is connected and the other end of the shunt is passed subcutaneously to either the atrium of the heart or the peritoneum and the entire system is then connected, providing a bypass route for the CSF.

SPINA BIFIDA

Spina bifida is a developmental abnormality resulting in a malformation in which the bony casing of the spine fails to fuse allowing the spinal cord and meninges to protrude. The lumbar and occipital regions are the two most common sites. The following different types of spina bifida have been identified (Fig. 15.1):

Spina bifida occulta. This is the most common and least troublesome. There is often no external evidence of the deformity and many individuals are completely unaware of its presence as it does not cause them any problems. There is no external sac although some children may have a hairy haemangiomatous patch at the site of the hidden defect.

Spina bifida cystica. This presents either as a meningocele, in which there is protrusion

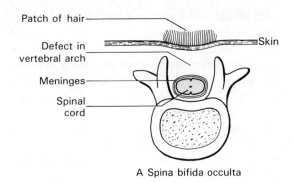

A Spina bifida occulta

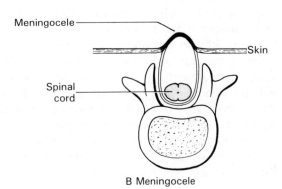

B Meningocele

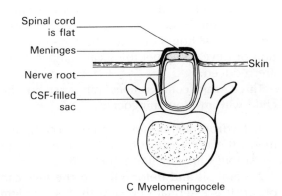

C Myelomeningocele

Fig. 15.1

of the meninges to form a sac containing CSF and covered with skin, or as a more severe form, myelomeningocele. This involves protrusion of the spinal cord and meninges often without a covering skin.

Diagnosis is by routine clinical examination of the newborn. Hydrocephalus often occurs in conjunction with spina bifida and its presence should raise suspicion. In the older child, weakened limbs and bladder and bowel incontinence are suggestions of a spinal lesion. Although difficult to elucidate in the newborn incontinence may also be a feature, e.g. faecal incontinence is recognised as a continual flow of faeces as opposed to a more regular normal pattern.

Treatment is by surgical resection. In a child with a meningocele this involves excision of the sac and repair of the dura. Following this the skin is closed over the defect. These children make a good recovery although some may be left with a residual deficit, e.g. incontinence if the lesion is sacral.

The child with a myelomeningocele presents a major medical and ethical problem. Despite surgical treatment, up to 25% of the children will be dead within 1 year of life and those who survive may develop further neurological problems; 80% will develop hydrocephalus, and urological and orthopaedic complications for the rest of their lives. In contrast there are those who will embark on an aggressive treatment programme having consulted with the child's parents, and sympathetically explained the situation. If the child is operated on early, i.e. within 48 hours of birth, the risks of infection or developing neurological complications are reduced.

Three main complications can arise in the child with myelomeningocele:

1. Hydrocephalus is a common accompaniment, the usual cause being the presence of an Arnold-Chiari malformation.
2. Paralysis and deformities to the legs can occur. It is essential to deal with this problem as it arises, i.e. the child's ability to walk may be enhanced by the use of splints and calipers. The child's quality of life will be improved dramatically if he is independently mobile as opposed to being confined to a wheel chair.
3. Impaired innervation of the bladder and bowel leads to the development of incontinence.

The incidence (1–4:1000 of live births) has been reduced since the introduction of screening for alphafetoprotein. This is a plasma protein, the level of which will be elevated in the maternal blood serum if the mother is carrying a child with a neural tube defect. This diagnosis can be confirmed by proceeding to amniocentesis, with a view to establishing a more accurate level of alphafetoprotein.

The initial blood screening would be indicated in those women who have a family history of spina bifida and indeed is performed in some centres as part of their routine prenatal diagnostic programme for all pregnancies. If the alphafetoprotein level in the amniotic fluid is raised, a decision will be made whether to abort the fetus or not. This is essentially a decision for the parents to make. A clear explanation of the facts and considerate and continual support must be provided by the health carers involved. Complex situations like this may be governed by other factors such as religious or cultural backgrounds.

Despite the reduction in the numbers of children born with spina bifida, advancing technology and better care of the handicapped child has now created a new set of problems. These children now live longer and so new social and psychological problems are arising for the first time.

The birth of a handicapped baby at what should be a happy time for the parents can have a profoundly devastating effect on them and their family. It is possible that not all the complications are evident at birth, therefore continual reassessment of the child and repeated explanation to the parents is essential. If a good rapport is established between the parents and the medical and nursing staff any decision to be made regarding treatment can be undertaken in a trusting and supportive atmosphere. The strange and unreal world in which the parents find themselves can lead to confusion as to what they consider is best for their child. In the past, many parents and health care staff have found themselves caught up in an ethical dilemma in relation to the level of treatment.

Nursing management of a child with spina bifida and hydrocephalus

Maintaining a safe environment

During the pre- and postoperative phase the child is nursed in an incubator or baby therm. Both these devices enable the maintenance of an appropriate external environment and provide warmth and protection from noise and infection. Reduction of noise either from staff conversing or the use of equipment associated with the incubator must be achieved. The baby with raised intracranial pressure will be sensitive to excessive noise. As the newborn baby has not yet developed an effective auto-immune system additional precautions will be necessary, e.g. good preventive cross-infection techniques particularly when handling the lesion prior to surgery.

Meticulous checking procedures are required prior to the administration of medication. In the pre-operative period, this will include vitamin K given as the newborn has not yet begun to manufacture his own and which is essential for blood clotting, particularly if surgery is imminent. Other drugs which may be given include antibiotics and analgesia, though not all centres advocate the use of analgesia in the newborn as the level of actual pain felt is debatable.

The child will be at risk due to the loss of sensory information as a result of poor circulation. This will necessitate regular turning and is dealt with in more detail under mobilising.

Observations and the provision of safety during a seizure will be necessary. Prevention of injury is achieved with the use of padding around the child's head. Access to oxygen and suction apparatus is also essential.

Controlling body temperature

It is well established that the newborn child is unable to maintain his own body temperature and is more sensitive to the fluctuation of the environmental temperature. For this reason, these babies are nursed in an incubator or baby therm. Modern incubators have alarm systems which should be utilised; however, they should not be viewed as a substitute for diligent nursing observation. Regular checking of the baby's core and peripheral temperature is essential.

Breathing

Observation of the child's breathing pre- and postoperatively will be performed as part of the routine monitoring of the vital signs. Respiratory rate, depth, volume and colour of the child are noted. An alteration in these normal parameters may be indicative of rising intracranial pressure, the onset of infection within the respiratory tract, or possibly the presence of an anomaly in the lungs.

If intracranial pressure is increasing, either in the pre-operative period due to hydrocephalus or in the postoperative period due to shunt failure, this will affect the respiratory vital centres located in the medulla. This will produce a decrease in the respiratory rate eventually leading to apnoea, if left unchecked. Any downward trend in the respiratory pattern should be reported immediately. The use of effective infection control, as already discussed, will contribute to the prevention of this breathing problem.

Personal cleansing and dressing

The child with an exposed spinal lesion will have this covered with saline-soaked gauze swabs to prevent drying out of the delicate nerve tissue pre-operatively.

In the postoperative period either following resection of a spinal anomaly or the insertion of a shunt, all dressings should be observed for the signs of leakage. Escaping CSF presents a major infection risk to the child, and this may be disguised with blood. Sutures are removed from the child's back at 10–12 days and from the head, at 3–5 days. Any drains which may be in place should be observed.

The child's regular personal hygiene will

also require attention. In particular, incontinence will increase the risk of skin breakdown in a child who is already at risk due to poor circulation. The condition of the skin over the hydrocephalic child's head should be regularly checked. Frequent turning will prevent the development of pressure sores. Again this can serve as a useful teaching point for the parents.

Eating and drinking

Where possible the child is fed orally, and failing this an intravenous infusion would be commenced. Nursing activities are performed prior to feeding to allow the child to rest after the feed. The hydrocephalic child is fed with his head well supported probably by the use of a pillow. If this is impractical, then cot feeding may be necessary. As a lengthy period of time may be necessary when feeding the child the nurse should position herself in a comfortable, well supported sitting position. Once the child is fed, he is placed on his side, in a slightly head-up tilt to avoid aspiration. If surgery is contemplated, then the baby will require to be fasted for a few hours.

Initially following surgery a nasogastric tube will be in situ and left on free drainage, possibly with hourly aspiration, to prevent abdominal distension. Feeding will recommence 4–6 hours later with a dextrose solution gradually progressing to milk feeds.

Eliminating

Pre-operatively the newborn baby with spina bifida is continually incontinent of both urine and faeces. The appropriate personal hygiene will be performed.

Postoperatively, observation of bowel and bladder function continues. Regular cultures of urine may be taken. Intravenous pylography may be indicated in the older child with urinary problems. Manual expression of the bladder may be necessary again in the older child. The opportunity should be taken to teach this technique to the parents. If urine collection and measurement prove difficult, then a urine bag may be used. If the child's condition permits, the cot may be elevated slightly to prevent backflow of urine. In the long-term, ileal conduit may be considered.

Communicating

The benefits of stimulating the newborn child verbally and by gentle touch are well established although this must be limited bearing in mind that this particular child is sensitive to excessive noise and disturbance.

The parents should be kept informed of progress or changes in the child's condition. This is best achieved through a caring and trusting relationship between medical staff, nurses and the parents. Where appropriate they may wish to participate in the child's care. It is important that the health care staff establish the degree of the parents' understanding of the condition.

Sleeping

Assessment of conscious level, preferably with a standardised paediatric coma scale is crucial. The level of consciousness is an accurate indicator of brain function and therefore would alert carers to a rise in intracranial pressure. Assessment would be performed along with regular measurement of the occipital-frontal circumference in the hydrocephalic child. The results are tabulated on a graph and this along with signs of bulging fontanelles and a deterioration in conscious level would confirm a rise in intracranial pressure. Other parameters which may be measured include pupillary changes, apex heart beat, respirations and limb movements.

On return from surgery observations would be maintained. A lack of progress may be indicative of a non-functioning shunt. Some centres advocate 'pumping' the shunt's reservoir to encourage drainage but it is recommended that departmental policy on this should be clearly established.

Another potential problem in the postoperative period which may affect conscious level is the development of a subdural haematoma. This may occur as a result of rapid drainage of CSF in the child with a shunt, leading to release of pressure on a previously slowly bleeding blood vessel. The additional space now created leads to the formation of a haematoma which needs evacuation. In this instance the fontanelles are found to be sunken.

Mobilising

During the pre-operative period, the degree of limb movement and muscle strength will be assessed.

The child is nursed flat, on either side and position is changed frequently. The development of skin breakdown is a constant threat both in hydrocephalus and spina bifida; a combination of both conditions increases the risk factor.

In the postoperative period the patient continues to be nursed flat. The hydrocephalic child is nursed on the side opposite the operation site initially, and put on a regular turning schedule. Spinal surgery demands that the child is nursed in the prone position prior to embarking on a turning schedule. Nursing the child prone avoids pressure on the back wound, until healing begins to take place.

Gentle passive range of movement exercises are performed within the limitations of minimal handling.

PSYCHOLOGICAL CARE

Support of the parents and family of a newly diagnosed handicapped child cannot be over emphasised. The uptake of information during what is an emotionally traumatic period can be diminished. The nursing staff must observe the parents and try to assess their level of understanding. Decisions based on the available knowledge need to be made by the parents with regard to the extent of treatment. A trusting and caring relationship needs to be developed between the parents and health care team. The shock of the birth can stun and confuse the parents, who have to make decisions when time is at a premium. The extent of future problems should be explained to the parents and may have to be continually repeated. Acceptance and understanding in the early stages are important as the child will meet with emotional problems later in life and will need their support. These problems will centre round society's indifference to disabled persons. Mildly handicapped children are now being integrated into normal nurseries and schools which greatly helps in the development of the child, relieves some of the burden on the parents and it is hoped helps to educate society, particularly tomorrow's adults into acceptance of handicapped people.

A great deal of time will be spent in hospital for revision operations and the child can easily become institutionalised. The provision of mother and child accommodation will help to ease the strain on the family, although problems such as jealousy, can arise within the family. Advice and help from a support group may also be beneficial.

Teaching the parents how to care for their child will allow the child to remain at home for longer periods of time, also maintain the family unit, and lessen the strain of separation during hospital stays. Topics included in the teaching plan would be:

- skin care including the importance of turning schedules
- importance of touch, speech, play and stimulation
- use of exercises to aid muscle tone
- feeding techniques and emotional care and support.

Other problems would be dealt with as they occurred as not all physical and psychological are apparent at birth.

Dying

Despite the advances in surgery or in those cases in which surgery is not deemed appropriate, some children born with hydro-cephalus and/or spina bifida die. The care appropriate to any dying child and his family would be provided. This is beyond the scope of this book and the reader is referred to the many specialised textbooks which deal with this aspect.

BIBLIOGRAPHY

Brunner L S, Suddarth D S 1986 Manual of paediatric nursing, 2nd edn. Harper and Row, London
Gamstrop I 1985 Paediatric neurology, 2nd edn. Butterworths, London
Purchese G, Allan D 1984 Neuromedical and neurosurgical nursing, 2nd edn. Baillière Tindall, London

16

Care of the patient with epilepsy

INCIDENCE

Epilepsy represents one of the most common neurological disorders in the world. It is difficult to determine the exact number of people who have an epileptic disorder. Seizures can be concealed, and except during an attack, a person may show no indication of the disorder. Some people may have epilepsy but do not consult their doctor and so the condition is not diagnosed. The statistics which do exist depend on the diagnostic skills of physicians, the willingness of people to consult medical advisors when they have an epileptic disorder, and the accuracy of record keeping.

The incidence of epilepsy (nonfebrile seizures) in a general population has been estimated at 20–50 cases per 100 000 per year, and patterns do not follow any particular national or racial difference. Most studies have found a slightly higher incidence among males. The prevalence rate of epilepsy varies depending on where the study was conducted, i.e. hospital or community, as well as how the condition was defined. Prevalence rates are highest among children, particularly in the first 5 years of life. Estimates of the prevalence of epilepsy in Britain and USA range from 6.57 to 18.6 cases per 1000 population. There are around 300 000 people with epilepsy in England and Wales, about 8 per 1000 of the population and it is more common in men than in women (Jeavons & Aspinall, 1985).

CAUSES OF EPILEPSY

Epilepsy is a symptom, not a disease — the seizure is a physical manifestation of excessive electrical discharges in the neurones of the brain. Anything that affects the cortex of the brain where most of the neurones are, can cause changes which produce one of the epileptic disorders. Some people are more liable to seizures than others. Perhaps in some people the brain cells are less able to suppress electrical discharges. In some instances a definite cause can be found, while in most people who do have an epileptic disorder, no definitive cause is found; medically this is known as idiopathic epilepsy. An important factor which is considered when investigating the cause of epilepsy is the age of onset of the problem, because injury at birth, or in the school playground, or a childhood illness could be significant, whereas strokes, a brain tumour or head trauma could be more relevant in older people with epilepsy.

When both the cause of seizures and the origin of the electrical discharges are understood, the person has symptomatic epilepsy (see Table 16.1). If an irritation of the surrounding cells in a specific area of the brain produces electrical discharges, these spread and a fit occurs. Such a 'focus' may be

Table 16.1 Symptomatic epilepsy

Disease of the brain
Tumour
Head injury
Cerebral vascular disease
Inflammation of the brain or its coverings (encephalitis or meningitis)
Intracranial surgery
Abscesses

Disease of the body affecting the brain
Tuberous sclerosis
Lipidoses
Febrile convulsions
Hypoglycaemia
Hyperglycaemia
Chronic alcohol abuse
Dementia
Stroke
Angioma
Kidney disease

Table 16.2 Classification of seizures

Partial (focal) seizures
Simple partial seizure
  motor
  sensory
  automatic
Complex partial seizure
Partial seizure evolving to secondarily generalised tonic-clonic convulsion

Generalised seizures (convulsive or nonconvulsive)
Absence seizures (typical and atypical)
Myoclonic seizures
Clonic seizures
Tonic seizures
Tonic-clonic seizures
Atonic seizures (astatic)
Unclassified epileptic seizures

caused by a head injury, an infection of the brain or diseases of the blood vessels of the brain. Symptomatic epilepsy may also result from a vascular or pulmonary disease which interrupts the flow of oxygen to the brain causing seizures. Kidney disease causing unfiltered blood to reach the brain may also precipitate an epileptic seizure.

CLASSIFICATION (Table 16.2)

The classification of epileptic seizures has been the subject of continual debate in recent years. In 1969, an internationally agreed classification was formulated, which has been recently revised and laid out in an easily understood manner (Shorvon, 1984). This scheme is now generally used in specialist practice, so that nurses need to learn these new terms which are more explicit than the former clumsy anatomical descriptions. The scheme is based on clinical and electroencephalographic findings divided into partial and generalised attacks.

DESCRIPTION OF SEIZURES

The new categorisation of seizures provides a framework for description. Seizure activity, when it occurs, does not always necessarily follow a classical textbook pattern. As already outlined, seizures are divided into partial or generalised. Partial seizures are produced as a result of a localised disturbance confined to a small area of the brain, whereas generalised fits are caused by a widespread disturbance of brain activity.

Seizures can manifest themselves in various presentations ranging from a momentary loss of concentration through to complete loss of consciousness.

Simple partial seizures

A focus within a particular part of the brain, usually the motor strip is irritated, producing a disturbance in function of the affected area of the body. Hands and face are two common sites affected. A focal seizure typically manifests itself as a twitching of the thumb or the side of the face. The patient remains aware throughout the seizure. The twitching in a focal seizure remains isolated but when it spreads to affect other parts of the body it is described as a Jacksonian fit or a simple partial seizure with marching, e.g. a twitch may be noticed in the patient's right thumb, This becomes progressively worse involving initially the arm and then spreads (or marches) to include all the affected side of the body.

Complex partial seizures

These originate in the temporal lobe where an irritant may produce a characteristic and distinctive type of seizure. It may be preceded by an aura, e.g. pins and needles, followed by an episode of altered behaviour in which the patient performs a number of peculiar movements and/or sequences and yet remains in communication with those around him. Automatism often occurs in which the patient may continually rub his hands together, pluck at his clothes or demonstrate distorted facial expressions. This type of seizure activity is also characteristically accompanied by sensory experiences. The patient may hallucinate, or state that he can smell something or complain of unusual gustatory experiences. The halluci-nations may comprise, typically, a feeling of déja vu, in which the person experiences familiarity with an unfamiliar situation.

Absence seizures

These comprise a brief alteration in consciousness, which onlookers often do not notice. It occurs in childhood and is termed as simple. In complex absences, the brief alteration of consciousness is also accompanied by a process termed automatism. In this the patient persistently repeats a movement, e.g. nodding of the head or rhythmical jerking of the arms.

Myoclonic seizures

Sudden, repeated jerking movements of one or more of the limbs occur during which there is a momentary loss of consciousness. This most often occurs in the early morning, within 1 hour of waking. Myoclonic jerks can occur in clusters and continue for hours at a time. If standing, the person would fall to the ground.

Tonic seizures

These may occur alone or as part of a tonic-clonic seizure. It commences with a sudden loss of body posture, characteristically the arms flex and the legs extend. Loss of consciousness usually occurs and respiration may cease for a time.

Tonic-atonic seizures

This seizure has the element of the tonic episode in which the muscles stiffen but atony also occurs, i.e. loss of tone. This stiffening/slackening routine can be repeated several times during which there is loss of consciousness.

Tonic-clonic seizures

This is the type of seizure that most people associate with epilepsy. It comprises several distinct stages; the first is the aura. This does not occur in everyone having a tonic-clonic fit, but when it does it can take the form of a strange feeling or taste in the mouth. It essentially acts as a warning of the impending fit. This is fortunate, as those patients who are able to recognise the warning can place themselves in a position of safety. As the seizure proper commences there is sudden loss of consciousness and if the patient is standing, he falls to the ground. The body stiffens as the seizure enters the tonic phase. The jaw closes tight shut and the patient may utter a cry as the thoracic muscles contract and air is forcefully ejected via the vocal chords. Cyanosis is evident as the patient is often apnoeic at this stage. Urinary and/or faecal incontinence may occur.

The tonic part of the seizure is characterised by rhythmic jerking of the limbs and stertorous breathing. Excess production of saliva during this stage is manifested as frothing at the mouth. The patient is usually tachycardic and sweating. The jerking movements

gradually slow down and the patient usually lapses into coma. The clonic phase lasts 1–3 minutes. The patient will now sleep for a number of hours and on wakening is usually amnesic for the events that have occurred and may be very drowsy and confused.

MEDICAL TREATMENT OF EPILEPSY

Anticonvulsant drugs (Table 16.3) can suppress seizures by either abolishing or reducing the amount of abnormal electrical activity in brain cells. In order to be able to do so they must reach the brain tissue where the convulsive activity begins. When a drug is swallowed it is absorbed from the bowel into the bloodstream where it is carried by protein molecules. When it reaches the brain, the drug diffuses into the fluid surrounding each nerve cell. The drug moves freely between the bloodstream and the brain. If the level of the drug in the blood increases, more moves into the brain and vice versa if the level is reduced.

Table 16.3 Drug treatment for epilepsy

First line drugs		
phenytoin (Epanutin)	Average daily dose 200–400 mg Once or twice daily	Generalised tonic-clonic and partial fits; serum level monitoring essential
carbamazepine (Tegretol)	Average daily dose range 600–1200 mg two or three times daily	Generalised tonic-clonic and partial fits
sodium valproate (Epilim)	Average daily dose 600–1500 mg once or twice daily	Generalised tonic-clonic and partial fits and absences
ethosuximide (Zarontin)	Average daily dose range 500–1000 mg on mg/kg basis for children and adults, two or three times daily	Effective against absences only
Second line drugs		
clonazepam (Rivotril)	Average daily dose range 1–3 mg twice daily	Partial fits, absences and myoclonic jerks
clobazam (Frisium)	Average daily dose range 10–30 mg once daily	Generalised tonic-clonic and partial fits, but tolerance frequently develops
primidone (Mysoline)	Average daily dose range (adults) 500–1000 mg twice daily	Generalised tonic-clonic and partial fits
phenobarbitone	Average daily dose (adults) 60–120 mg once or twice daily	Generalised tonic-clonic and partial fits

This means that, for most drugs, the anticonvulsant activity is related to the level in the blood.

The body detoxifies drugs by metabolism in the liver and subsequently excretion into the urine. The faster the breakdown, the less the drug will accumulate and the lower will be the blood level. It is not possible to predict the way a person will absorb and then eliminate a drug as this varies from person to person. Therefore, effective and toxic doses of the same drug may vary greatly from patient to patient. The rate of breakdown of an anticonvulsant in an individual varies with age, state of health, other drug treatment and sometimes with alcohol intake.

It has been known for years that excessive amounts of anticonvulsive medication can cause toxic side-effects. The unwanted symptoms are dose related: they can usually be abolished by reducing the dose. Before anticonvulsant blood level estimation was available, it was not uncommon for patients to take high doses of anticonvulsants, often to the point of developing toxic symptoms, in order to achieve seizure control.

With the development of technology for estimation of anticonvulsant blood levels, it became possible to determine more precisely the necessary dose for each individual patient. Measuring blood levels provides an estimate of the amount of the drug in the brain and of the resulting anticonvulsant effect for the person investigated. The most significant thing which has been learnt from the estimation of serum anticonvulsant levels is that the many drugs which doctors traditionally prescribed for their patient with epilepsy may have been less successful in achieving its aims than careful monitoring of serum levels of fewer drugs. The aim of treatment is to prescribe enough medication to balance the continuous elimination by the liver and kidneys. Sometimes monitoring plasma levels offers the only way of ensuring optimal dosages of drugs or of avoiding toxicity (Reynolds & Zander 1982).

In the past, if a patient's seizures were not well controlled with a standard anticonvulsant regimen, it was customary either to increase the dose with the risk of inducing toxic serum levels or add a second drug. Polypharmacy (the prescription of more than one drug simultaneously for the treatment of a given condition) has many disadvantages. When estimations of serum anticonvulsant levels became available, it was clear that some of the 'failures' of single drug therapy were due to poor patient compliance, while in other cases, satisfactory seizure control could be achieved by increasing the dose to give levels at the top end of the therapeutic range. Serum levels are most useful for monitoring therapy with phenytoin, barbiturates (including primidone) and carbamazepine. Serum levels will also usually incriminate the offending agent should toxicity occur when a patient is being treated by a combination of anticonvulsants.

Richens (1980) explains that determination of serum drug levels will improve the quality of medical care for patients taking anticonvulsants. When a drug dosage is being increased, the additional amount is more easily determined when the drug serum level is known, particularly for phenytoin, for which small increases in dosage can result in dramatic increases in blood level which would be toxic. In many patients drug levels remain low, in spite of a large dose being prescribed. Knowledge of the blood level enables the doctor to identify the cause of the effects of medication, either metabolic absorption rates, poor compliance or toxicity. When drug levels suddenly change in spite of no alterations in prescriptions, this could be due to drug interactions or to the presence of some other disease.

Monotherapy versus polytherapy

Disadvantages of polytherapy

1. The complex interrelation between the various compounds results in a less predictable response. The administration of several drugs together makes monitoring the situation and maintaining an optimal blood level very random.

2. The more drugs a person has to take daily, the more he will rebel and either take them sporadically or not at all. There is a risk of confusion between tablets.

3. It is depressing for people to feel that their epilepsy is so bad that they have to take 'all those drugs'. A person may feel that the number of drugs prescribed indicates the severity or difficulty of his or her epilepsy.

4. The sedative effect of a combination of anticonvulsant drugs may be more than the sum of each drug if it was taken separately. The effect of combining two or more drugs is not simply additive, one drug enhances or retards the action of another.

5. In some patients polytherapy exacerbates seizures, as seen when they are weaned off the multiple therapy, and seizure frequency falls.

Benefits of monotherapy

1. Fewer risks of drug interaction.
2. Improved cognitive function and mood. One study found that a year after the reduction of treatment the control of seizures was improved in 16 patients out of 40 (55%) and their mental function was improved (Shorvon & Reynolds 1979).
3. The less drugs one has to take, the more likely the person complies with the prescription, than if there are several to remember to take.
4. The more rapid establishment of a therapeutic blood level, the greater ease of maintenance of the blood level is possible.

Having established beyond doubt that the patient has epilepsy, the decision to treat is based on the number of attacks, their severity and type, the presence of other disorders, triggering factors and the person's domestic and social circumstances. A compromise may have to be made between seizure control and the potential harmful effects of therapy which would be for some years.

When anticonvulsant treatment is begun or doses are changed, it usually takes several days or weeks for plasma and brain levels to stabilise, and further seizures may occur during this time. A drug is introduced in the lowest generally effective dose in order to minimise side-effects which are often worse at the onset of therapy. The dose may have to be increased until fits are controlled, or side-effects become evident. Where facilities exist (in hospital clinics) the blood levels of drugs are taken to confirm that they are in the therapeutic range, and to check on compliance (see Table 16.3 for details of anticonvulsants commonly used).

Maintaining treatment

If, despite gradually increasing doses of a drug, the patient still has seizures, it is necessary to ensure that he or she is actually taking the drug as prescribed. Some discussion may be necessary to ascertain how rigorously the doctor's advice is followed. We must never be judgemental towards patients, and it helps to remember that taking prescribed medications may be a threat to a person's feeling of self-control. Having ascertained that the drug is being administered as required, the drug level is investigated. If the level is almost at the optimum therapeutic range, or if toxic effects have begun to appear, then a decision may be made to discontinue the drug very gradually and substitute another first-choice drug simultaneously. The aim of anticonvulsant therapy is to keep the drug regime as simple as possible in order to minimise drug side-effects, reduce chronic toxicity and to encourage people to take the drugs which are prescribed for them.

Most anticonvulsant drugs increase the amount of the liver enzymes that are responsible for the metabolism of steroid hormones. The oral contraceptive pill is also metabolised by these enzymes and so may be ineffective in preventing pregnancy. Sodium valproate does not induce hepatic enzymes, and is the anticonvulsant of choice for women on the pill. If they must continue on another anticonvulsant, a pill containing high doses of oestrogen may be prescribed, and the woman is advised that it may be ineffective.

Should a woman become pregnant while taking an anticonvulsant, there is a small risk that the baby will develop a congenital abnormality. This is about 3% for phenytoin but the risk of other anticonvulsants has not been assessed. As both mother and fetus may be harmed by hypoxia during an uncontrolled seizure, most neurologists would recommend that a person with epilepsy should continue on anticonvulsants (preferably monotherapy) during pregnancy as the risks of congenital abnormalities are very low. Seizures occurring for the first time during pregnancy are treated in the usual way.

Anticonvulsant metabolism is altered during pregnancy and serum levels should be checked frequently during the first and third trimester so that the appropriate changes in dose may be made.

Recent studies of the natural history of epilepsy suggest that 50% of patients who have not had a seizure for 2 years will remain free of attacks. It would seem reasonable to discontinue therapy if a patient has been free of attacks for 2 years, with the understanding that treatment will need to be reinstituted if seizures recur. The current legal requirement is that a patient should be free of all daytime seizures whether on or off therapy for 2 years before holding a driving licence. Therefore, if a patient needs to drive, he or she may be better advised to continue therapy rather than run the risk of a further seizure.

The current recommendation is that anticonvulsants should be withdrawn slowly over a series of months, as it is observed that patients tend to have recurrent attacks if their medication is withdrawn abruptly.

Side-effects of anticonvulsant drugs

In anticonvulsant medication, side-effects are caused by:

- idiosyncratic hypersensitivity (allergic) reactions
- acute (dose-related) effects
- chronic effects.

1. **Hypersensitivity** is experienced usually within the first few days or months of commencing medication. Toxic effects are seen in about 5–10% of patients started on phenytoin or carbamazepine, but are less with sodium valproate therapy. An idiosyncratic reaction is one that cannot be predicted from one patient to another. Idiosyncratic effects of anticonvulsant drugs affect primarily the skin. Occasionally the capacity of the bone marrow to form blood cells is affected.

2. **Side-effects** that are dose-related may appear in patients whose anticonvulsant level is in the toxic range. They include fatigue, transient sleepiness, severe lethargy, ataxia (balance problems), slurred speech and all the appearances of alcoholic intoxication. These dose-related side-effects can be reversed by lowering the dose, or prevented, by monitoring the serum levels of the drug being taken by each patient.

3. **The long-term toxic side-effects** of anticonvulsant medication are not clearly dose-dependent, They may be insidious and only slowly progressive, which means that it may take some time for the patient, relatives, nurses or doctor to identify the changes taking place. Shorvon (1984) states that 'many of these toxic side effects remained unrecognised for many years and no doubt many remain to be discovered.' Side-effects vary in degree with each individual person receiving prolonged medication, so that people taking phenytoin for some years can experience gum swelling, drowsiness or unsteadiness; other drugs may cause behaviour changes such as aggression and irritability.

STIGMA TOWARDS PEOPLE WITH EPILEPSY

There is evidence that individuals with epilepsy are regarded with hostility and denied adequate medical and social care, in a wide variety of cultures. In pre-technological societies, people with epilepsy have been subject to ridicule and outcast and to beliefs about aetiology, which imply social rejection (Levy et al 1964, Dada 1968).

The importance of public attitudes for people with a disability

Whether or not epilepsy itself prevents people who have it from working, other people's attitudes may. Generally speaking, a handicap is not just a condition, but a relationship between an individual human being and society, so that a handicapped person is as handicapped as society makes him or her. The capacity for functioning is therefore dependent on the attitudes this person encounters. Public and professional ignorance of epilepsy can be even more disabling than the condition itself. Rejected by society and deprived of essential life opportunities, the person with epilepsy may live-down to expectancy which confirms the prejudice and misunderstanding of the non-epileptic person and reinforces discriminatory attitudes and behaviour.

Public attitudes towards people with epilepsy

The first systematic study of the opinions and attitudes toward epilepsy was made in the United States in the late 1940s (Caveness 1949). The study has been repeated at 5-yearly intervals on representative samples of the total population (Caveness et al 1974). The practice of monitoring attitudes toward epilepsy has spread widely. By the 1960s, several countries had produced reports of public attitudes to epilepsy.

Bagley (1972) investigated the extent to which these hostile attitudes to epilepsy are manifest in western cultures, and to what extent individuals can be free from prejudice about epilepsy. He found that people with epilepsy are rejected not only in pre-technological societies, but in technological ones as well. A more recent study claimed that 'even highly developed societies contain a certain degree of prejudice and superstition, resulting in serious problems for persons with epilepsy' (Loyning 1980).

German public opinion polls conducted in 1967 and in the early 1970s revealed the gloomy view that 'whether most places of work in the Federal Republic are truly ready to employ people with seizures is still an open question' (Diehl 1976). People with epilepsy were often regarded as 'bad tempered, suspicious, outsiders, moody and aggressive' (Remschmidt 1973). A Norwegian doctor concluded that: 'As long as physicians are unable to prevent the development of unpredictable bursts of epileptic brain activity, the very nature of epileptic seizures is bound to create psychosocial problems and some prejudice and suspicion in any society of the world, regardless of its general level of knowledge and understanding' (Loyning 1980).

In the United Kingdom, Bagley (1972) found evidence that social prejudice occurred at all levels — in the fields of employment, education and even in medical care. He found that people with epilepsy are regarded with more hostility than the mentally ill and than people with cerebral palsy.

It may be claimed that people with epilepsy are more disabled by the ignorant attitudes of other people than by the disorder itself. Scambler & Hopkins (1986) found that there is a lay belief that a person with epilepsy is bad and that 'being epileptic' is what disturbs people, rather than having seizures. The experiences recounted by people with an epileptic disorder include such comments as: 'I was made to feel like an "untouchable" by the medical personnel, before being passed fit for employment.' A young woman explained to her potential employer: 'I certainly have not contracted a disease', but he replied; 'We can't employ you here, you have epilepsy.' She was devastated, even more so when she applied for similar jobs and was turned down for the same reasons. She had not had a fit for 5 years (Floyd 1983).

Bagley (1972) considered a hypothesis of fear as the basis of prejudice in different kinds of cultures and directed to different groups of people. Fears of homosexual's behaviour may be due to our own fears of homosexual aspects of our own natures. Fears of coloured people may stem partly from a fear that the black man is primitive and savage, whose reactions to any given situation are unpredictable, someone who could act with irrational savage strength. The person with epilepsy is feared because, without warning, and in any situation, he may unpredictably lose control of his movements, and loss of control is something we are afraid of happening to ourselves. A person who reverts to the 'primitive' is punished by social rejection and ostracism, which then appears to be justified. Prejudice against people with epilepsy and coloured people has, according to Bagley, its basis in an irrational fear of the unpredictable.

RECEIVING THE 'BAD' NEWS — DENIAL

When a patient, and his family, are faced for the first time, with the diagnosis of epilepsy, there is almost invariably a feeling of intense shock of inevitable disaster. They go through a painful period of adjustment. The idea of having something wrong with the brain immobilises many individuals. Some are afraid to ask questions or are afraid to listen to what the doctor or nurse is telling them. Parents refuse to admit that their child has epilepsy, that a product of themselves is imperfect. In many cases, the parents or the patient will insist that they do not have epilepsy, but a seizure disorder. The sadness and dismay aroused by a diagnosis of epilepsy lead parents to search for a different diagnosis. The consequences of having epilepsy, as the patient sees it, are distorted by misconceptions, ignorance, mood disorder or misunderstanding by others. People who are told that they have epilepsy may consider this a dreadful diagnosis which has to be resisted at all costs.

If the patient feels that the word 'epilepsy' means disaster, his or her reaction is based on irrational fears. It is only those of us who know the facts about epilepsy who can recognise the common misconceptions as being irrational. The diagnosis may remind the patient of a convulsive, brain-damaged village idiot, and he therefore assumes that this means that he will be less intelligent or that his personality will be less than perfect. On the other hand, denial of the diagnosis of epilepsy may be just the initial stage of adapting to chronic illness, a necessary process for everyone who has to face up to an altered self-image and identity.

It must be acknowledged, however, that some misconceptions of epilepsy are so frightening that people are never able to accept the diagnosis, the grieving process is blocked. These people talk about their 'turns', 'fainting attacks' or 'dizzy spells'. Denial may continue long after the process of adaptation should have been completed. Long periods of time between seizures tend to support the denial response. The nearer the patient's anticipation of the diagnosis is to reality, the lower the level of fear, and the greater the possibility for adjustment.

The word 'epilepsy' still conjures up the idea of an hereditary degenerative stigmatising condition. The denial may have its roots in the historical association of epilepsy with insanity, infection or evil forces.

DECLARING OR DENYING AN EPILEPTIC DISORDER

Some people have a tendency to conceal information about epilepsy because of their experiences of being outsiders, and their own belief that they are severely handicapped and so they tend to hide any adverse information about seizures. Professional people may not accept their epileptic disorder, because of worries about it impeding their career (Scambler & Hopkins 1980). Older people, conscious of adverse social implications of the label, may adopt a policy of strict secrecy. There are many examples, particularly in the developing countries, of people with epilepsy being ignored or concealed by their family, because of the evil spirits that are thought to be involved. Occasionally a husband in Britain may deny his wife's epilepsy, preferring to describe her condition as 'hysterical'.

The person who has seizures will face the problem of being found out, both at the work level and at the level of interpersonal relations. This constant anxiety that epilepsy will be revealed, or they will have a seizure which may cost them a job, can itself trigger the occurrence of seizures (Honbridge 1981, Floyd 1983).

VICTIMS OR INSTIGATORS?

Despite all the efforts that have been directed towards investigating community attitudes towards people with epilepsy, very little effort has been devoted to evaluating how patients see their own condition or their role in society, or society's expectations of them. A person's observations of how others react to him or her modifies all the person's internal psychological processes, especially the person's self-image. One theory (symbolic interaction) suggests that children and adults with epilepsy may come to internalise views which other people hold about them and have more behaviour problems than individuals who do not have epilepsy (Rutter et al 1970, Bagley 1972).

The stigma of epilepsy self-perpetuates vicious cycles similar to the stigma attached to other differences among people, such as race, religion or physical attractiveness. The situation of people with epilepsy is characterised less by the experience of actual stigmatisation than by a largely false belief that others hold negative attitudes and are ever ready to discriminate. A belief that employers discriminate against epilepsy or fear of rejection by other workers can be self-fulfilling prophecies. Self-denial of opportunities is at least as important as either stigma or sensible discrimination as a cause of employment difficulties. Some people with epilepsy may seem insecure and defensive. It has often been said that behavioural, psychological and social problems may all be greater barriers to employment than the actual seizures (McGuckin 1980, Scambler & Hopkins 1980, Anderson 1981, Antonak & Rankin 1982).

It is usual for individuals who have failed to establish themselves socially or at work, to attribute their failure to other people's preju-dice. There are many cases when the prejudgement is on the part of the patient, when he anticipates non-existent difficulties and adopts a scratchy abrasive mien to those around him. His associates are not put off by his epilepsy but by his own attitude to it and to them (Laidlaw & Laidlaw 1976). Although in one study 90 people referred to epilepsy as stigmatising, only one-third of them could actually give details of even one incident when they suspected another of stigmatising them. Only 23 of the sample with epilepsy who had full-time employment since the onset of their epilepsy, recollected such an incident at work (Scambler & Hopkins 1980).

'We do not need to change the world's view of epilepsy as much as we need to change the world view of those with epilepsy' (McGuckin 1980). Too often problems of those with epilepsy are presented as factors over which they have no control. People with epilepsy are even encouraged to expect bad treatment — they learn a 'victimised' role and are expecting to be at the receiving end of many injustices.

The pattern of examining public attitudes towards epilepsy encourages attention to focus on those cruel people 'out there'; the problems are said to originate in society and rejection of people with an epileptic disorder. Perhaps it is now time to readjust our focus of attention towards the individual whose life has now to include epilepsy. The world is not going to change in order to make life more comfortable for those who feel victimised by cruel stigmatising attitudes. Concentrating on positive aspects of the person with epilepsy may prove to be more constructive, if it means that the self-esteem of the individual is preserved and even strengthened as they re-educate others about their experience of living a full life, even though they also happen to have an epileptic disorder.

WHAT TO DO WHEN A PERSON HAS AN EPILEPTIC FIT

- Stay calm — do not try to restrain or revive the person.

- Help the person into the recovery position on the floor and protect them by putting something soft under the head.
- Remove glasses and loosen any tight clothing. Remove hazards such as hard objects that could cause injury if the person falls or knocks against them.
- If respiration continues to be laboured after the movements have stopped, gently check that saliva, vomit or dentures are not blocking the back of the throat.
- There will be no memory of the seizure activity and the person should not be left alone until fully alert. Some people are quite able to resume their normal routines after a period of sleep or quiet rest. Calm reassurance is needed as the person may feel embarrassed or disorientated after an attack.

WHAT NOT TO DO

- Do not try to revive the person. A seizure cannot be stopped once it has begun.
- **Never** attempt to force anything between the person's teeth — it is impossible to swallow the tongue. Cut tissue on lips or tongue heals, but broken teeth are a social embarrassment.
- There is no need to call a doctor if the seizure ends in under 15 minutes, if consciousness returns without further incident and if there are no signs of injury, physical distress or pregnancy.
- Do not give anything to drink until the person is fully awake.

WHAT TO DO WHEN SOMEONE WITH EPILEPSY HAS A MINOR SEIZURE (NON-CONVULSANT)

Seizures take many different forms, if prolonged confusion occurs:

- Gently protect the person from obvious dangers (wandering into a dangerous area).
- Keep other people from crowding round.

- Speak gently and calmly to the person to help reorientate to surroundings as quickly as possible.
- Stay with the person until he/she is fully orientated. As a convulsive seizure can occur at the end of a minor fit, it is necessary to be prepared for this.

WHAT NOT TO DO

Do not keep asking the person to decide how they need to be helped — their confusion prevents them from being able to respond during the seizure.

RECORDING AN OBSERVED SEIZURE

An important aspect of a patient's time spent in hospital is the observations made by nurses caring for patients 24 hours a day. Detailed records of witnessed seizure activity are necessary for medical staff to plan the treatment of a person with an epileptic disorder.

1. Did the person cry out or attract the nurse's attention in any way?
2. What was the patient doing when the seizure commenced?
3. Did the position of the body change after the onset of the seizure?
4. Did the eyes deviate in one direction? Did the pupils change in size, were they equal or did they react to light during the attack or after?
5. Did the face and lips change colour?
6. Was there frothing at the mouth, flecks of blood?
7. Was there a tonic phase? How long did it last and what parts of the body were involved?
8. Was there twitching or jerking of any particular part of the body? Where did it begin? How did it spread and how long did it last?
9. Was the patient unconscious, and for how long?
10. How was the patient after the attack? Was

he confused or did he have difficulties with speech, or complain of having a headache?

11. How long did the attack last?

12. Did the patient have incontinence of urine or sustain any injury from the attack?

NURSE/PATIENT DISCUSSIONS ABOUT EPILEPSY

The treatment of epilepsy does not end with a diagnosis and a prescription — it really just begins at this stage. From this point on information and knowledge, specific and even broad, concerning a symptom which carries connotations of superstition and prejudice must be directed to the patient, and his or her family and close friends. Because it may be chronic in nature, epilepsy requires thoughtful responses to long-term medication, where a balance has to be struck between the need to control seizures and to minimise side-effects of such medication.

It is necessary for nurses to avoid the pitfall of developing 'patient education' programmes derived from what the nurse thinks the patient should know about his or her medical condition rather than what the patient has identified as personally determined needs. An assessment of each patient and the patient's close family or friends should evaluate the educational, emotional and psychosocial needs of the people concerned (see Fig. 16.1). The information needs of other family members who are concerned about the patient, may also have to be considered. If correct information is not substituted for the misconceptions which family and friends have about epilepsy, the adjustment period for the patient can be very difficult and prolonged and perhaps never fully resolved.

A nurse with particular interest in epileptic disorders, who listens and talks with patients, can assess the educational, emotional and psychosocial needs, concerning these specific themes:

— coping with epilepsy in family and social and occupational life

1. Coping with a threatened self-image
  (i) How do you feel about having epilepsy?
  (ii) How has epilepsy affected your life?
  (iii) Do you experience any special problems as a result of epilepsy?
  (iv) Do you have any particular concerns related to epilepsy?
  (v) How do you cope with the problems which you may have had or do have now?

2. Seizures
  (i) In your opinion, what information should people with epilepsy have available?
  (ii) Are there specific topics regarding your seizure disorder that you would like to know more about? What are they?
  (iii) What type of seizure disorder do you have?
  (iv) What is your understanding of the cause of seizures?
  (v) What does the EEG tell the doctor?
  (vi) What kind of things can bring on a seizure for you?
  (vii) Are they any foods and or beverages that a person with epilepsy should avoid?

3. Medications
  (i) Do you see any benefit from taking your medication?
  (ii) What would happen if you stopped taking your medication?
  (iii) Have you ever had a bad experience related to taking tablets?
  (iv) Do you have any questions, worries or difficulties about your medication?
  (v) Do you feel that you would benefit from additional information about your medication, side-effects, blood tests or any specific theme?

4. Social resources
  (i) Do you know of any voluntary, or statutory agency which you could turn to for help?
  (ii) What is available in your local area if you have specific difficulties relating to epilepsy?
  (iii) Have you ever had any difficulty in getting a job and/or insurance? What were these difficulties and do you know why they occurred?
  (iv) What would you do if you had such difficulties again?

Fig. 16.1 Assessment questionnaire.

— knowledge about seizures
— medications
— occupational problems which patients associate with epilepsy
— topics on which patients feel they need to have more information etc.

A questionnaire may help the busy nurse to identify particular themes to focus on, in helping patients and families to come to terms with epilepsy.

A suitable check list for nurses might include some or all of the following:

Activities
Sports should be encouraged, with the activity selected dependent on each individual's particular seizure pattern.

Alcohol
Warn about dangers of drugs and alcohol interacting.

Denial
Discuss when denial is positive and when it is negative.

Diagnosis
Explain how it is reached, significance of tests and evaluate what this diagnosis means for each patient and family.

Driving
Define the legal position at home and abroad.

Drugs
Discuss why they are needed, how they work, interactions with other drugs; how to take them and how often. Warn about the risks of sudden stopping of medication. Inform about exemptions of prescription charges. Discuss drug levels if this information is required.

Employment
Interviews, attitudes, educating work colleagues. The emphasis should be on using the strengths of each person, rather than teaching him/her to expect rejection and promoting self-denial of opportunities.

Fears
Passing-it-on, mental deterioration, all the ancient stigmas.

Fits
Simple precautions: safety pillows, shower or shallow bath; photosensitive people sit 3 metres from the TV with a light on above the set.

Heredity
The risk to a child born to a parent with epilepsy depends on the nature of the parent's epilepsy and the seizure threshold of both parents. Everyone has a seizure threshold level and is capable of having a fit in appropriate circumstances. A high threshold level can be passed on in a person's genetic structure.

Insurance
Employers must be told that people are not high risks for accidents. Information about the British Epilepsy Association, and the insurance scheme this includes, should be provided for newly diagnosed patients.

Marriage
Fears of marriage may need to be discussed, and then to help the person and their relatives to concentrate on a normal full life.

Pregnancy
Discuss medication, breast feeding. When asked about teratogenic risks, refer to current research findings which show that risks of damage to unborn babies are present but statistically very low.

Risk and precautions
Pillows, bathing, heights and other reasonable precautions. Trigger factors — TV, stress, hunger, hyperventilation, overtiredness, premenstrual state, fever, alcohol, photic and other reflex stimuli. Each individual person has to identify his/her own triggers.

Some of the myths and misconceptions which should be corrected may include:

— brain-damaged
— criminal
— devil possessed
— dying in a fit
— quack remedies
— sexual intercourse dangerous
— insurance impossible
— insane
— infectious 'catching'
— marriage and pregnancy impossible
— someone's fault
— stigma — everyone hates me!

REFERENCES

Anderson R A 1981 Training and placement services: an employment services model program for persons with epilepsy. Advances in Epileptology: XIIth Epilepsy International Symposium, p. 245

Antonak R F, Rankin P R 1982 Measurement and analysis of knowledge and attitudes toward epilepsy and persons with epilepsy. Social Science and Medicine 16:1591

Bagley C 1972 Social prejudice and adjustment of people with epilepsy. Epilepsia 33

Bell M 1979 Some social problems of adults with epilepsy. Perspectives (93) British Epilepsy Association, London

Caveness W 1949 A survey of public attitudes toward epilepsy. Epilepsia 4:19

Caveness W, Merritt H H, Fallup G H 1974 A survey of public attitudes toward epilepsy in 1969 with an indication of trends over the past twenty years. Epilepsia 15:523

Dada T 1968 The social problems of epilepsy in Nigeria. Rehabilitation 27

Diehl L W 1976 Changes in popular attitudes to epilepsy in the Federal Republic of Germany and the USA. In: Janz D (ed), Epileptology (Proceedings of the 7th International Symposium on Epilepsy). Georg Thieme Verlag, Stuttgart, p 97

Floyd M 1983 Draft report on an exploratory study of epilepsy and employment. Tavistock Institute of Human Relations, London, Tavistock Centre, p 49

Honbridge E 1981 Epilepsy: how social workers redress the balance. Community Care 368:12

Jeavons P M, Aspinall A A 1985 The epilepsy reference book. Harper & Row, London, 33

Laidlaw J, Laidlaw M V 1976 People with epilepsy — living with epilepsy, A textbook of epilepsy. Churchill Livingstone, Edinburgh p 359

Levy L, Forbes J, Parirenyatwa T 1964 Epilepsy in Africans. Central African Medical Journal 10:7

Loyning Y 1980 Comprehensive care. In: Wada J A, Penry J K (eds) (Advances in epileptology. Xth Epilepsy International Symposium) Raven Press, New York p 363

McGvckin H M 1980 Changing the world view of those with epilepsy. In: Canger R, Amgeleri F, Penry J K (eds) (Advances in epileptology: XIth Epilepsy International Symposium) Raven Press, New York p 209

Remschmidt H 1973 Psychological studies of patients with epilepsy and popular prejudices. Epilepsia 14:347

Reynolds F, Zander L I 1982 Anticonvulsants: why monitor plasma levels? Modern Medicine 27(12):14

Richens A 1980 Drug Information Sheet. British Epilepsy Association, Crowthorne, England Leaflet

Rutter M, Tizard L, Whitemore K 1970 Education health and behaviour, London

Scambler G, Hopkins A 1980 Social class, epileptic activity and disadvantage at work. Journal of Epidemiological and Community Health 34:129

Scambler G, Hopkins A 1986 Being epileptic: coming to terms with stigma. Sociology of Health and Illness March, 8(1): 26

Shorvon S D 1984 Clinical pharmacology. Epilepsy Update Publications, Postgraduate Centre Series, London, p 20

Shorvon S D, Reynolds E H 1979 Reduction in polypharmacy for epilepsy. British Medical Journal 2:1023

Shorvon S D 1984 Epilepsy update. Hospital Update June: 541

Sletmo A 1982 Rehabilitation in epilepsy. In: Atkimoto H, Kazamatsuri H, Seino M, Ward A (eds) Advances in epileptology. XIIIth Epilepsy International Symposium. Raven Press, New York, p 433

17

Care of the patient with an infection or inflammation of the nervous system

Infection of the meninges is known as meningitis and that of the brain as encephalitis. Sometimes both structures are involved and this is called meningo-encephalitis. Myelitis is an infection or inflammation of the spinal cord.

MENINGITIS

The pia mater and arachnoid mater are acutely inflamed and in pyogenic types, exudate accumulates in the sulci and cisterns which may lead to hydrocephalus. The causes are many, though the Gram-negative Meningococcus is the commonest cause of bacterial meningitis in the UK. All strains are sensitive to penicillin though an increasing number have become resistant to sulphonamides. Other organisms which may cause meningitis include *Neisseria meningitidis*, Pneumococcus, *Haemophilus influenzae*, Streptococcus, Staphylococcus and *Listeria monocytogenes.*

Certain features occur in all types of meningitis. The illness starts with a few days of pyrexia and vague aches and pains throughout the body and a cold or sore throat. This is followed by severe headache causing neck stiffness, vomiting and photophobia, restlessness and irritability. The neck rigidity can be demonstrated by attempting to flex the neck

Table 17.1 Changes in CSF in meningitis

CSF	Type of meningitis Pyogenic	Acute aseptic
Appearance	Yellow	Clear, sometimes turbid
Cells	Polymorphs 1000–2000 per cubic mm or more	Mononuclear 50–1500 per cubic mm
Protein	Increased 1.0–5.0 g/l	Normal or slight increase
Chloride	110–115 mmol/l	Normal 120–130 mmol/l
Glucose	Much reduced or absent	Normal 4.0–6.0 mmol/l
Organisms	Present in smear or on culture	Absent in smear and ordinary culture media. May be demonstrable by special virological methods
Pressure	Elevated	Varies

to place the chin on the chest. If the hip is flexed and then an attempt is made to straighten the knee the movement is restricted and very painful (Kernig's sign). In infants there may be opisthotonos and convulsions. Some patients may display drowsiness, confusion and a decrease in conscious level.

Diagnosis is based on examining the CSF obtained at lumbar puncture. Prior to performing this it needs to be established that it is safe to do so. The changes seen in CSF are outlined in Table 17.1. Other investigations include, chest and skull X-rays, blood cultures and syphilitic and viral serology.

Other types of meningitis

Tuberculous meningitis

This is much less acute than bacterial meningitis and is usually spread from the lungs, glands or bones via the bloodstream, to the meninges. Treatment is of a long duration and of a combination of antituberculous therapy for a period of 9–12 months. Rifamycin, isoniazid, ethambutol, pyrazinamide and para-aminosalicylic acid (PAS). Pyridoxine may also be given; this is vitamin B$_6$ and is used to prevent peripheral neuropathy asso-

ciated with isoniazid therapy. Prednisolone may also be prescribed. Various combinations of these drugs will be used, according to medical preferences. Any of these drugs may produce a hypersensitivity reaction consisting of pyrexia and erythematous skin eruption which usually develops 2–4 weeks after treatment has started. Other specific side-effects include optic neuritis from the ethambutol.

The CSF will show fewer cells than in bacterial meningitis with polymorphs and lymphocytes present. The glucose and chloride levels are also very low.

Meningovascular syphilis

The meninges may be covered by an exudate which damages the cranial nerves. The pupils are small and irregular and do not react to light but respond to convergence (Argyll Robertson pupil). The CSF shows an increased lymphocyte count, a moderate rise in protein and in the gamma globulin fraction. Serological tests are usually positive in 90% of cases.

Viral meningitis

This is the most common type of meningitis occurring in epidemics in children and young adults. The illness is usually less severe than in bacterial meningitis and may develop as a complication of viral infections involving other organs, e.g. mumps, measles, herpes zoster, hepatitis, glandular fever etc. CSF shows a raised lymphocyte count with a slightly elevated protein level. The glucose and chloride levels are normal.

Poliomyelitis

This is now rare in the UK due to the successful immunisation programme for children using the Salk and Sabin type vaccines. It results from an acute attack on the anterior horn cells of the spinal cord and cells of the brain stem nuclei. A few people develop paralysis during the meningitic stage involving acute damage to the lower motor neurones. The most serious cases have bulbar paralysis and require artificial ventilation and nasogastric tube feeding. One in 10 will die from bulbar complications and permanent disability may be expected in about 20% of cases.

Cryptococcal meningitis

The yeast-like fungus *Cryptococcus neoformans* usually affects patients who have an underlying disease involving the immune system and causing a chronic lymphocytic meningitis. Treatment consists of oral fluorocytosine and amphotericin B by intravenous and intrathecal injection.

Malignant meningitis

This is usually due to secondary spread from elsewhere in the body giving rise to multiple cranial nerve lesions and malignant invasion of the meninges. Current evidence suggests that many of these complications are due to a hypersensitivity reaction on the part of the nervous system to the presence of a neoplasm.

Complications of meningitis, although rare, may include hydrocephalus due to an obstructed CSF outflow from the fourth ventricle; blindness either due to hydrocephalus or chronic arachnoiditis affecting the optic chiasma; spastic paraparesis due to arachnoiditis of the spinal meninges interfering with the blood supply to the spinal cord.

Encephalitis

All the viruses and bacteria which cause meningitis may also cause encephalitis. The brain is diffusely affected and cell changes vary from swelling to necrosis. There is perivascular infiltration at first with polymorphs and later lymphocytes and a widespread microglial reaction.

Virus particles may reach the brain by the bloodstream, along nerves or the olfactory route to the temporal lobes. Head injury and otitis media have also been implicated.

Viral encephalitis occurs in all parts of the

Table 17.2 Neurotropic viruses

Japanese Type B encephalitis
St Louis Type encephalitis
Russian Spring-Summer encephalitis
Murray Valley encephalitis of Australia
Rabies
Herpes simplex — temporal lobes
Encephalitis letargica
Inclusion encephalitis
Herpes zoster

world and is particularly common in the tropics. The neurotropic viruses known to man are listed in Table 17.2.

The commonest neurotropic virus in the UK is *Herpes simplex encephalitis*. The onset is acute and associated with marked behavioural disturbance often lasting 2–3 days before other features develop. The organism has a predilection for the temporal lobes and because of this disorders of behaviour, memory and hallucinations are common. Epilepsy is frequent. The patient may have herpetic eruptions on the skin or in the throat. The patient is acutely ill with headache, drowsiness and confusion. Speech disorders, hemiplegia or cranial nerve palsies may also be evident.

Investigations will comprise lumbar puncture, electro-encephalography and CT scanning. The CSF will reveal an increased lymphocyte count and protein and is often mildly blood stained. EEG will demonstrate a diffuse slowing of rhythms while the CT scan may reveal swollen temporal lobes. Other investigations include blood cultures and viral titres and throat and rectal swabs for viral culture. If the patient is deteriorating in the absence of a definite diagnosis, a brain biopsy may be performed. This is not without risk and a special immunofluorescent laboratory test can confirm the diagnosis in most cases.

Encephalitis lethargica (von Economo's disease, sleeping sickness)

In this the brain stem is affected causing paralysis of the eye movements. The patient may display a reversal of his sleep pattern in which he is drowsy during the day and wakeful at night. Parkinsonian features are evident hence the name post-encephalitic Parkinsonism.

Rabies (hydrophobia)

This is transmitted to humans by a bite from an infected animal. The virus enters the nervous system along the peripheral nerves and attacks the nerve cells. The incubation period is from 28–60 days. The patient displays restlessness, apprehension, and depression followed by pharyngeal spasm which extends to respiratory and then trunk and limb muscles producing opisthotonos. Any attempt to drink induces spasm, salivation and later paralysis. Death may occur during a spasm as a result of respiratory or cardiac failure.

Treatment is with human rabies immunoglobulin or human diploid cell strain vaccine.

Measles encephalitis

There are three types:

1. **Acute post-infectious encephalomyelitis** due to an immune response to the virus. Incidence is less than 1 in 1000.
2. **Sub-acute sclerosing pan-encephalitis** which is thought to be due to infection by a myxovirus which is either measles virus or a very closely related agent. It occurs in children and adolescents and the onset is usually insidious with intellectual deterioration, apathy, clumsiness and myoclonic jerks. This is followed by fits, ataxia and finally spasticity and mutism. The disease is nearly always fatal with death occurring within 2–6 months. The measles antibody titre is abnormally high in the serum and CSF, and EEG demonstrates characteristic bursts of triphasic slow waves.
3. **Epidemic myalgic encephalitis** occurs in closed communities such as schools and hospitals; an epidemic in the Royal Free Hospital led to the name 'Royal Free Disease'. The outcome is favourable.

Symptoms include, headache, muscle pains, exhaustion, lymphadenopathy and paraesthesia. Cranial nerve palsies sometimes occur.

Jakob-Creutzfeldt disease

Of the slow viruses listed in Table 17.3 Jakob-Creutzfeldt is perhaps the best known. The others are scrapie, kuri and mink encephalopathy. It is a disease of the grey matter of the brain and spinal cord and there is neuronal degeneration in the cerebral cortex, basal ganglia, thalamus, cerebellum, brain stem nuclei and the anterior horn cells of the spinal cord. The average age of onset is between 50 and 60 years and the disease is not familial.

Table 17.3 Slow viruses

Creutzfeldt-Jakob disease
Kuru
Subacute spongiform encephalopathies
Subacute sclerosing leucoencephalopathy
Progressive multifocal leucoencephalopathy

In a retrospective study over a 10-year period an incidence of 0.09 per million was noted and it is estimated that no more than 20 new cases per year are identified in the UK. A transmittable agent has been identified and it can infect non-human primates and other animals from an affected patient. Iatrogenic patient to patient transmission has occurred in cases following a neurosurgical procedure. It is not known at what stage of the disease it becomes possible for transmission to occur.

A definitive diagnosis can usually be made on clinical evidence. A rapidly progressive form of dementia, it is accompanied by myoclonic jerking and progressive paralysis and epileptiform fits leading to death within a few months to 1 year. The EEG shows characteristic periodic sharp waves against a background of slow wave activity.

Cerebral abscess

This is a collection of pus within the cerebrum

or cerebellum usually caused by an extension of an infective process from another part of the body. Chronic infections of the middle ear, mastoids and sinuses are common causes. Lesser causes may include trauma or surgery. In up to 20% of cases, no cause is detectable.

The signs and symptoms may mimic a tumour and include headache, malaise and an elevated temperature. More specific neurological signs may be seen depending on the site and extent of the abscess and these include seizures, speech disorders, visual field deficits, inco-ordination, confusion and drowsiness.

The investigation of choice is CT scan on which the abscess will be demonstrated. An elevated white blood cell count and ESR may be noted. Contradictions exist as to the usefulness and safety of a lumbar puncture. If CSF is obtained there is typically a raised protein level although this is not necessarily diagnostic.

Treatment is with antibiotics, usually intravenously and in large doses. Penicillin, chloramphenicol and metronidazole are often used. Surgical intervention may comprise excision and drainage of the abscess cavity. The mortality rate is about 25% and sequelae such as focal deficits and epilepsy are common.

Nursing care

Maintaining a safe environment

The patient is nursed in a quiet, darkened side room, if possible. Failing this, consideration should be given to the reduction of as much external noise as possible. Dark glasses may be worn if the patient prefers. The patient should be barrier nursed if the meningitis is of an unknown or unidentified organism or if an epidemic is ongoing. The patient with cryptococcal meningitis requires reverse barrier nursing in order to protect from further infection, as a result of the patient's immunosuppressed state. If the patient is suspected of having Jakob-Creutzfeldt disease, barrier nursing is not necessary, but plastic aprons and disposable gloves should be worn when handling blood or CSF or treating wounds. Again, a quiet environment is essential because of the high degree of startle myoclonus which these patients have.

Seizures pose a threat to the patient. Precautions are adopted prior to and during the seizure. The patient should be protected from injury and an accurate record maintained.

Communicating

A balance needs to be struck between keeping the patient informed of his progress and orientating him to his surroundings particularly if he is confused and maintaining a quiet environment. The patient should be spoken to quietly and forewarned of any procedure. Verbal stimulation is used during observation of conscious level and this should be kept to an absolute minimum.

The relatives should be provided with information regarding the need to nurse the patient in the particular fashion being used. Proper explanation will avoid any misunderstanding. Relatives should be provided with regular updated reports of the patient's condition.

Breathing

The position often adopted is one in which the patient lies curled and therefore adequate pulmonary function is compromised. The patient should be encouraged, where appropriate, to participate in deep breathing exercises. Drowsiness and confusion will compound the problem.

Eating and drinking

Initially, fluid intake is maintained with an intravenous infusion both to administer i.v. drugs and fluids in those instances of vomiting. Gradually oral fluids are introduced as the patient is able. The patient with muscle wasting, as in Jakob-Creutzfeldt disease, benefits from a high protein diet. An accurate record of fluid balance is needed and a minimum daily intake of 2500 ml should be achieved. If there is a delay in implementing an oral intake, an alternative method of feeding is needed, e.g. nasogastric feeding.

Eliminating

If feasible, the patient is toileted at frequent intervals. Drowsiness and confusion may preclude this and catheterisation may need to be considered. A record of output is needed in order to assess fluid balance.

Personal cleansing and dressing

Often, many of the activities of personal cleansing and dressing need to be performed for the patient. In particular, the patient who is vomiting will need additional attention to oral hygiene. The restless, confused patient and those in whom muscle wasting is evident are particularly at risk of skin breakdown.

Controlling body temperature

Many of the infections of the central nervous system produce a pyrexia and therefore an accurate method of measuring body temperature is needed. If the temperature is markedly elevated, measures are adopted to reduce this, such as tepid sponging, cool fanning and the administration of aspirin suppositories. This will result in the patient feeling more comfortable and will avoid using up reserves of oxygen which are utilised in pyrexia.

Mobilising

The adoption of appropriate positions in bed to achieve maximum comfort for the patient and avoid problems in relation to skin breakdown and the development of contractures is essential. The patient must be handled with care and sensitivity and forewarned of any sudden movement or painful procedure.

Sleeping

Accurate serial neurological observations are performed on a regular basis.

Dying

Sensitive care of the dying patient and his family is paramount. Provision of adequate pain relief is crucial

BIBLIOGRAPHY

Bannister R 1985 Brains's clinical neurology, 5th edn. Oxford University Press, London
Behan P O, Currie S 1978 Clinical Neuro-immunology. Saunders, London
Department of Health and Social Security 1981 Advisory Group on Creutzfeldt-Jakob Disease. HMSO, London
Hickey J V 1986 The clinical practice of neurological and neurosurgical nursing, 2nd edn. Lippincott, Philadelphia
Moir-Bussy B 1983 Creutzfeldt-Jakob Disease. Journal of Infection Control Nursing 23:16 in Nursing Times 79(35).
Mathews W B, Glasser G H 1984 Recent advances in clinical neurology — volume 4. Churchill Livingstone, Edinburgh
McFarlane J K, Castledine G 1982 A guide to the practice of nursing. Mosby, London
Ross-Russell R W, Wiles C M Neurology. Heinemann, London

18

Care of the patient with a neuromuscular disorder

MUSCULAR DYSTROPHY

Muscular dystrophy is a progressive degeneration of certain muscle groups. Several types have been identified, the commonest being the X-linked pseudohypertrophic types, i.e. Duchenne and Becker. Duchenne dystrophy is described below in more detail. Other types include facioscapulohumeral and limb girdle dystrophy.

One type, dystrophia myotonica and myotonia congenita, are distinguished by the addition of myotonia (lack of muscle tone). Duchenne dystrophy is the most frequent and severe type of muscular dystrophy. It affects only boys and is inherited in the female line so that their mothers, sisters and female relatives may be carriers. The condition is progressive and eventually fatal after a period of many years of disablement.

The onset is usually within the first 3–5 years of life. The child who walked at a normal age becomes clumsy in walking and running, has difficulty in climbing stairs, falls frequently and rises from the supine position by climbing up his legs (Gowers' sign). He walks with his abdomen protruding and typically with a waddle.

There is progressive weakness of the proximal upper and lower limb muscles with an enlargement (pseudohypertrophy) of the calves, glutei quadriceps, deltoids and infraspinate muscles. Often the child is unable to walk by the time he is 8–12 years old. Death is due to respiratory infection or cardiac failure due to cardiomyopathy often before the age of 20 years.

The increased level of the serum phosphokinase is indicative of the disease. The test is also used for identification in the preclinical stage in male siblings and in the diagnosis of the carrier state of their mothers and sisters. Electromyography may demonstrate myopathic changes and may reveal atrophy. Electrocardiographic studies may display a typical tracing showing wave abnormalities. An accurate diagnosis after investigations is usually made by a neurologist or paediatrician.

In Duchenne muscular dystrophy the progression is fairly predictable and almost standardised treatment schedules can be undertaken.

The neurologist will first see the parents and explain the results of the investigations and their implications for the child. This is a very traumatic experience and the parents will need time and help to accept the diagnosis. There may be initial disbelief and refusal to accept the diagnosis and they will need time and several interviews with the neurologist before they can accept the diagnosis. They may initially blame each other, then father may blame mother and if the family do not get the correct genetic counselling right at the start then the future management of the child may be difficult.

The senior ward staff should always be available to answer the relatives' questions after they have seen the neurologist and been given the diagnosis. It is then important for the child to be brought into the discussion so that his care profile can be agreed by all persons concerned.

Facioscapulohumeral dystrophy affects the muscles of the face and shoulders. Onset is usually in adolescence.

Limb-girdle dystrophy affects the shoulders or pelvic girdle muscles. Later onset occurs between 20 and 35 years of age.

Nursing care

Mobilising

As the boy will cease to walk independently at about 9–13 years of age it may be necessary to give him a spinal support and calipers to aid walking. This will help to maintain the upright posture for as long as possible and give a much needed psychological boost to both patient and parents.

Regular daily stretching of limbs will help to delay development of flexural contractures. It will also be necessary to supply the boy with a wheelchair. Initially a hand-propelled one will suffice but as the child becomes weaker he may need an electric one.

Clothing should be carefully chosen so that there are no seams which will press on pressure areas. Sheepskin pads in the wheelchair will help to reduce discomfort as will alternating compartment air-filled cushions (Row/hoe) or gel-filled cushions. Firmly-based cushioning is essential. Dependent oedema of the lower limbs due to immobility can be a problem leading to skin ulceration, therefore elastic stockings and elevating leg rests attached to the wheelchair may help to reduce the oedema.

Foot deformity. Initially regular physiotherapy will prevent flexion deformities but as walking ceases the deformities occur with inversion of the foot and planter flexion of the ankle. If not exercised this will become fixed and immobile. The use of sheepskin bootees will prevent pressure sore formation and polythene night splints will help to delay the contractive stage.

Spinal deformity. This usually commences with a slight pelvic tilt to one side and progresses to form a gross kyphoscoliosis with rotation of the spinal column. This can lead to respiratory embarrassment.

The child should be measured and fitted with a block leather spinal jacket in an attempt to control or prevent deformity and this may be renewed every 6 months during the growing years. This will delay the formation of spinal deformity providing it is worn when the patient is sitting upright.

Pain. Pain in the legs especially at night is a frequent finding and means the nurse or the family should change the child's position every few hours and give appropriate analgesia.

Obesity. Excessive weight gain may lead to considerable problems with lifting, patient transferring and respiratory function. It is often very hard to suggest the need to lose weight to the child or the parents as the parents see the psuedohypertrophied muscles as being a sign of great strength and thus prolonging the child's life expectancy. However obesity may lead to problems in home nursing as a heavy teenager cannot easily be lifted by his parents and frequent toileting and bathing will quickly tire the parents and often necessitate the child's admission to hospital or a young persons' disabled unit. It is advisable to start the child on a low carbohydrate, high fibre diet and ask the dietitian to see the parents.

Eating and drinking

Impaired motor mobility in the upper limbs leads to the inability to cut up food and weak grip causes difficulty in handling cutlery or lifting cups. It is advisable to ask the occupational therapist to assess the child and provide suitable padded cutlery and lightweight cups with large handles to enable the child to maintain his independence for as long as possible. Plastic drinking straws will provide a statisfactory solution to a drinking problem. With the provision of supports greater independence may be maintained as the child will not like being fed by his parents or a nurse.

Personal cleansing and dressing

As the child becomes more disabled he will require help with bathing. He may find it possible to bath with the aid of a seat or bath board or alternatively a mechanical hoist may be used.

As the boy gets older and more disabled he will still want to dress in clothes which are fashionable and it may be that minor adjustments, e.g. Velcro fastenings will lead to greater independence.

Eliminating

It is advisable to train the bowel to evacuate at approximately the same time daily in order to avoid embarrassment from faecal incontinence. This can usually be achieved by giving a high fibre diet with added bran and aperients when necessary. The child should be taken to the toilet where 'grab rails' are used to transfer the patient and help him balance on the toilet. He should be left alone to evacuate his bowel, but he may require some assistance to wipe the anus following defaecation.

Educating

Due to severe physical disabilities the child will usually be receiving tuition at schools for the physically handicapped. As the child usually suffers from intellectual impairment an individual teaching programme must be devised.

Dying

It is unusual for the child to show signs of anxiety or depression about his physical handicaps or the knowledge of his early death though his parents do need full support from medical, nursing staff and social workers. Coming to terms with the tragedy of the death of a child may also mean parents spend much time and effort looking for cures. Intermittent admission to hospital for a grossly handicapped child will give the mother a much needed rest and enable her to carry on caring for him for much longer at home than might otherwise be the case.

In the later stages of the disease the health team will provide support for both patient and family as they would for any dying child.

DYSTROPHIA MYOTONICA

This disorder is characterised by the features of muscular dystrophy in combination with myotonia. Other dystrophic changes might be present including cataract. Onset is between the ages 15–40 with the peak occurring around 20–30 years. The presenting symptom is usually mytonia in the face, shoulder girdle, forearms and hands and the lower legs. Typically, the face is expressionless.

MYOTONIA CONGENITA (Thomsen's disease)

Following a voluntary movement, the patient displays a prolonged tonic contraction of the affected muscles followed by retarded relaxation. Onset is usually in childhood and the child can become profoundly handicapped. Myotonia congenita is not associated with muscular wasting. Treatment is very limited. Quinine or procainamide hydrochloride may relieve the myotonia.

MYASTHENIA GRAVIS

This is an uncommon, but important, disease characterised by excessive muscular fatigue and weakness on sustained or repeated contraction, with recovery at rest. The name comes from the Greek, myasthenia meaning muscle weakness and the Latin, gravis meaning severe.

A population of 100 000 will produce one new case in 2 to 3 years. It most commonly affects young women, but it may occur in either sex at any time from infancy to old age. It tends to fluctuate in severity and remissions of months or years are common in the early stages but infrequent in the later stages.

The clinical picture is one of diplopia, ptosis of one or both eyelids and weakness of neck flexion. Later, the patient may suffer from weakness of the shoulder muscles followed by weakness of the face and tongue with difficulty of speech. In severe cases, dysphagia is also apparent. Any skeletal muscle may also be involved.

Pathology

Transmission of motor commands from the nervous system to the skeletal muscle requires liberation of acetylcholine from the motor nerve terminals into the synaptic cleft of the endplate of each muscle fibre. It attaches to specialised acetylcholine receptors causing the generation of an endplate potential. If this potential reaches an adequate voltage, the action potential mechanism of the muscle is triggered and the fibre contracts. A surplus of acetylcholine and acetylcholine receptors constitutes a safety factor so that transmission is preserved despite decreasing output by the nerve terminals during sustained effort. To respond to each action potential in the motor nerve, each jet of acetylcholine must be destroyed by an enzyme (acetylcholinesterase) in the endplate. In myasthenia gravis a high proportion of the receptors are damaged or blocked by antibodies directed against part of the receptor, reducing the safety factor and eventually preventing neuromuscular transmission in an increasing proportion of endplates in some or all of the skeletal muscles hence the patient appears weak.

Diagnosis is by clinical history and measurement of the antibodies in the blood and electromyelography, in which there is evidence of reduced neuromuscular transmission and brief remission following injection of endrophenium, but this is non-specific.

Treatment is aimed at promoting power in the muscles by raising the safety factor for neuromuscular transmission. The primary immunological disorder is then treated. Drugs used in the treatment programme include pyridostigmine and neostigmine, both anticholinesterase drugs. If the optimum dose of pyridostigmine has been reached without maximum effect, anti-immunological agents may be considered, e.g. azathioprine. It produces gradual improvement over a period of 1 to 2 years. Plasma exchange may also produce a temporary improvement. Steroids are commonly used, but if over a prolonged period of time, consideration must be given to long-term side-effects.

Thymectomy may be considered for most myasthenia sufferers unless they have had

Table 18.1 Drugs used in the treatment of myasthenia gravis

Anticholinesterase drugs
Administered in an attempt to enhance neuromuscular transmission which they do by prolonging the action of acetylcholine by inhibiting the enzyme acetylcholinesterase.

Pyridostigmine (Mestinon) Dose 0.3–1.2 mg orally, in daily divided doses. Effect lasts longer than other anticholinesterase drugs therefore used overnight.
Neostigmine (Prostigmin) Dose 75–300 mg daily in divided doses. Effect lasts up to 4 hours.

Side-effects include diarrhoea, gastric discomfort, excess salivation and bronchospasm. Atropine may be given to diminish these parasympathetic side-effects.

Ambenonium (Mytelase) Dose 5–25 mg in daily divided doses.
Edrophonium (Tensilon) Test dose of 2 mg intravenously followed after 30 seconds by 8 mg. Used as a means of diagnosing myasthenia gravis or for the detection of under- or overdosage of cholinergic drugs. Very short acting.

Corticosteroids
May be indicated when thymectomy is not advised and the drug of choice is usually prednisolone in high daily doses. May produce a deterioration prior to improvement therefore only administered under direct hospital supervision.

well controlled myasthenia for more than 10 years. The thymus gland may be abnormal. Some patients have a thymoma (a tumour) while others have germinal centres, which are collections of lymphocytes, arranged in a way that suggest they are secreting antibodies.

NURSING CARE

The patient may be admitted to hospital for:

— diagnosis and evaluation
— alteration of drug regime in particular for the introduction of steroid drugs
— intercurrent infections, i.e. pneumonia
— myasthenic or cholinergic crisis
— thymectomy.

Often the patient will have been referred to the neurologist only after she has been around many doctors and psychiatrists, so that when she is admitted her psychological state is often the major obstacle. She should be given a full explanation of the nature of the expected diagnosis and all tests particularly those likely to fatigue her as it is essential to get the patient's and family's co-operation at the earliest stage in the medical and nursing management.

The patient should be welcomed to the ward by a friendly face and, if at all possible, given a bed close to another young person or perhaps a patient with the same disease who has adjusted well and will be able to help her to come to terms and understand the reason for compliance to any drugs which may be prescribed.

All patients' drugs have to be individually titrated and after the drugs, and their use and side-effects, have been fully explained, self-medication should be permitted. The patient should be instructed to keep a diary concerning the fluctuations of the symptoms. The timing and height of dose should be adjusted with special attention to meals and peak activities.

She should be warned not to increase the dose of her drugs without medical advice as this may lead to cholinergic crisis. An individual care plan should be formulated between the patient and nurse paying particular attention to dietary needs and the fluctuating nature of her weakness. She should be given a form signed by the doctor and advised to wear a Medi-alert bracelet at all times.

If diplopia and ptosis cannot be corrected by anticholinesterases other simple measures, e.g. a thin adhesive tape over the upper eyelid, a lid crutch fixed to the inner side of spectacles or a steel wire loop (Lundrie loop) can be fitted to the spectacles. Covering the spectacle glass and alternating the eye covered on alternate days is a simple way of correcting the diplopia.

Eating and drinking

As chewing and swallowing are often very

difficult initially, a high protein diet should be given either in the form of a minced or puréed diet or, if bulbar symptoms are present, a nasogastric tube may need to be inserted in order that adequate nourishment can be given. This is also a means of giving the anticholinesterase and other drugs needed.

Careful timing of drugs is essential if the patient is to enjoy a meal without fatigue and ideally pyridostigmine should be given 30–45 minutes before the meal.

Hot meals may induce weakness of throat muscles and some patients prefer cold food and perhaps suck an ice cube prior to eating. Wearing a soft collar helps weak neck muscles. A table of the correct height so that the patient does not have to bend the head forward, will save muscle work and thus less fatigue for the patient. The chair should have a head rest so that the patient may take frequent breaks during the meal. Small meals at 2–3 hourly intervals are preferable to 3 large meals a day.

Eliminating

Very occasionally the patient may experience incontinence of urine, thought to be due to weakness of pelvic floor muscles and usually transitory, though very distressing for the patient. Great understanding on the part of the nurse will help to reduce the patient's embarrasment. Constipation is not usually a feature of myasthenia gravis as anticholinesterase usually causes frequent bowel actions. Enemas have a bad name in the history of myasthenia gravis as they may precipitate a crisis in severely ill patients.

Personal cleansing

Hot baths and sunbathing should be avoided if muscle weakness is increased following them. While the patient may seem to get easily into a bath unaided she should have a communication bell so that if she is too weak to get out of the bath help will be readily at hand.

Observations

These should include peak flow recordingss immediately prior to and 1 hour following a dose of pyridostigmine. Measurement of forced expiratory volume may be indicated if the patient is very weak and ventilation is expected. Taking a deep breath in and counting out quickly is often a more reliable measurement of lung function, particularly if the patient has any cranial nerve weakness which is most often the case. Pulse and blood pressure readings 4 hourly will detect early signs of crisis.

Psychological support

It is vitally important to explain the *peaks* and *troughs* which may occur either in an acute exacerbation or while introducing new drugs, e.g. steroids. The patient should be told that artifical ventilation may be necessary and if it is at all possible she should visit the intensive care unit and meet the staff and be shown the machinery.

If thymectomy is performed most patients will go back to the intensive care unit for a period of 48 hours or longer. Tell her that the reason for this is that due to the surgical incision in the sternum she will experience pain and this may hinder her breathing but that it is temporary. As she may only be ventilated for a short time she may not need a tracheostomy so it is vital to tell her that the tubes will be in her mouth. While she is fully alert, she will be unable to speak. A non-verbal communication board must be available so that she is able to make her needs known. Analgesics should be given regularly for the first 48 hours then as required by the patient.

Myasthenic crisis

The patient develops increasing weakness of the bulbar muscles causing dysphagia and inability to cough vigorously. In this state some aspiration of food or saliva or a mild upper respiratory infection causes further exhaustion.

Other crisis-precipitating mechanisms include:

— brittle myasthenia
— i.v.diazepam
— commencement of steroid therapy
— surgery
— hyperthyroidism.

An impending crisis should be recognised by a fall in vital observations, occurrence of short attacks of dyspnoea with inspiratory stridor and short losses of consciousness, increasing bulbar weakness, restlesssness and insomnia, tachycardia and hypertension due to CO_2 retention. Patients with a myasthenic crisis frequently have signs of autonomic disturbance: sweating, salivation, urgency of micturition and defaecation, tachycardia and dilated pupils.

Treatment

The patient requires artificial ventilation and anticholinesterase should be omitted until the cause of the crisis is established. The most effective way to terminate a crisis is to combine plasma exchange with a high dosage of prednisone daily (1.5–2.0 mg/kg). Improvement usually starts after the second or third exchange. Prednisone may be withheld from patients whose crisis was due to intercurrent infections, thyrotoxicosis, emotional stress and obvious under- or overdosage of anticholinesterase.

Cholinergic crisis

Cholinergic signs are salivation, bronchor-rhoea, diarrhoea, vomiting, sweating, lacrimation, bowel and bladder incontinence muscle weakness, fasciculation and cramps if bulbar signs are present but there is no ptosis. Miosis will help to distinguish it from the myasthenic crisis. Restlessness, anxiety, headache and vertigo are signs of cerebral dysfunction. Other central nervous system signs include confusion, coma and convulsions.

Cholinergic crisis is due to overdosage of anticholinesterase and the patient may require artificial ventilation in order to preserve life.

BIBLIOGRAPHY

Behan P O, Currie S 1978 Clinical Neuro-immunology. Saunders, London
Bickerstaff, E 1987 Neurology, 4th edn. Hodder and Stoughton, London
Green J H 1976 An introduction to human physiology, 4th edn. Oxford University Press, London
Greenwood R, Newsom-Davis J, Hughes R A C et al 1982 In: Tindall R S A (ed) Therapeutic apheresis and plasma perfusion. Liss, New York
Hickey J V 1986 The clinical practice of neurological and neurosurgical nursing, 2nd edn. Lippincott, Philadelphia
Lyons J B 1974 A primer of neurology. Butterworths, London
Mathews W B, Glasser G H 1984 Recent advances in clinical neurology — volume 4. Churchill Livingstone, Edinburgh
MacLeod J 1984 (ed) Davidson's principles and practice of medicine, 14th edn. Churchill Livingstone, Edinburgh
Oosterhuis Hans J G H 1984 Myasthenia gravis. Clinical neurology and neurosurgery monographs. Churchill Livingstone, Edinburgh
Osserman K E 1968 Myasthenia gravis. Grune and Stratton, New York
Shore A, Limatibul S, Dosch H M, Gelfand E W 1978 Identification of two serum components regulating the expression of T-lymphocyte function in childhood myasthenia gravis. New England Journal of Medicine 301(12):625
Simpson J A 1960 Myasthenia gravis: A new hypothesis. Scottish Medical Journal 5(10):419

19

Care of the patient with a nerve root or peripheral nerve disorder

NEUROPATHY

Neuropathy is a disease process of nerve degeneration and loss of function. Two characteristics are often associated with neuropathy: axonal degeneration and demyelination.

If one peripheral nerve is affected this is termed a *mononeuropathy*; if more are involved, it is known as *mononeuritis multiplex*. If all the peripheral nerves are diseased this is called a *polyneuropathy*.

Pressure neuropathies

Median nerve

The nerve is compressed as it travels along a tunnel in the wrist, hence the name carpal tunnel syndrome. It innervates the pronators, long flexors and in the hand the two radial lumbricals and the short thumb muscles.

Causes include leaning on a hard surface, osteoarthritis, and fracture of the elbow or wounds of the wrist. It often develops without obvious cause but may be associated with rheumatoid arthritis, diabetes mellitus or trauma to the wrist.

The patient will complain of pain in the wrist and arm which is severe at night. There is also persistent tingling in the outer three fingers and later the thumb becomes weak making coarse, gripping movements and pincer action of the thumb and index finger difficult.

Analgesia is tried in the first instance and if this does not produce relief, a non-steroidal, anti-inflammatory agent may be given along with a supporting wrist splint. The disorder may be relieved by an intra-articular injection of cortisone into the carpal tunnel, but these treatments may only bring about temporary relief of pain. Surgical decompression may eventually be indicated.

Ulnar nerve

This nerve innervates the flexor carpi-ulnaris and the inner half of the flexor digitorum profundus and adductor pollicis and the remaining intrinsic muscles of the hand. It also conveys sensation from the little finger and the adjacent side of the ring finger. The nerve is often affected where it travels along through a fibrous tunnel in the inner margin of the elbow.

The patient will complain of tingling of the inner two fingers and find that delicate movements are impaired. On examination the hand shows wasting of the interosseous muscles. The thumb is flexed due to inaction of the adductor pollicis, the ring and little finger are clawed and the little finger abducted by the unopposed pull of the extensor tendons. The nerve can be palpated at the elbow, and by tapping the point over the nerve with a tendon hammer, the unpleasant sensation of paraesthesia may be produced (Tinsel's sign). The patient will be referred to an orthopaedic surgeon for transposition of the nerve to the front of the elbow thus freeing it and preventing further damage.

Femoral nerve

This can occur as a result of a penetrating wound or compression by a pelvic neoplasm. The patient complains of hip flexion and an inability to extend the knee.

On examination the quadriceps muscle is paralysed and a weakness of hip flexion and sensory impairment is noted over the medial and anterior aspects of the lower two-thirds of the thigh. If the saphenous nerve, a branch of the femoral nerve, is also affected the patient will complain of analgesia and anaesthesia down the inner side of the leg and foot. Treatment will vary, depending on the cause.

Meralgia paraesthetica

This is a mononeuropathy of the lateral cutaneous nerve in the thigh due to trapping of the nerve in its fibrous tunnel in the groin (fascia lata).

The patient will complain of intense burning and tingling sensation on the outer aspect of the thigh. It often occurs in overweight people.

If obesity is the cause, the patient will be given dietary advice as the symptoms often subside when the patient loses weight. If symptoms persist dissection of the nerve may be required.

Sciatic nerve

Lesions here usually result from gunshot wounds or other penetrating injuries to the buttocks or thigh and may also be caused by pelvic injury or femoral fracture, or by lateral prolapse of an intervertebral disc (see Ch. 14).

The sciatic nerve enters the buttock via the sciatic notch and then passes into the thigh midway between the greater trochanter of the femur and the ischial tuberosity. A complete nerve lesion produces paralysis of hamstring muscles and results in an inability to flex the knee and paralysis of all muscles below the knee.

The patient complains of difficulty in walking and of pain shooting down the leg from the buttock making sitting very uncomfortable and he will also complain of numbness due to sensory loss over the whole foot except for a small area on the medial surface of the heel. On examination the ankle fork and plantar responses are absent and sensory loss is noted over the foot and lateral and posterior aspects of the leg below the knee. Treatment is dependent upon the cause.

Lateral popliteal nerve (*common peroneal*)

This is a division of the sciatic nerve. Lesions here usually result from trauma to the nerve as it curls around the neck of the fibula.

The patient will notice that he trips up steps and has to pick his feet up high in order to walk properly. On examination, he will be found to have a complete paralysis of the dorsiflexors of his foot and toes and of the peroneal muscles. This results in foot drop with inversion. Sensory loss will be noted over the anterolateral aspect of the foot and leg extending medially to the cleft between the fourth and fifth toe.

Treatment will depend on the cause. The patient can be provided with a plastic foot splint to be worn inside his shoe to help correct the foot drop. Physiotherapy may also be advised.

Medial popliteal nerve

This is also a division of the sciatic nerve. This lesion usually only results after a penetrating wound. The muscles of the calf and the sole of the foot are paralysed and the foot is partially dorsiflexed and everted. The patient complains of loss of sensation on the sole of the foot and the plantar surface of the toes.

Posterior tibial nerve (*tarsal tunnel syndrome*)

This nerve is compressed behind and below the medial malleolus. It is characterised by burning pain in the toes, the sole of the foot and sometimes extends up the leg. The patient may complain of loss of sensation in the distribution of the posterior tibial nerve and tenderness over the nerve. The symptoms are worse at night and eased by moving the leg or letting it hang out of the bed. Surgical decompression is the treatment of choice.

Peripheral neuropathies

These can be classified, in an arbitary fashion, according to cause as follows:

- infections, usually via an indirect source
- metabolic, which may be the result of:
  — vitamin deficiency
  — poisons
  — unwanted side-effects of drugs
  — porphyria
  — renal failure
  — diabetes
- generalised disorders such as polyarteritis nodosa and systemic lupus erythematosis
- genetically determined disorders including peroneal muscular atrophy.

Landry-Guillain-Barré syndrome

The onset is acute or subacute and the patient presents with a generalised polyneuropathy. The cause is unknown but often follows a viral infection lending support to the idea that this syndrome may be an auto-immune response of the peripheral nervous system. Presentation is variable and might include muscular weakness, sensory changes and some disturbance of autonomic function, e.g. hypotension. Cranial nerves may also be involved. The onset may be over several hours or days and it can take up to 6 months to recover. Improvement usually begins within days of the maximum deficit being reached. The incidence is equal amongst both sexes, peaking within the decade 16–25 years. Frequency is 1.6 per 100 000 of the population.

Investigations centre on the clinical history and CSF findings, as outlined in Table 19.1 Viral studies of blood may prove useful. Treatment is supportive. The patient is at risk of developing respiratory failure and intercurrent infection. Mechanical ventilation via tracheostomy is often needed and therefore the nursing care of this patient plays a significant part.

Drug therapy has included immunosuppressive agents and steroids although their use has

Table 19.1 Changes in CSF in Guillain-Barré syndrome

Protein	Raised 2.0–3.0 g/l
Colour	Yellow
Cells	Within limits
Pressure	Raised

now been discontinued. Plasma exchange, in which the patient's plasma is removed and replaced has been tried. The theory is that if the circulating antibodies are removed from plasma, the patient will enter a remission phase. Some patients did show a degree of improvement but evidence is now mounting that plasma exchange is not beneficial. The mortality rate is about 10–15%.

Nursing care

The patient is highly dependent, paralysed, possibly apnoeic and fully alert.

Maintaining a safe environment

The patient with impaired motor and sensory function is at risk from several problems, e.g. skin may be at risk of breakdown or the patient's ability to feel heat may be compromised. It is necessary for the nurse to predict when and how the patient may be in danger and institute avoiding action, e.g. frequent turning and repositioning or disallowing the use of heating devices. Measures should also be adopted to prevent the spread of infection.

Communicating

Any difficulties which the patient might have with speaking require attention. The presence of a tracheostomy or prolonged speaking in an easily fatigued patient necessitates the use of alternative communication. Pencil and paper messages may work but that is unlikely due to motor weakness. Picture boards, which are limited in their use, and sophisticated electronic communications aids may be all that is available. Some patients may have a disposable speaking tracheostomy tube in place. Improved communications will lead to a decrease in anxiety without resorting to the use of drugs.

Breathing

Assessment of the patient's respiratory status will highlight the need for additional support.

Assessment will include checking respiratory rate, depth, volume and the patient's colour. Equipment to measure tidal volume should be made available. Arterial blood gases may also be monitored. If any deterioration is noted, this should be reported immediately.

Tracheostomy is an easier way of managing respiratory failure. If it is performed early on in the course of the illness it is more comfortable for the patient. The appropriate care for the management of a tracheostomy tube is performed. Likewise, should it prove necessary to ventilate the patient, the appropriate measures for this should be adhered to. Access to, and familiarity with, oxygen and suctioning is essential. Chest physiotherapy is performed on a regular basis.

Eating and drinking

Modification of dietary intake will almost certainly be required. Most often, this will involve the passage of a nasogastric tube and implementation of an appropriate feeding regime. This should be devised taking cognisance of the patient's needs and the advice of the dietitian.

Eliminating

Despite the acknowledged dangers, urinary catheterisation is usually necessary initially. This demands the implementation of an aggressive catheter management protocol. The long-term aim should be to remove the catheter as soon as possible and replace it with an alternative system such as an external collection device.

Personal cleansing and dressing

As the patient is normally fully dependent, all the activities in relation to personal cleansing and dressing will need to be attended to by the nurse.

Mobilising

Proper positioning and regular passive range

of movement exercises will assist in enhancing mobility once the patient begins the recovery phase.

Working and playing

A return to work should happen eventually, but in the meantime the patient and his family may suffer financial hardship. The help of the medical social worker may prove beneficial.

Sleeping

Regular assessment of neurological status will provide an indication of progress.

METABOLIC NEUROPATHY

Subacute combined degeneration of the cord

This disorder is caused by vitamin B_{12} deficiency resulting in a gradual degeneration of the posterior columns (concerned with touch, vibration and joint position sense) and that part of the lateral columns transmitting the corticospinal tracts. The disease process often also involves the posterior roots and peripheral nerves, giving the clinical features of a predominantly sensory axonal polyneuropathy.

The patient complains of numbness and tingling in the fingers and toes, soreness of the calves and unsteadiness, especially in the dark, and soreness of the tongue.

Commonly patients will describe the sensation as if it were a tight band of constriction around one toe, limb or the waist. On examination, vibration sense in the limbs is impaired and Romberg's sign is positive. The patient does not know where his fingers or toes are in space. In an advanced stage, sensory ataxia develops so that walking and maintenance of posture in the dark becomes impossible. The tendon reflexes are either impaired or absent. If the pyramidal tracts are involved the patient complains of stiffness and slowness in walking which eventually develops into a spastic paraparesis. Investigations will include a full blood count and bone marrow puncture although the most important test will be to measure the serum vitamin B_{12} level.

The Schilling test might reveal histamine fast achlorhydria in the gastric juices.

Treatment will consist of replacement vitamin therapy. The patient is given hydroxocobalamin 1000 μg daily for 1 week, then weekly for 3 months followed by monthly thereafter for life. The patient will require outpatient physiotherapy. It must be stressed to the patient that it is important to maintain therapy.

Prognosis depends on how early the diagnosis has been made and treatment commenced. The signs due to peripheral neuropathy often recover completely. Ataxia may markedly improve but if there is a spastic paraplegia and moderately severe dementia prior to commencement of treatment some persistent disability will remain.

Other causes of neuropathies

Poisons. Lead is known to cause neuropathy but its incidence is now falling.

Drugs. The commoner drugs known to cause neuropathy include phenytoin sodium, penicillin, isoniazid and nitrofurantoin.

Porphyria. Acute intermittent porphyria is characterised by severe abdominal pain with a fairly acute onset. The porphyrias are a series of conditions associated with abnormal porphyrin metabolism and in some patients this produces a neuropathy.

Renal failure. The metabolic disturbance in renal failure has been recognised as causing neuropathy.

Diabetes. This is usually mainly sensory and found in long standing diabetics. The patient often notices ulceration of the foot as the first sign. Improvement of the diabetic state does not usually improve the neuropathy.

Nursing implications

The nurse should be aware of the extent of the patient's sensory and motor loss and give advice regarding potential dangers. Should a splint or cast be prescribed it is important that this fits properly and that the patient is aware of the correct method of application.

BIBLIOGRAPHY

Bannister R 1985 Brains's clinical neurology, 5th edn. Oxford University Press, London

Behan P O, Currie S 1978 Clinical Neuro-immunology. Saunders, London

Dowling P C, Menonna J P, Cook S D 1977 Guillain Barré syndrome in greater New York — New Jersey. Journal of the American Medical Association 238(4):317

Lesser R P, Hauser W A, Kurland L T, Mulder D W 1973 Epidemiologic features of the Guillain-Barré syndrome. Neurology 23:1269

Lyons J B 1974 A primer of neurology. Butterworths, London

Macleod J 1984 (ed) Davidson's principles and practice of medicine, 14th edn. Churchill Livingstone, Edinburgh

Medical Research Council 1976 Aids to the examination of peripheral nerve injuries. HMSO, London

Walton J 1982 Essentials of neurology 5th edn. Pitman, London

20

Care of the patient with a chronic neurological disorder

DEMENTIA

Dementia is the name given to an illness whose characteristic clinical features are failing memory, intellectual deterioration, personality changes and behavioural problems. It is always due to an organic cause. Most sufferers are over 70, but people of over 40 can also be affected. It is one of the most feared diseases of modern medicine — feared especially by older people, and those who have seen a friend or relative affected.

The incidence of dementia increases with age, 10% of people over 65 years are affected, and this increases to 20% of those over 80. At present in Britain, we have an 'ageing population', as people live longer. At the turn of the century, less than 5% of the population of Britain was over 65, by 1977 this percentage had increased to 15%. It is estimated that by 1995, there will be 1.76 million people in Britain over 80 years. From current statistics we can expect 20% of these to suffer from dementia, which gives some idea of the significance of the disease.

Dementia has a tremendous social impact. Most affected individuals live in the community — either alone, or with relatives — and as the illness progresses, need an increasing amount of support from various sources. Inevitably, some sufferers are eventually admitted to psychiatric hospitals, and 27% of the deaths in mental hospitals are due to dementia.

Hence it is important for us to learn about dementia, to enable us to help sufferers to live as fully and independently as they can and to understand the stress and grief the disease causes to both the patients and also their friends and relatives, so we can help to support them effectively.

In this chapter we shall be considering the presentation and causes of dementia, the reasons for admission to hospital, the nursing care which may be required in hospital and ways in which the hospital team can help to arrange support for the patient and his family when he returns home.

Presentation of dementia

Dementia is a progressive disease which causes deterioration of the memory, intellectual powers and the ability to reason things out. It starts insidiously; initially, those people involved with the patient may be puzzled by slightly odd decisions, or behaviour which is out of character. He may make errors of judgement, or make mistakes which previously would have been unthinkable for him. Later in the illness, the memory becomes more unreliable — affecting short-term memory in the beginning, but later becoming more general. Some articulate patients can camouflage the gaps in their memory for a long time; it only becomes apparent with careful testing how defective their memories are. Concentration also becomes poor and the patient may be unable to finish his sentences. Personal hygiene may become neglected, and dressing and self-care become very erratic. A person on his own may take to living on biscuits because preparing a meal is beyond him. The sufferer frequently loses all sense of time, and may get up in the middle of the night. Very often, the patient starts to wander aimlessly, as he sets off to do something, but quickly forgets what it is.

At this stage a lot of help will be needed to cope with daily living, and looking presentable. Personal care and hygiene are extremely sensitive areas to us all and the patient may resent help, especially if it comes from a younger member of his family. It is difficult to advise a person on personal care without appearing to be critical and the relatives often bear the brunt of the patient's anger and frustration. Relatives also suffer by seeing the person they knew as a capable and respected individual become more and more dependent and handicapped. They also feel guilty that they are unable to help more.

Other patients show no insight at all into their condition, and try to carry on as usual. This can be equally hard on the relatives. Their acquaintances and friends do not see the stress they are living with and brand them uncaring if they try to talk over their problems.

Eventually, the patient can become totally dependent on others. He may become incontinent, need help at mealtimes, and need assistance with washing and dressing and all aspects of life. His speech can be affected. Even thus handicapped he may still be able to walk and may wear himself out with continual aimless wandering.

The exact course of the illness, and the speed of the deterioration, varies, but dementia does shorten the patient's life expectancy. A study in 1970 which followed up dementia patients found that 17 had died after 4 years, against 7 in the control group. This, then is the picture — a very distressing illness which affects the patient, his friends and relatives.

Causes of dementia

Some types of dementia have a treatable cause; the brain damage can be stopped and in some cases reversed if treatment is prompt. Treatable causes of dementia include certain metabolic disorders, for instance, myxoedema, and parathyroid disease; also deficiency states, particularly deficiency of the B group vitamins: for example, Wernicke's encephalopathy, pellagra and vitamin B_{12} deficiency. These are relatively easy to investigate and treat.

Sometimes, dementia can be a feature of other neurological diseases. Jakob-Creutzfeldt disease is an example of this. This is a trans-missible slow virus infection, which causes a rapidly progressing dementia, associated with myoclonus. Middle-aged people are normally the victims of this rare disease and death usually follows about 18 months after the first symptoms are noticed. Huntington's chorea is another disease where dementia is one of the symptoms.

Diseases with dementia as the primary or sole symptom can be basically divided into 2 groups:

- Alzheimer's disease
- arteriosclerotic dementia.

Alzheimer's disease

Also known as 'senile dementia', this type of dementia can occur in younger people (over 40) but normally affects people over 65. Although either sex can be affected, it seems more common in women.

At first, the person's memory for recent events is lost. There is a steady insidious deterioration and, after 2 or 3 years, the dementia becomes much worse; the patient can develop dysphasia and apraxia. In the later stages, fits are fairly common. Personality and insight are affected quite early in the disease.

There are no neurological signs, except occasional coarse muscular twitchings in the later stages of the illness. It is clear, from post-mortem examination of brains of sufferers, that there is both shrinkage of brain tissue, and disintegration of grey matter. On average, 25% of brain cells may be lost. The frontal and temporal areas are particularly badly affected by cell loss, although it is not exclusively confined to these areas. The cerebral ven-tricles appear larger, but the increase in size is not necessarily correlated with the degree of dementia.

Degenerating brain tissue forms micro-scopic plaques, which are scattered in large numbers throughout the cortex, and to a lesser extent, through the deeper grey matter and brain stem. These have an amyloid core, and contain degenerating neurites and presyn-aptic terminals. Another microscopic feature is the neurofibrillary tangle — paired helical filaments which originate from a brain protein form tangles by winding themselves round cell nuclei. Although both plaques and tangles have been found on examination of a normal brain, they are very much more numerous in the brain of a dementia sufferer, and it appears that the more severely the patient is affected the more plaques and tangles there will be.

Research has not yet established whether these lesions are actually responsible for the brain damage, or cause the cerebral symp-toms by interrupting nerve pathways. Since there are reduced numbers of dendrites in parts of the temporal lobes of sufferers and less branches in those present, it is possible that there is interference with transmission at the synapse.

Research is still continuing into the causes of Alzheimer's disease. Until recently, it was regarded as an accelerated form of ageing but this is now disputed. Some of the ideas under investigation are:

1. Whether it could be due to a slow virus infection like Jakob-Creutzfeldt disease (and hence transmissible). At present, this does not seem to be the case.

2. Whether a genetic defect could predis-pose an individual to Alzheimer's disease.

3. Whether there is a soluble toxic substance responsible for the degenerative changes. Research in 1978 found a factor in a brain sufferer which induced some changes in brain tissue in the laboratory.

4. Whether aluminium acts as a neurotoxic agent. Increased concentrations of the metal have been found in the brains of sufferers, and there is some evidence to suggest a correlation between high aluminium levels and formation of neurofibrillary tangles.

One biochemical finding is that choline acetyl-transferase, an enzyme important for the synthesis of acetylcholine, appears to be less active in dementia victims and becomes further reduced as the disease progresses.

Arteriosclerotic dementia

Sometimes known as 'multi-infarct dementia', in this type of dementia the brain damage is caused by impairment to the blood supply and small infarcts. Naturally, the presentation varies widely depending on which and how many blood vessels have been affected. There can be multiple tiny infarcts, or more devastating damage if a larger artery obstructs.

Typically, the patient has a history of 'little strokes' and hence the deterioration is in steps. For example, the history could be one of several episodes of sudden confusion, possibly associated with neurological signs such as hemiparesis, slurring of speech and dysphasia, which then resolve to at least some degree in a day or so when the circulation is at least partially restored by compensation from other cerebral vessels. Eventually, recovery is less complete after each episode, and the patient becomes worse after each deterioration.

Although this can occur in younger people, it is more common in the over 60 age group, and men are more commonly affected. Insight into the illness is not usually impaired until quite late, although the patient may be quite handicapped some time before this, which is a major source of frustration to him.

Presenile dementia

This is a term applied to dementia affecting a younger person, e.g. 40–60 years old. Alzheimer's disease can occur in this age group. Pick's disease is a focal cerebral atrophy, which affects localised areas especially in frontal lobes. Often more than one member of a family is affected. Because of the focal nature of the disease, it can cause neurological signs and can present like a localised brain lesion.

Because of the younger age group affected, the implication of a presenile dementia on the sufferer and his family are terrible. As a person of 45 may still have young children, all the responsibility for family life, as well as the stress of caring for a person with dementia, falls on their partner.

Investigations

These should seek to exclude a reversible cause for the dementia. Blood tests can easily exclude dementia caused by metabolic disorders and deficiency states.

Sometimes, the clinical psychologist is asked to test the patient to assess the degree of dementia. Many patients, especially those with some insight, find this deeply distressing, as it brings home to them how much their memory and other abilities have deteriorated. They will need gentle support and understanding from the nurses — after all, none of us likes to fail a test in front of others, however tactfully it is handled.

Drug treatment

Use of drugs in dementia can be approached in two ways — the first is to attempt to improve the brain function, and the second to attempt to treat the troublesome symptom; for example, agitation, nocturnal restlessness.

Trying to improve brain function

At present, this area is still under investigation. It has been demonstrated that use of vasodilators to improve the cerebral blood flow is not really helpful in dementia and can cause unpleasant side-effects. However, products are being tried which are thought to act by improving the way in which the brain utilises oxygen and glucose. Hydergine, originally developed as a peripheral vasodilator, is such a drug. It is now thought to help brain cell metabolism, and transmission at the synapses, although how it acts is not fully clear. Clinical trials of this drug indicate that it appears to help with some of the problems of dementia, particularly with mental performance and mood, although the improvement normally takes a few weeks to be apparent. The usual dose is 45 mg daily, and it is well-tolerated normally.

The continuing research into dementia is also trying to find out more about the action of these drugs. The loss of activity of choline acetyltransferase could imply that drugs with an anti-cholinergic action would worsen dementia. Similarly, it is possible that in future a drug to stop the degeneration and perhaps even improve things could be found.

Treatment of symptoms

Drugs can be used to control the more distressing symptoms of dementia such as agitation, aggression, behavioural disturbances and mood changes (usually depression). Obviously, use of drugs must be considered carefully, and usually they are prescribed because the patient and his relatives are finding the symptoms very disturbing. Although tranquillizers and sedatives may relieve the troublesome symptoms, the medication can cause more problems, e.g. night sedation to control nocturnal restlessness can cause daytime drowsiness and haloperidol can cause rigidity. Likewise, use of sedatives needs to be reviewed frequently to cope with changes. Here, the nurses, who are in constant contact with the patient, can help by being alert to and reporting changes promptly, and ensuring that sedation never becomes routine.

Nursing care in hospital

Reasons for admission to hospital

There are four main reasons for admitting a person with dementia to hospital.

For diagnosis and investigations. In this case, the person would probably be admitted to either a neurology ward or a geriatric unit. Not all patients with dementia need hospital investigation — in some, the diagnosis is obvious, and any investigations are done by their general practitioner or in the outpatient department.

To relieve the carer. Caring for a relative with severe dementia is very hard, and the carers need short breaks to help them cope. Sometimes, this is to enable the carer to have a holiday, sometimes it is because the carer is ill. It is better for the patient to keep him in his own home, and to get the other relatives, friends and social services to take over the care temporarily, but in practice, if there is a sudden crisis, the offer of a hospital bed may be the most practical assistance.

Other illnesses and accidents. People with dementia can be admitted to general wards if they suffer from other ailments such as broken limbs from falls or pneumonia. The sudden change caused by the illness can make them completely confused. When planning for nursing care, the nurses will have to take the dementia into account and also will need to consider preparations for discharge very carefully to ensure the patient really will be able to cope at home.

When constant supervision is required. Some patients are eventually admitted to hospital because they can no longer be supported at home, either because relatives cannot cope any longer, or because there are no relatives. Behavioural difficulties are often the last straw — continual disturbed nights from night-time wandering, faecal incontinence and personality changes are amongst the things relatives find most traumatic.

Nursing care of a patient with dementia

Nursing care of a patient with dementia can be effectively divided into two areas:

— the care which he will require in hospital, which is essentially very practical, involves a careful analysis of all the patient's problems and anticipation of his needs.
— planning for his return home, which involves co-ordination with other agencies and departments to make sure that from the moment he arrives home he will get the support he needs to help him to manage successfully.

It is obvious that the two areas blend and overlap, and it is not in the patient's best interests to let him become less independent while he is in hospital. The practical care may be tackled by encouraging him to try things, under supervision, so you can assess what he can do and see exactly what the problems are. As you observe these patients, and carry out the nursing assessment, it will be obvious that some patients are more dependent than others.

As changes or unfamiliar surroundings often baffle a person with dementia, it is very helpful to ask the person who brings him to hospital to stay and help him with the admission interviews. The gaps in the patient's memory may be so large as to give quite a different history to that given by the carer. Similarly, with large memory problems, the patient may not reveal a problem which is fairly major at home (such as incontinence) because he has completely forgotten about it. It is common for a person with dementia not to know why he is being admitted. It is also very helpful to the medical team if the relative is asked to stay and can be seen separately.

When a care plan has been formulated, it should be discussed with the patient and the relative so that everyone knows what will be happening in hospital.

Nursing assessment

When admitting a person with dementia, it is useful to establish what he is normally able to do by himself, so you can determine what features of the illness are causing more distress to him and his family. This will enable you to plan individual care concentrating on these problems and also to ensure that, while he is in your care, the patient does not lose any independence.

There are four main areas for assessment:

- degree of dementia
- physical problems
- psychological problems
- social problems.

Degree of dementia

To a certain extent, you will be able to assess how badly your patient is affected by the way in which he answers your questions on admission. This particularly applies to questions about his present illness, past medical history, medication and reasons for admission. He may remember and give you a previous address. It is advisable to check these details discreetly with a relative afterwards, both to ensure their accuracy and to illustrate the extent of the memory deficit and the patient's awareness of this.

Physical problems

Dementia affects most aspects of everyday living and you should check for these. Once again, it is also important to seek the relative's opinion, as the patient may forget a major feature. Personal cleansing, mobilising, eating and drinking and sleeping can all be adversely affected by dementia and we will look at these individually to see what likely problems are.

Mobilising. As well as assessing how the patient mobilises, and whether he uses any aids to mobility, it is helpful to ask about falls at home and about wanderings. Wandering is frequently a great problem and the sufferer may continue to walk up and down even when really too frail and hence may fall often. Sometimes, the patient goes off for long walks and can become lost, and sometimes more frail patients confine themselves to repetitive behaviour in the home, for instance, cleaning the carpet so frequently they wear the brush out.

Eliminating. You should establish whether the patient is normally continent, and if not, whether he realises it. If incontinence has been a problem at home, what have they been able to do about it and do they get any help, e.g. incontinence aids, special laundry service? It is helpful to find out if the family has any special routines to maintain continence, and if you can incorporate these into your care plan you will benefit the patient and relatives. If the patient suffers from constipation, what does he use to correct this at home?

The patient's bladder habits at night are quite important. It is useful to know how many times he needs to get out at night, and whether he uses a bedside commode. A forewarned night nurse can anticipate the reasons for restlessness and searching by the bed, and avoid an embarrassing episode of incontinence.

Personal cleansing and dressing. Can the

patient wash and dress himself unaided, and if not, how much help is required?

Eating and drinking. As well as finding out whether the patient is on a special diet, it helps to find out if he can eat and drink without supervision, or if his concentration is so poor that he needs constant reminders or even feeding.

Sleeping. You should establish the times the patient normally goes to bed and gets up and if he sleeps all night. Night wandering is one of the most trying facets of caring for a relative with dementia; the patient can take naps during the day, but the unfortunate carer gets night after night of broken sleep, which affects her health, morale and ultimately her ability to go on coping.

Psychological problems

If the patient has a fair degree of insight into his difficulties it is quite likely that he will be depressed, and frustrated. Some patients cope with this by abusing their nearest and dearest, who they know, deep down, will not abandon them. Some patients are oblivious to the problems caused by their illness and this can add to stress for their relatives. When the carer is driven to consult the doctor or social worker and the patient then denies all the problems it can make the carer feel extremely guilty and disloyal. The patients with no insight can also get into difficulties when they try to carry on as usual, for example trying to collect their pension several times a day, every day.

Judgement is often affected. This can be assessed by the patient's attitude to his admission; some patients will see it as an attempt to get rid of them, which will be very upsetting for both the patient and relatives. Another difficulty can arise if an elderly parent is cared for by a son or daughter. Although the parent needs help and advice, he may bitterly resent having to accept it from his offspring. This especially applies to the over 80s, who grew up with different ideas about the parent-child relationship. Whether this will improve in years to come, with the freer relationships of modern times, remains to be seen.

Social problems

It should be established whether the patient already sees a professional community worker — social worker, district nurse, health visitor — and a contact name should be obtained. This will be valuable when planning to send him home. You should also ascertain what services and help the patient gets at home — home help, meals on wheels, day care. Again, if possible, get a contact name, to simplify re-arrangement of services before discharge.

It is important to discover whether the patient lives alone, or with somebody else and if so, with whom. A person with severe dementia will not normally be able to cope alone, so you should establish who helps him, whether it is a relative or a friend or neighbour. If you can, it is worth casting an eye over the 'main carers' to see if they themselves are elderly and frail. (After all, a patient of 80 could have child of 60, who is experiencing individual health problems.) Any specific accommodation problems will be easily established on admission, but problems within the family may not be so obvious.

After all these enquiries, you will form a picture of the patient's abilities and daily routine and will be able to use this information when planning his nursing care. You will also have an idea of the home conditions — where he lives, with whom, who helps him, how fit he is and what services he is receiving. This will be valuable information when planning the patient's return home.

When planning nursing care, the patient should be encouraged to do the things he is capable of, so that he does not become more dependent while in hospital. It may even be possible to make him a little more independent.

After the assessment interview, the patient should be shown round the ward, especially to toilets. He should be told what to expect in the way of tests and ward routine and you should be prepared to repeat these.

Planning nursing care

Nursing care must be individually planned to allow for individual needs. What follows here are a few suggestions which could help a person with dementia. As previously discussed, the patient will benefit if you can find ways to incorporate his familiar routine into his hospital care. A slight change in routine can completely baffle the patient, whereas a few familiar elements may keep him more orientated.

Maintenance of orientation

The aim should be to ensure the patient does not become less orientated in hospital. He will need to be kept informed of ward routine, investigations and similar events. A very forgetful patient will need regular reminders.

Sometimes, a person with dementia is extremely attached to his main carer, or another relative, so that he is literally lost without them. In this case, it is helpful to find out when this person is likely to visit, to reassure the patient, who may wander around aimlessly looking for this relative.

Careful judgement is needed to decide how far in advance to warn the patient about investigations — the relatives and friends may be able to offer advice here. Some patients will remember and worry if they know too far in advance, and others will panic if things are sprung on them. As a general rule, it is best to keep life at a slow pace and free from panic. Attempting to hurry a person with dementia is usually counterproductive; rush and panic added to confusion will often completely immobilise the patient.

Mobilising

With regard to mobilising, it is most important to ensure the patient does not lose independence in hospital. The physiotherapist may be able to help immobility with exercises. However, in dementia, wandering is more common than immobility and this is sometimes associated with falls. If falls are frequent, it pays to check the surroundings and footwear — slipping shoes can cause falls as can furniture on wheels. The physiotherapist can also advise which aids, if any, are most suitable for the patient.

Eliminating

If incontinence has not occurred at home, you should aim to prevent it happening in hospital. Since the patient is in unfamiliar surroundings he must be shown where the toilets are, and if necessary discreetly reminded to visit them regularly.

If incontinence has occurred at home, it is worthwhile to take a urine sample to check for infection. Regular toileting may help to promote continence. You should check that the patient's fluid intake is adequate — older people's solution to incontinence is to cut back the intake, with a view to reducing the output, which leaves them more prone to infections.

If constipation has been troublesome at home, it is worth increasing the amount of fibre in the patient's diet. Wholemeal bread, high fibre cereals and bran in the soup or stew are easy to do, not too expensive, and not too unpalatable. It is important to observe bowel habits in hospital, as the patient may not remember them for long, so that constipation can be treated before it leads to other problems.

Constipation and a full bladder can both be a cause of agitation in a person with dementia, and simple practical steps to alleviate both problems should be taken before resorting to drugs.

Personal cleansing and dressing

There will be great variation in the amount of supervision each patient needs, and in the first instance the nurse should discreetly observe and assess what the problems are, rather than take over. It takes a great deal of tact to help another person with personal hygiene and dressing without embarrassing him. A person with dementia can spend 30 minutes repeatedly washing his face, but never moving on to other parts. It sometimes helps to let the patient wash himself, while reminding him what to wash. Most people can wash something themselves, even if you do all the rest, and thus semi-independence is achieved.

As regards dressing, the occupational therapist may be asked to carry out a dressing assessment, or may suggest ways around particular difficulties with clothing, e.g. shirts with Velcro fastening that are easy to put on. If it is possible, the patient should dress himself, however long he takes.

It is much better for morale to be dressed in normal clothing rather than pyjamas. Keeping the patient in nightwear will not curtail wandering, so he might as well be warmly dressed for his travels. If you suspect he may wander off there are other steps to cope with this, such as noting what he is wearing and warning neighbouring wards and hospital porters.

Eating and drinking

Careful observation is required to ensure that diet and fluid intake are adequate. Wanderers particularly require a good calorie intake to replace all the energy they burn off on their travels. If the patient is not eating well, the nurses should investigate this — it could be he cannot cut the food up, or would benefit from adapted cutlery or a plateguard, or the food may be something he dislikes. A person with really poor concentration may need feeding, either to start him off, or when he gets bored and tired. Fluids can easily be forgotten by a person with dementia — he may leave his tea to cool slightly and not find it again until it is cold and unpalatable. In hospitals where a housekeeper gives out meals and drinks, it is very important that somebody watches to see the patient eats and drinks and reports to the nurse in charge.

Sleeping

In this area incorporating parts of the patient's

normal routine can help. If he can get up, go to bed and bathe, at his usual times, he is more likely to feel on familiar ground. Many people with dementia get up in the small hours, refreshed and completely oblivious to the fact that others are asleep and hope to stay that way. The dementia sufferer may get up and rummage around, which can be a great trial for others, both at home or in hospital.

Medication can sometimes help, but it is usually difficult to induce sleep without unwanted side-effects, such as daytime drowsiness. Drugs may also cause incontinence and falls. If it is practical, it is better to let the patient prowl around the day room, or keep the night staff company for a while, if it can be done without waking the whole ward.

Maintenance of morale

It is essential to the patient's wellbeing to treat him as an important individual, and to discuss his present and future care with him, even though he may not retain what has been said. Daily discussions of what is likely to happen to him may help to keep him orientated. Some patients, especially those with some insight into their illness, find interviews with doctors most distressing, as it reminds them how much their memory has deteriorated and not being able to answer the questions makes them feel useless and embarrassed. The nurses can help by discussing the reasons for these tests with them and emphasising how they help the doctors make the diagnosis. If the patient's judgement is affected, he may completely misconstrue the motives for the tests and feel the doctor is trying to catch him out or make him look ridiculous. These feelings are best expressed — feeling that the doctor is out to get him will make the patient depressed, miserable and possibly uncooperative.

A person with dementia who realises how forgetful and handicapped he has become, may get very depressed, and the depression can make the dementia appear worse. Antidepressants may be useful.

Maintaining a safe environment

Individual needs are very important here. Very badly affected patients will need the nurse to anticipate potential dangers; others will resist attempts to mollycoddle them. Wanderers, particularly, can be difficult to cope with. It is almost impossible to stop them wandering, and it helps to warn neighbouring wards and porters, so they can intercept. This, plus careful observation from the nursing and ancillary staff on the ward, should ensure you manage to keep them on the ward. At home, where it is completely impossible to stop a person wandering, it helps to ensure that the wanderers carry a card in their coat pocket, with their address and phone number on it, and a coin for the phone. The theory is that if they are lost, they can find a phone box, ring home, say what street they are in, and be collected.

Restriction inevitably produces more problems than it solves. Getting out of a 'geriatric' chair can cause more damage than a simple fall, and cot sides on the bed can be very frightening. It is better to watch the patient carefully, ready to step in if he needs help, rather than to depress and frustrate him with unneccessary restrictions.

Simple safety points which protect the very frail include not giving drinks which are too hot, or meals on very hot plates, checking the bath temperature and watching for trailing flexes and other potential hazards.

Careful observation and daily reviews with the patient and family should ensure that the nursing care is exactly what the patient requires.

Preparation for discharge

Since there is no curative or preventative treatment for dementia at present, the sufferer is dependent on supportive care from friends, relatives and health and social services. Most people with dementia continue to live in the community, either alone or with relatives, while others are cared for in residential homes, geriatric hospitals and psychiatric hospitals. The demand for services exceeds the supply. As the ageing population increases, the demand on support services will also increase.

Probably the most important point in preparing to send a person with dementia home is to ensure that there is good communication between all interested parties, including the patient, his relatives, his general practitioner and any official support services. The hospital team must not work in isolation; the successful survival of the patient in his own home depends on his getting the right kind of help, so it is most important to co-ordinate all parties and to start all services on discharge, with no time lapses or confusion.

While in hospital, both patient and relatives should be kept involved in progress and informed of new developments. If the occupational therapist and physiotherapist have been helping the patient, they could also meet the relatives, especially if one relative is the main carer, to show them the exercises and ideas which have been used. Then the relatives will know the capabilities of the patient, and can encourage him to persist with exercises. Relatives can also be taught new techniques of caring, especially helpful in dressing, walking and transferring.

The discharge date should be planned well in advance to give time to arrange all the services and support required, and to keep everybody informed. The nurse, especially the ward sister, becomes the linchpin, who passes on information to others, and ensures that all the interested parties get together. Communication with the outside world is vital — the general practitioner especially should know the discharge date, so he can take up supervision of the patient again.

The social worker should interview the patient and his relatives about their feelings and needs. She can advise about the availability of financial assistance, e.g. attendance allowance. One of the major problems of caring for a relative with dementia is lack of information about available services and help. When you are caring for a dependent relative, you lack the opportunity to go out and search for the information yourself, and find it hard to meet anybody in a similar situation to compare notes. Attempts to discuss your difficulties with others not in a similar situation are usually unhelpful as others do not realise what stresses are involved, and may think you are complaining unnecessarily, or trying to evade your responsibilities.

The social worker can be very helpful to these people arranging more practical aspects such as home help and meals on wheels. A social worker will also have information about sitter services, day care and carer support groups, which enable the carer to have some time off, and let her know she is not isolated.

Hence, hospital admission provides a valuable opportunity to review the services and support the patient receives, and check there is nothing new on offer from which he could benefit.

Arranging outside services

Provision of services will vary according to the individual needs of the patient and the availability of services. Services will differ widely in different geographical areas, varying particularly between town and country areas. Likewise, a person living alone will have different needs compared to a person living with relatives.

If you are discharging a person with dementia who lives alone the general practitioner must be informed prior to the event. It is also important to ensure that somebody will be at home to receive him, and to see he has some food in the house. A relative is best, but there will normally be a friend or neighbour willing to do this. The patient will tell you who he will trust to do this. Services which might be required include a home help, meals on wheels and bath helpers. Home helps play a very important role in community care: as well as attending to housework and shopping, they become trusted supporters who notice changes, and can alert other agencies if things start to go wrong.

There will be different criteria if the patient lives with a relative, depending on whether the relative is young and fit, or older and less fit. A patient living with another elderly relative may need the same services as a person on his own, plus a careful watch kept on the elderly carer to see how he is coping. The district nurses and health visitors can be very useful here. Where the patient lives with a younger relative, contact with a social worker at intervals can be useful and provides someone to turn to in time of crisis.

Support for the carers

Dementia is a grim illness, which alters the personality of the sufferer. The carer, especially if a relative, will remember the old days, when the patient was well and independent and cannot help but grieve to see him as he is now. In some patients, the personality change is so absolute that the family feels as if the person they once knew no longer exists.

If there is only one person living with the patient, that person will be continually 'on call'. Regularly disturbed nights quickly make the carer depressed and exhausted and reduces her ability to go on coping. Some patients, even if this would have been out of character previously, can be extremely difficult to their relatives; an elderly parent may resent his daughter advising him and become abusive, violent or storm out of the house. Repetitive behaviour can also be very stressful — to be asked the same question fifty times a day is extremely trying. The carers may feel very guilty and disloyal if they complain, or ask for help and may feel that they should be able to cope alone.

A social worker can help to provide regular relief and support. Just talking over the problems may help and in some areas, there are support groups for carers — a group of people all in the same situation who can be mutually supportive and listen to each other's problems. Naturally, to enable the carers to attend, somebody else has to look after the patient, and if no other friend or relative can help, a volunteer agency may be able to arrange a sitter service. The social worker will be knowledgeable about what is available in that area.

Occasional relief to give the carer a day off or a holiday is very welcome; sometimes, the patient can attend a day centre. In some areas, a care assistant will go in and help the patient in his own home, to enable the carer to take a holiday. At least, then, the patient is still in his familiar surroundings, and can follow his normal routine, even if it is a different person helping him. In other areas, temporary accommodation may be arranged in a residential home or hospital. If there is a choice, the wishes of the patient should be considered.

It is only recently that the needs of carers have been considered at all. Talking to them occasionally is not enough — they need to know that if they need help, they will get it, and should know whom to call in a crisis. If the carers are looked after, they will be able to continue looking after their relatives. Without their support, the patient may not be able to remain at home. Some patients eventually come to the point where they need constant supervision, and either because they have no relatives able to do this, or the relatives are unable to cope any more, need to live in a residential home or hospital.

PARKINSON'S DISEASE

Parkinson's disease was described in 1817 as an involuntary tremulous motion with lessened muscular power in parts not in action and even when supported; with a propensity to bend the trunk forwards and to pass from a walking to a running pace; the senses and the intellect being uninjured.

It is thought to be due to the loss of melanin pigment and degeneration of neurones in the substantia nigra part of the basal ganglia (extra-pyramidal system). Neurones from the substantia nigra pass to the corpus striatum which has the lowest dopamine content of the brain.

The patients are usually middle-aged or older but occasionally younger. The disease commences insidiously with shaking of a hand or foot which is most marked when resting and the so-called 'pill-rolling' movements are an early feature. The tremor ceases during sleep. It is most obvious in the hands and wrists but may affect any part of the body. It is rhythmical and regular at rest but stops as soon as the limb is put into action. The speech is rapid and monotonous.

Rigidity can be felt by moving a joint, e.g. wrist, when it gives a jerky sensation. This is known as cog wheel rigidity. The patient is stooped with a flexed position of the hands, arms and trunk. The presence of akinesia (an inability to initiate movements or to perform them quickly enough) is responsible for the poverty of facial expression and movements such as blinking, resulting in the so-called Parkinsonian facies or mask-like face. The patient has difficulty in walking and fails to swing his arms. The Parkinsonian shuffle is a short, variable, accelerating one.

Autonomic nervous system involvement is seen by the excessive saliva, sweating, greasiness of the skin, intractable constipation and, on occasions, retention of urine. In the late stages of the disease the memory may deteriorate and obsessional trends may develop. Treatment is with drug therapy.

It is vitally important that the patient is given his medication on time and that the effects and side-effects are carefully noted. The patient will often prefer the dyskinetic movement seen with overdosage in order to remain mobile and relatively independent. The dyskinesia is often more of an embarrassment to the relative than to the patient.

At certain periods during the day the patient loses the benefit of dopamine and will suddenly 'seize up' becoming rigid and immobile for varying periods of time. This can be corrected by fine titration of the drug regime, with the drug being given every 2 hours in order to keep the patient mobile. If the on-off phenomenon is evident the doctor will want to know when the patient becomes akinetic following the drug and also how long it takes for the next drug dose to act before the patient is mobile. This is very often a striking feature of severe Parkinson's disease. It is

Table 20.1 Drug treatment in parkinsonism

Dopaminergic preparations
These attempt to increase the amount of dopamine within the basal ganglia by the administration of its precursor dihydroxy-phenylanine (dopa).

Levodopa with carbidopa (Sinement, Sinemet Plus) Dose 100–125 mg, 3–4 times daily.
Levodopa (Brocadopa) Dose 125–500 mg in divided daily doses
Levodopa with Benserazide (Madopar) Dose 50–100 mg twice daily

All these drugs are adjusted according to the desired response and should be given following meals to reduce their gastric irritant effect.
Levodopa improves bradykinesia and rigidity more rapidly than tremor.
Side-effects can include nausea, vomiting, confusion, involuntary movements and postural hypotension.
Dopamine agonist
These act by direct stimulation of surviving dopamine receptors.

Bromocriptine (Parlodel) Dose 1.25 mg daily, gradually increasing until 10–80 mg in three daily divided doses is reached

Side-effects are as for levodopa.
Bromocriptine may be prescribed for patients on the maximum therapeutic dose of levodopa although this would need to be gradually reduced as the dosage of bromocriptine was increased.
Anticholinergic agents
These block the muscarinic receptors and attempt to correct the cholinergic excess which is thought to occur in parkinsonism as a result of dopamine deficiency.

Benzhexol (Artane) Dose 1 mg daily gradually increasing to 5–15 mg in daily divided doses
Benztropine (Cogentin) Dose 0.5–1 mg daily increasing to a maximum of 6 mg daily
Orphenadrine (Disipal) Dose 150 mg daily gradually increasing to 400 mg

These drugs are particularly effective against tremor.
Side-effects may include dryness of the mouth, blurring of vision, nausea, palpitations, constipation, retention of urine, confusion and hallucinations.
Anti-viral agents
Amantadine (Symmetrel) Dose 100 mg daily to a maximum of twice daily. Used as a complementary therapy, and may improve mild bradykinetic disabilities as well as tremor and rigidity.
Side-effects, which are rare, include nervousness, inability to concentrate and insomnia.

often helpful to devise a drug regime chart showing times and mobility acquired by treatment.

The use of surgery in Parkinson's disease was first tried in 1952, when it was noted that

accidental occlusion of the anterior choroidal artery causing infarction involving the globus pallidus and ventrolateral thalamic nucleus resulted in improvement of the tremor. This led to the use of stereotaxic surgical methods. Thermocoagulation of cells of the globus pallidus or thalamus decreases rigidity and tremor but akinesia is unaffected. It is now rarely performed and usually only on young people who have severe unilateral tremor only.

Nursing care

The aim is to promote maximum independence. The patient is usually admitted to hospital for drug adjustment or to allow relatives to have a holiday.

Maintaining a safe environment

In order to pre-empt dangerous situations within the patient's environment, the nurse should assess the extent of the tremor, rigidity and bradykinesia. The layout of the patient's immediate bed area or ward may need to be altered in order to prevent accidents. Any precautions taken at home will need to be implemented, where applicable, in hospital. The patient's reaction time will be impaired which will prevent him from taking avoiding action in the event of colliding with an object. The immobile patient is at risk from the development of skin breakdown and appropriate precautions should be adopted to avoid this.

Communicating

The patient's disability can make communication difficult and frustrating.

Aids for communication with the nurse, e.g. a hand bell or call system, must be available at all times, having ascertained that the patient is able to use the system. This will help to reduce the feeling of helplessness and panic if he suddenly wishes to go to the toilet or alter his position in bed or chair.

The patient will often withdraw from company due to embarrassment as the voice is often very weak and faint. The nurse must sit down with her patient in a quiet area of the ward and listen carefully to what he has to say thus preventing frustration and possible anger. The loss of normal eye contact and body language should be borne in mind. It is not necessary for the nurse to use a loud voice unless the patient is deaf.

It is vitally important that the patient has adequate explanations about all his care and if possible the care is best given by the same nurse as she can build up a relationship of mutual trust and understanding.

Agitation and confusion may be due to drugs, constipation or frustration on the part of the patient, therefore the nurse and the family must work together and communicate all information, however trivial, in order to relieve the patient's distress.

The opportunity should be taken to implement a patient teaching plan, with a view to eventual discharge. This might include:

— providing information about the disease and the help available, including self-help groups such as the Parkinson's Disease Society
— outlining the problems and hazards of immobility
— the role of drugs and their effects in the treatment
— advice on how to deal with urinary problems.

The teaching plan must also include the relatives and should be an ongoing process.

Eating and drinking

The problems related to eating and drinking are those associated with physical dependence as a result of the extent of the patient's abnormal posture, tremor and swallowing difficulties.

Feeding is a slow process due to the patient's difficulty with swallowing and excess salivation. Feeding by the nurse should not be started until absolutely essential. It may be that the patient is able to feed himself but cannot cut his food. The consistency of the food requires consideration and the advice of the dietitian should be sought. A minced or puréed diet may be advocated but it is important to tell the patient what it is. The use of specially adapted cutlery and crockery and other aids such as non-slip mats may prove helpful. A nurse should always be available to supervise the meal and assist in feeding the patient if he tires. Simple measures, such as holding the elbow close in to the body while lifting a spoonful of food, may help to overcome spillage due to tremor. The use of a bendable straw may aid drinking. Attention should be paid to oral hygiene following a meal.

Eliminating

Limited mobility in conjunction with urinary frequency or hesitation can lead to embarrassing episodes of incontinence. Offering to take the patient to the toilet at regular intervals may avoid this. Adaptation of clothes to permit easier access may avoid 'accidents' and location of the patient's bed within the vicinity of the toilet may be beneficial.

Constipation, which is common, can be helped by using faecal softeners or bulking agents regularly. The patient should be taken to the toilet at the same time each day rather than being offered a commode at the bedside. Dietary intake of fibre and extra fluids should be encouraged, but this sometimes requires a good deal of persuasion on the part of the nurse as the patient may fear urinary or faecal incontinence and so be very reluctant to take advice.

Personal cleansing and dressing

Immobility may result in physical dependence for personal cleansing and dressing. The degree of disability will determine the extent of help required. Particular points to note are skin care, provision of tissues to deal with excess salivation and additional personal hygiene to deal with the excessive greasiness of the skin. Adaptations to clothing may be necessary.

Mobilising

A major feature of Parkinson's disease is the multifaceted one of immobility. Problems can include difficulty in initiating walking, shuffling, tottering, being unable to stop, 'freezing' and stiffness leading to difficulty in rising from a chair, getting out of bed and turning.

The physiotherapist and the drug regime should assist in getting the patient mobile. Passive range of movement exercises are instituted and continued in the absence of the physiotherapist. A low bed with a firm mattress will help the patient to get out of bed and a spring assisted chair may solve the problem of rising from a chair. The patient should be instructed to sit in a high backed chair rather than the 'lounge' type chair. Assistance may need to be provided for regular turning and repositioning in bed.

Once standing, several techniques can be used to assist the patient. Gentle rocking of the patient to initiate walking may be helpful. If the patient 'freezes' tell him to imagine that there is a step in front of him and that he needs to step over it; this often gets the patient going again. If the patient starts to shuffle he should be stopped and restarted.

Working and playing

A chronic disabling disorder such as this will affect the patient's ability to socialise and continue in employment. The intervention of the medical social worker, occupational therapist and disablement resettlement officer may be considered appropriate.

Expressing sexuality

There may be anxiety about the performance of intimate procedures particularly if the patient is incontinent. It is vital that the nurse respects the patient's dignity at all times and minimises his embarrassment. Some difficulties may be experienced with the act of sexual intercourse. Professional guidance should be given and if the nurse feels unable to provide this, arrangements should be made for a trained counsellor to see the patient.

HUNTINGTON'S CHOREA

This was first described by George Huntington, a physician in New York, in 1872 when he described an inherited condition of chorea and dementia in a group of families.

The characteristic features are progressive dementia, facial grimacing and uncontrollable choreiform movements of the limbs. It may occur very rarely in childhood or early adulthood with generalised rigidity of the limbs.

The patient walks with wide-based lordotic gait, lurching from heel to heel with variable steps, starting and stopping and marked by vigorous movements of fingers and wrist and respiratory irregularity. The symptoms of the disease usually present between the ages of 30–50 years. The age of onset influences the rate of progression. Early development of symptoms is associated with rapid deterioration. It is transmitted by a dominant gene which, when present, will always produce Huntington's chorea. As the gene is transmitted on an autosome, it is an autosomal dominant disease. Both sexes are equally affected and each child of an affected parent has a 50% chance of developing the disease in later life.

It has been shown biochemically that gamma-aminobutyric acid (GABA), an inhibiting neuro-transmitter substance, is greatly reduced in the substantia nigra with a resultant fall in the activity of the enzyme GAD. Therefore it appears that there is death of the nerve cells producing GABA. Experiments suggest that GABA pathways exist between the basal ganglia and the substantia nigra.

Approximately seven people per 100 000 of the population in the UK are affected with Huntington's chorea. The disease occurs in all racial groups. There are about 5000 sufferers in this country. For every affected individual there are about two more who carry the abnormal gene and will later develop the disease.

Huntington's chorea appearing before the age of 20 years is passed from the father in 80% of cases and in those of very late onset the abnormal gene is more commonly transmitted by the mother. The nature, course and prognosis of the disease should be very carefully explained to the family and they should be offered genetic counselling and encouraged to join the Association to Combat Huntington's Chorea, a self-help group.

Diagnosis is made from the evaluation of symptoms and signs and the positive family history. EEG may show abnormally low voltage waves believed to be characteristic of Huntington's chorea. CT scanning may reveal atrophy of the caudate nuclei.

The progressive deterioration in the patient's physical and mental condition results in him/her being unable to work. This often leads to awkward, demanding and aggressive behaviour which can seriously disrupt the family. These unprovoked outbursts of physical aggression towards the family and their belongings often make it impossible for the patient to be nursed at home.

A genetic marker has been found in the DNA sequence of polymorphisms. A bacteriophage clone, code named G8, contains a sequence of human DNA that maps to chromosome 4. These particular polymorphisms show two variant forms and together form a halotype comparable with that seen in the HLA system. Unfortunately, these real advances have far-reaching effects on the patients and their families. Early detection of gene carriers may lead to untold agony for those who are told they carry the abnormal gene. On the other hand those family members who are cleared of carrying the abnormal gene can then marry and produce families without the fear of transmitting the disease to their offspring.

Nursing care

The patient ultimately requires long-term hospital care and will need expert nursing skills. The nurse must adopt a good rapport with the patient and his family.

Eating and drinking

Eating and drinking and smoking may become hazardous due to the choreic movements and the patient will eventually need help in order to get adequate nutrition. Swallowing is often difficult and the nurse must spend a long time with the patient and encourage a high calorie diet with frequent glucose drinks between meals. When the patient is no longer able to swallow, feeding via a nasogastric tube will be required and the patient given a high calorie diet. Drugs can be given by this route which obviates the need for intramuscular injections in the emaciated patient.

Eliminating

Constipation is often a problem and the use of an aperient and suppositories may be needed.

Communicating

As the disease progresses the patient's speech will deteriorate and loud grunting noises will be audible. This may lead to difficulty with communication and thus outbursts of aggression due to frustration. The family are often the key link in communication and should be consulted at all times especially when a difficulty with nursing arises.

Mobilising

The patient will eventually become totally dependent for nursing care. He will become emaciated, immobile and display rigid limbs and an abnormal posture. Care must be given to prevent the development of skin breakdown.

Dying

The patient will eventually die of exhaustion or hypostatic pneumonia but relief of symptoms at all times must be achieved so a peaceful, dignified death is achieved, preferably with the patient's family in attendance.

Drugs which may be used during the course of the illness include phenothiazines, e.g. chlorpromazine. These are dopamine receptor blocking agents and are designed to reduce the choreic movements. Tetrabenazine is now widely used. It acts by preventing the storage of dopamine thus reducing the amount available to be released when the nerve cells are stimulated. One of its side-effects is depression which may prove to be a bigger problem than the chorea. Diazepam may be given to relieve anxiety, and depression may be treated with the use of tricyclic antidepressants. Any psychotic aggressive behaviour may respond to phenothiazines. There is no treatment to prevent the progressive dementia. Antibiotics may be given for the treatment of intercurrent infections.

MOTOR NEURONE DISEASE

Motor neurone disease is a chronic progressive neuromuscular disease affecting the motor nuclei of the brain stem and the anterior horn cells of the spinal cord. The disease usually occurs in middle life and affects men more commonly than women. It generally occurs sporadically but in isolated instances it may occur in typical form in several members of the family. The cause is unknown but cases have been described as occurring many years after an attack of paralytic poliomyelitis, but the significance, remains doubtful. Four distinct clinical syndromes have been described, though most cases eventually show the features of more than one variety.

Progressive bulbar palsy

The lower motor nerve nuclei in the medulla are predominantly affected. The bulbar muscles become affected resulting in a wasted, shrunken and wrinkled tongue with visible fasciculation. At the same time the palate soon becomes affected as do the extrinsic muscles of the pharynx and larynx. The patient finds difficulty in protruding his tongue and finally is unable to do so. Speech becomes difficult due to paresis of the lips, tongue and palate and swallowing becomes increasingly difficult as the patient cannot propel the food to the back of the mouth and often the food is regurgitated through the nose.

Amyotrophic lateral sclerosis

The pyramidal tracts are predominantly affected causing a degree of weakness which is disproportionately great in comparison with the severity of wasting.

The patient complains of difficulty in walking because of stiffness of the legs and of dragging of one or both limbs. There is hyper-reflexia throughout all limbs with extensor plantar responses. Fasciculation in the shoulder girdle and thigh muscles is present and subsequently muscular atrophy appears. Symptoms and signs of bulbar paralysis are a late manifestation usually resulting in death. The diagnosis is made with clinical examination and the EMG results.

Progressive muscular atrophy

Anterior horn cells of the spinal cord are predominantly affected. The patient may present with a unilateral foot drop or weakness of muscles in one hand or the forearm which progresses insidiously. The patient may complain of difficulty with fastening buttons, sewing or writing and will eventually develop a wrist drop. As the disease progresses, extensive involvement of the muscles of the limbs and trunk becomes evident and the bulbar palsy develops with the patient complaining of difficulty with speech and swallowing. Widespread fasciculation of the muscles may be evident.

Bulbar-pseudobulbar palsy

Upper and lower motor neurone degeneration of corticospinal tracts above the medulla causes weakness of the bulbar muscles and leads to dysarthria and dysphagia. The weak muscles are spastic. The patient may develop the emotional lability often seen with inappropriate laughing and crying. The subcutaneous fat disappears as the muscles waste and marked emaciation characterises the later stages of the disease.

No medical treatment improves the outlook of the patient with motor neurone disease. Implicit in the diagnosis of motor neurone disease is the brief life expectancy of an average of 18 months to 5 years although in progressive muscular atrophy some cases have been known to survive 10–15 years from diagnosis.

Treatment is aimed at maintaining independence and morale of the patient for as long as possible. Death usually results from pneumonia and respiratory failure in a patient who is anarthric, aphagic and has widespread weakness and wasting of all muscle groups but who is mentally alert right up to the time of death. This is a very distressing illness not only for the patient but also for his family and nurses who may have been involved in giving care and support since the initial diagnosis was made.

Nursing care

Communicating

It must always be remembered that these patients are mentally alert and therefore the nurse must be especially careful not to show annoyance or irritation, if it takes a long time for the patient to make himself understood. He may wish to write notes asking about his care and expressing his anxieties about death and his sense of isolation. A pencil and note pad should be at hand at all times so that as he thinks of a problem he can jot it down.

Patients suffering from advanced motor neurone disease often feel sudden and frightening panic if they have an episode of choking or difficulty with breathing and it is for this reason that they should never be left alone without some means of communication. They are particularly frightened at night so, if at all possible, they should not be left alone.

The speech therapist can contribute to the patient's care by providing communication aids, a one finger typewriter and visual display board. She will advise the nursing staff as to to which communication aid is best suited to the patient's needs.

Breathing

Respiratory distress can be minimised by nursing the patient upright and slightly forward. Intermittent oxygen may also give some relief. Small doses of opiates may be prescribed to relieve distress and suppress coughing.

Eating and drinking

Dysphagia is a very distressing feature of the illness and one which causes the patient great embarrassment especially when in company as he chokes and drools over his meal. A puréed diet is better tolerated than a liquid one, as the latter tends to be regurgitated down the nose. The nurse should be sensitive to the needs of the patient during mealtimes. He may wish privacy to eat and this should be afforded. Any assistance requested should be rendered, e.g. providing a serviette or a supply of tissues to protect clothes from saliva and food.

Suction should be on hand in case of a choking episode and the patient may feel safer if a nurse stays with him throughout the meal. A piece of ice to suck prior to the meal often helps swallowing. When swallowing becomes impossible it is sometimes possible to perform a cricopharyngeal myotomy operation. This gives temporary relief to this very distressing problem and therefore it may be necessary to pass a nasogastric tube and then feed the patient this way.

Eliminating

As constipation is a common feature in this disease, the use of aperients and, if necessary, suppositories or enema may be indicated.

Personal cleansing and dressing

During the terminal stages of the disease the patient will become bedridden and as there will have been a significant weight loss throughout the illness, extra care will be needed to prevent skin breakdown.

Mobilising

Both the nursing staff and physiotherapist will perform exercises with the patient in order to maintain some degree of independence. A Hartshill support may be supplied. This is a plastic splint worn inside the shoe to support the foot in cases of foot drop. These are very lightweight and give patients a psychological boost by preventing them from tripping and injuring themselves. Active chest physiotherapy will also be applied.

Other walking aids include walking sticks and Zimmer frames and eventually a wheelchair may need to be supplied.

Working and playing

The medical social worker should be introduced to the patient and his family as she can provide the vital link to the care of the patient at home. She can also advise on the entitlement of the patient to financial help and alterations to the home to make life easier.

DEMYELINATING DISEASE

Multiple sclerosis, also known as disseminated sclerosis, is the most common neurological disorder in temperate climates but is exceedingly rare in the tropics. It is a disorder characterised by recurrent patches of demyelination in the nerve fibres of the brain, spinal cord and optic nerves. In order to make a firm diagnosis there must be dissemination in time and place. Therefore, it is not possible to attach the multiple sclerosis label to a patient on his first admission to hospital. The disease usually occurs in people aged 20–50 years and rarely begins after the age of 50. It is slightly more common in females.

Optic nerve

Acute demyelination of one or both optic nerves results in retrobulbar neuritis. The patient may complain of impaired vision which rapidly worsens and total blindness may occur. There is often pain on moving the eyes from side to side. In most cases the vision improves and is back to normal in about 4–6 weeks.

If ophthalmoscopy is performed, the optic disc is red and inflamed. However, when the attack has subsided the disc may look abnormally pale.

Spinal cord

The posterior columns are concerned with joint position sense, vibration and touch. Thus a plaque in this area could impair all three sensations. The patient will complain of loss of touch sensation in an arm, leg or in difficulty in knowing where his limbs are in space.

The most important fibres travelling in the lateral columns are the pyramidal tracts, the spinocerebellar pathways and the intermingled fibres concerned with bladder control. Plaques in this area will therefore cause pyramidal tract signs in the limbs below the level of the damage, i.e. spasticity, weakness, hyperreflexia and extensor plantar responses. The patient will complain of stiffness in the limbs when walking and a tendency to drag the leg and is subject to frequent falls due to tripping over trivial projections. Damage to the spinocerebellar tracts results in a wide-based gait, incoordination, clumsiness in control of hand and arm movements and intention tremor.

The impairment of bladder fibres results in frequency, hesitancy or urgency of micturition followed by incontinence or retention as the disease progresses.

Brain stem

This includes the eye muscle nuclei (cranial nerves 3,4 and 6), the pathway concerned with coordination of eye muscles and the corticospinal pathways. Disturbance of cranial nerves 3,4 and 6 results in diplopia often occurring abruptly but resolving in a few weeks. Malfunction in cerebellar pathways results in slurred, jerking speech (scanning dysarthria) and nystagmus when the patient attempts to look to one side. The combination of nystagmus, scanning speech and intention tremor (Charcot's triad) is a hallmark of the disease.

Euphoria may occur in up to one-third of the patients due to demyelination within the frontal lobes. Depression is a very common occurrence.

The cause of the disease is, as yet, unknown though many factors have been suggested and researched. These include infection, allergy, diet, climate, toxins, thrombosis of the small veins, and hereditary predispositions. None seems to bear any constant relationship although familial incidence of the disease is not uncommon and work on identical twins has shown that one twin may develop the disease several years before the other.

Patients with multiple sclerosis have been shown to have a deficiency of blood linoleic acid, a polyunsaturated fatty acid normally present in the myelin sheath and that linoleic acid deficiency leads to abnormal myelin sheath. Another possibility is that it may be an auto-immune disease in which antibodies are formed against the myelin sheath.

It is very important how and when a patient is told that he has multiple sclerosis and it must always be followed up by counselling sessions with the nursing staff. The patient must realise what a variable disease it is and that it can be very benign in many cases.

Many treatments have been tried including diet e.g. gluten free, fat free; drugs, e.g. immunosuppressives, cytotoxins; hyperbaric oxygen. The latter is based on the theory that multiple sclerosis is caused by fat globules which are trapped in small blood vessels of the brain and spinal cord cutting off the blood and oxygen supply. None of these treatments has been found to arrest the disease. ACTH may be helpful in the acute phase (during relapse) but does not benefit chronic cases.

Investigations include the clinical history. A history of relapses and remissions, retrobulbar neuritis, weakness and dragging of limbs and extreme fatigability are highly suspicious. Lumbar puncture may reveal a mild rise in cell count, an elevated total protein and gamma globulin fraction. The gamma globulin is a protein particularly concerned with antibody production and is elevated in approximately 60% of cases. It is said that the CSF is active for the first 5 years of the disease and thereafter returns to normal.

Other investigations include visual evoked responses, brain stem auditory responses and somatosensory evoked responses.

Nursing care

Maintaining a safe environment

Walking difficulties, visual disturbances and sensory loss may place the patient in danger. Precautions should be taken to prevent the patient from harming himself either within his home or in hospital. The integrity of the patient's skin should be inspected regularly. Simple measures to avoid cross-infection should be adopted; these patients are particularly at risk of developing chest and urinary tract infections.

Communicating

Communication does not normally present any major problems. However, the patient should be kept informed of his progress. Choosing the appropriate time to tell the patient his diagnosis is very difficult. This usually cannot be done until at least the second admission to hospital and this serves to increase anxiety.

An effective teaching plan would include:

— advice on care of the skin and any urinary problems
— advice on drug therapy
— the importance of maintaining social contact
— availability of the medical social worker regarding the availability of financial help and welfare benefits
— information on self-help groups, e.g. Multiple Sclerosis Society
— advice regarding sexual activity.

Eating and drinking

Advice may be sought on the use of special diets. As already stated these diets have not proved to alter the course of the disease. However, the patient may wish to try one of these dietary measures.

Eliminating

Assessment of any urinary problems, e.g. hesitancy or frequency, will allow the nurse to develop a programme to assist the patient. Retraining the bladder may be feasible along with the use of drugs. Continence aids, e.g. external penile collection sheaths, may be useful. Urinary catheterisation may eventually have to be considered. Provided that an aggressive catheter management protocol is adopted, the dangers associated with this can be minimised. Dietary advice should be provided with regard to the patient's bowel movement pattern. If necessary, aperients may be used.

Personal cleansing and dressing

The patient's skin is at risk and needs to be regularly inspected for breakdown. Regular position changes and the use of aids may be advocated. Assistance is needed, depending on the degree of disability, to cater for the needs of personal hygiene.

Controlling body temperature

Warn the patient to avoid extremes of temperature. They should not have hot baths or holiday in warm climates. Advice about how to deal with pyrexia should be given.

Mobilising

Moderate physical exercise only should be participated in. A daily schedule may be devised with the physiotherapist; the objective is to maximise mobility and reduce spasticity. Proper positioning in bed and the use of muscle relaxants may also be considered to reduce spasticity. The patient is encouraged to achieve independence within limitations. Various mobility aids may be used. To achieve the maximum effect it is important that the appropriate aid is recommended.

Working and playing

Changes in ability will affect the patient's social and working life. The intervention of the medical social worker may assist in developing an altered lifestyle to the patient's satisfaction.

Expressing sexuality

Problems may arise due to impotence. Professional counselling may need to be sought to deal with this and other similar problems. The patient should be allowed to express his feelings on his altered sexuality. Early advice should be sought regarding the risks of pregnancy.

BIBLIOGRAPHY

Bannister R 1985 Brains's clinical neurology, 5th edn. Oxford University Press, London

Bickerstaff E 1987 Neurology, 4th edn. Hodder and Stoughton, London

Cooksley P A 1979 A patient with multiple sclerosis. Nursing Times 75(45):1925

Durston J H J 1977 Motor neurone disease. Nursing Times 73(35):1352

Godwin-Austen R B 1984 Parkinson's disease handbook. Sheldon Press, London

Harper P S 1983 A genetic marker for Huntington's chorea. British Medical Journal 287:1567

Harrison M, McGill J I 1969 Transient neurological disturbances in disseminated sclerosis: a case report. Journal of Neurology, Neurosurgery and Psychiatry 32:230

Illis L S, Glanville H H, Sedgwick E M 1982 Rehabilitation of the neurological patient. Blackwell, Oxford

Kocen R S 1976 The neuromuscular system. Churchill Livingstone, Edinburgh

Lyons J B 1974 A primer of neurology Butterworths, London

Macleod J (ed) 1984 Davidson's principles and practice of medicine, 14th edn. Churchill Livingstone, Edinburgh

Walton J 1982 Essentials of neurology, 5th edn. Pitman, London

Wells N E J 1980 Dementia in old age. Office of Health Economics, London

21

Control of pain — the neurosurgical viewpoint

And a woman spoke, saying, Tell us of Pain.
And he said:
Your pain is the breaking of the shell that encloses your understanding.
Even as the stone of the fruit must break, that its heart may stand in the sun, so must you know pain.

Kahlil Gibran *The Prophet* (1926)

How can pain be defined? It is a sensation with which almost everyone is familiar — both from personal experience of pain and, as nurses, the pain expressed by patients. Consider, for a moment, how you would describe pain . . . it is very difficult to put into words, because pain varies. It may be mild or severe, a discomfort or an unbearable sensation. If it is difficult to describe your own pain, how much more difficult it is to describe someone else's pain.

The Concise Oxford Dictionary defines pain as 'suffering or distress of body or mind'; it can be deduced from this definition that pain is not just a physical sensation. Through the ages, many people have attempted to describe pain, and it has been associated with factors such as emotions, fear, guilt and punishment. The spiritual link with pain is quite pronounced in many cultures, i.e., pain related to divine or demoniacal intervention.

The word 'pain' is derived from the Greek 'poine', meaning penalty. In the Christian religion, the idea of pain being related to punishment is predominant, e.g. Eve's punishment for eating the fruit which was forbidden by God was 'with pain will you bring forth children' (The Holy Bible, Genesis 3:16), the pain suffered by Jesus, and His ultimate sacrifice in death, is central to the Christian religion — 'Pilate took Jesus and had Him flogged. The soldiers twisted together a crown of thorns and put it on his head . . . and they struck Him in the face . . . Finally, Pilate handed Him over to them to be crucified' (New Testament, John 19).

The relationship between pain and punishment may become associated with feelings of guilt which can be distorted. A person may believe that his pain (or illness) is some form of retribution for something which he has done wrong in his life. He may say, 'What have I done to deserve this?'.

Many people fear that death will be a painful experience —. associating it with physical pain — but these fears need not be justified. As nurses, our aim should be to prevent and relieve the suffering which pain can bring — not only for the dying patient, but also for the patient who has to live with his pain.

Perhaps it is so difficult, at times, to deal with pain because it is not a purely physical sensation. Aristotle said that pain, like pleasure, was 'one of the passions of the soul'. The physical, psychological, sociological and spiritual aspects have to be taken into account in order to achieve effective pain control.

Pain is a very personal and subjective experience. It differs from one individual to another and is expressed in a variety of ways in different cultures. In answer to the question at the beginning of this introduction, perhaps one of the best definitions of pain is that it is 'whatever the patient says it is, and exists whenever he says it does'. (The original source of this definition is difficult to trace, as it has been quoted in a number of works.)

WHY DO WE HAVE PAIN SENSATION?

Essentially, pain is a *protective* mechanism of the body. Humans learn to avoid or correct situations which provoke pain. For example, one learns (either by first-hand or second-hand experience) that fire burns and causes pain; an object which is causing pain, such as a small stone in one's shoe, can be removed. Pain is a major reason why people seek medical advice, and this often reveals an underlying problem. If pain sensation is lost, as in spinal cord injury, damage to tissues (such as burns, trauma and pressure sores) can occur.

Pain can also be viewed as a *plea* for help, sympathy or attention. As stated in the previous paragraph, pain often drives people to seek help. If the sufferer is ignored, or feels that his pain is not being adequately taken into account, criticism and resentment may build up.

A third consideration in relation to pain is that it may occasionally be used as a *pretence*. Situations where work is avoided, for example, or pain is used as an excuse to decline an invitation to go out — 'I have a headache'. Pain may be used to gain something, e.g. financial gain from an injury, where the pain is made out to be of greater significance than it really is. The latter, however, is quite rare; very few people are true malingerers.

PHYSIOLOGICAL MECHANISM OF PAIN

Pain sensation is initiated by the stimulation of *pain receptors*, transmitted via sensory nerve fibres to the central nervous system, and relayed to the sensory cortex of the cerebrum. Pain receptors (see Fig. 21.1) are free nerve endings located mainly in the skin and on the joint surfaces, and a few in the deeper tissues and some internal organs. It is thought that both mechanical and chemical stimuli may be involved in evoking the sensation of pain, either directly or indirectly. For example, stimulation due to injury, extremes of temperature, intense pressure or chemicals released by microorganisms may be responsible. One theory is that damaged cells release chemicals which initiate the afferent nerve

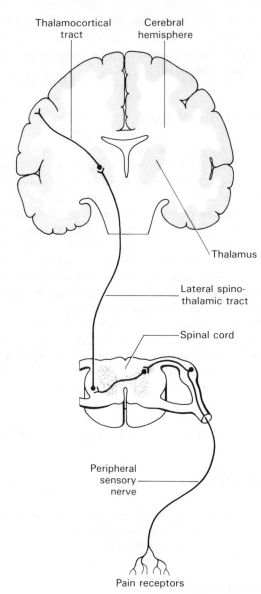

Thalamocortical tract

Cerebral hemisphere

Thalamus

Lateral spino-thalamic tract

Spinal cord

Peripheral sensory nerve

Pain receptors

Fig. 21.1 Psychological mechanism of pain (specificity theory).

impulses. A polypeptide resembling brady-kinin, and acetylcholine, have been shown to elicit pain (Keele & Armstrong, 1964).

Sensory nerve fibres

Peripheral nerves

The peripheral nerve fibres conduct the

impulses, which have been initiated by the pain stimulus, to the spinal cord or brain stem (depending upon where the stimulus originated in the body). It has always been accepted that sensory fibres enter the posterior nerve root of the spinal cord, but it is now believed that some may enter the anterior root.

Two main types of nerve fibres have been identified as pain fibres: 'A fibres' and 'C fibres'. 'A fibres' are larger in diameter and myelinated, and transmit impulses very rapidly. 'C fibres' are smaller in diameter and unmyelinated, and transmit impulses less rapidly than the others. The reasons for having the two types are not fully understood, but it is thought that the larger fibres deal with initial, intense pain and the smaller fibres deal with more diffuse pain and 'aches' associated with an injury.

Central nerves

Within the central nervous system, various mechanisms are involved. The most basic response to pain is the primitive *withdrawal reflex* (spinal reflex action). This is an involuntary response such as the withdrawal of the hand when a hot object is touched. It is a result of the sensory nerve impulse being transmitted directly to motor neurones within the spinal cord, to initiate an immediate motor response.

Impulses which are relayed to the brain pass across to the opposite side of the spinal cord and ascend the lateral spinothalamic tract to the thalamus and sensory cortex.

Areas within the brain — these are involved in *perception, interpretation* and *response* to pain. It is not known whether perception occurs in the thalamus or sensory cortex (i.e. awareness of pain). Interpretation of the site, quality and intensity of pain is at the cortical level. It is at this level that physical and psychological responses to pain are initiated.

The pain pathway described above is incorporated into what is known as the *specificity theory*, and is the basis for using surgical intervention in intractable pain. However, as new evidence comes to light, it is now known that the sensation of pain can invoke various responses before it is perceived.

INHIBITION OF PAIN

It is now accepted that pain impulses can be modified or inhibited before reaching the level of perception. Much of the research on this was based on a theory put forward in 1965 by Melzack & Wall, known as the *gate theory*. They suggested that a 'gating mechanism' was responsible for allowing pain impulses to ascend the spinal cord ('gate open'), allowing some impulses to be transmitted ('gate partially open'), or preventing impulses from being transmitted ('gate closed'). The original theory was modified by Wall (1976), as there was controversy about the actual location and mechanisms of the 'gate'. However, the basis of the theory may be accurate as it is known that there are areas within the central nervous system which inhibit pain impulses. The mechanism is much more complex than that stated in the original theory, and is still not fully understood.

The gate theory allows for certain measures in relation to pain relief, e.g., counter-irritation and electrical stimuli (other tactile stimuli decrease the perception of pain), reduction of anxiety (giving information about the pain and how to help to relieve it — inhibits the pain). Inhibitory descending fibres are known to exist in the brain stem, thalamus and cerebral cortex.

NEUROTRANSMITTERS

In 1975, certain pentapeptides were identified, which have a potent opiate agonist activity. The first two to be discovered were named *endorphins* and *encephalins*. Endorphins have a longer lasting analgesic effect, and encephalins a shorter effect. Both are produced naturally in the body (in the central nervous system). It is thought that these are conveyed in descending pathways of the spinal cord to the posterior horn cells, and inhibit the pain impulses. More chemicals with a similar action have since been identified.

PERCEPTION OF PAIN

The severity of the pain perceived depends upon the intensity and frequency of pain impulses (which ties in with the gate theory). The point at which a painful stimulus first elicits awareness is known as the *pain threshold*. The pain threshold, in physiological terms, is thought to be similar in everyone in relation to the same intensity and frequency of pain. However, individuals react in different ways according to physical circumstances and psychological make-up.

The pain threshold can be *lowered* — i.e., perception of pain is increased — by such things as inflammation or injury of surrounding tissues, and reduction of other stimuli. (Pain increases at night, when other stimuli are at a minimum.) The pain threshold can be *elevated* — i.e., perception of pain is decreased — by such things as shock, drugs and alcohol.

TYPES OF PAIN

Pain may be described according to where it is perceived as being located in the body, and classified as acute or chronic.

Location of pain

Superficial — pain arises from the stimulation of surface receptors (free nerve endings in the skin).

Deep — pain arises from stimulation of receptors in the deeper tissues and organs.

Localised — pain is perceived as being at the direct site of stimulation.

Referred — pain is perceived as being in a part of the body remote from the actual site of stimulation. There are several theories as to why referred pain arises, the main one being that some visceral and somatic structures share a common sensory nerve pathway in the central nervous system. This may result in misinterpretation in the cerebral hemisphere. Examples of referred pain are gall bladder pain referred to the right shoulder, and cardiac pain referred to the left arm.

Projected — pain is felt which logically should not be present, e.g. phantom limb pain, following amputation. The pain is probably perceived due to 'memory' of the nerve pathway which was once present.

Acute and chronic pain

Acute pain

Such pain is transmitted more rapidly than chronic pain; there is often an obvious cause, such as tissue injury. Anxiety related to the pain may be high, but the social effects are minimal if the pain is of short duration (e.g. postoperative pain).

Chronic pain

This is transmitted more slowly. The pain may not be related to any obvious tissue injury. Depression and anxiety are common and the social effects are marked.

Acute pain can often act as a warning and is usually manageable — the cause can be treated. Chronic pain, if continuous and unrelieved, becomes a threat to the patient. Pain which is persistent, severe, and cannot be controlled by conventional methods is termed *intractable*.

In some patients, there is no detectable organic cause of the pain. Although termed *psychogenic pain*, it is, however, very real to the patient. This type of patient presents a great challenge and should not simply be dismissed. He may benefit by referral to a 'pain clinic', where techniques complementary to medical practice are employed, e.g., relaxation, hypnotherapy.

Reactions to pain

An individual's response to pain involves both physical and psychological aspects. It will be affected by past experience, cultural attitudes and the person's present physical, mental and emotional state. The individual's reactions in coping with his pain will vary from time to time, as his perception of the intensity and the effect on his life changes.

PHYSICAL RESPONSES TO PAIN

Voluntary and involuntary responses to pain are evident:

Voluntary responses involve skeletal muscles, i.e., the withdrawal reflex (an immediate, protective mechanism), which can, in some instances, be overruled by the will; supporting or rubbing the affected part; adopting a position to provide relief; voluntary movement to distract from the pain, such as walking about, rocking, or tossing and turning in bed; removal of an offending object which is causing pain; seeking advice and assistance.

Involuntary responses include the withdrawal reflex, as mentioned above; actions related to the autonomic nervous system and increased output of adrenaline: superficial vasoconstriction (resulting in skin pallor); increased blood supply to the brain and skeletal muscles; increased cardiac output, with a resultant elevated blood pressure, tachycardia and more rapid respirations; decreased gastrointestinal activity; increased perspiration; dilatation of the pupils; cold and clammy skin and a dry mouth; involuntary muscle actions are contraction or increased muscle tone, which help to mobilise the affected part in injury.

If the pain is deep, severe or prolonged, other responses may occur. These include shock, low blood pressure, weak pulse, general weakness and debilitation, and nausea and vomiting.

PSYCHOLOGICAL RESPONSES TO PAIN

Individual differences in psychological make-up produce various reactions to pain. Factors mentioned earlier play a part, as do the threats posed by the pain and feelings of frustration which may accompany it. Some of the factors which need to be considered in relation to an individual's response to pain are summarised below:

1. **Social and cultural background** has a conditioning effect on the individual's response. It is acceptable, in some cultures, to display outward reactions such as moaning or crying. In other cultures, it is not expected that an outward show of emotions will be displayed. The nurses, and others, involved in the care of patients with pain should be careful not to judge by their own expectations.

2. **Emotions** such as anxiety, depression, frustration, anger and fear may exaggerate the individual's perception of his pain.

3. **The significance of the pain** must be taken into account. Apprehension is greater, and the pain intensified, if the patient does not know or understand the cause of the pain. Patient involvement and communication are important factors in the management of pain. If the pain results in a disruption of lifestyle, or is associated with certain parts of the body, such as the heart, these factors can be influential.

4. **Previous pain experience** may increase or decrease the individual's reaction to pain. If, for example, the patient has memories of previous suffering, he may have have a fear of this being repeated.

5. **The patient's physical condition** has an effect, for example, weakness and fatigue tend to increase the psychological reactions to pain.

6. **The intensity and duration** of the pain may pose more of a threat to the patient if severe and prolonged. Sometimes, however, the individual may become resigned to the pain and be able to accept and cope with it.

7. **Distraction** from the pain can diminish its severity. If attention is focused on the pain, it is perceived with greater intensity. The use of imagery and distraction can help the patient to focus away from the pain.

It is important to take into account the individual's reactions to pain, in order to deal with it as effectively as possible. An understanding of the causes and types of pain, the factors which can modify the pain threshold, and the physiological and psychological mechanisms which are involved, is essential.

ASSESSMENT OF PAIN

There is no easy method of understanding a patient's pain because it is an entirely subjective matter. Consequently, communication of information between the patient and people caring for him can present difficulties. Yet it is of great importance, for example, that the nurse communicates to the doctor how effective treatment is.

Several methods of helping in the assessment of pain have been proposed and put into practice. Some examples of assessment/observation charts are included here. They vary from a simple linear evaluation scale to the more detailed observation chart. Whichever method is used — and any is better than none — it is vital to include the patient in the assessment of his pain and his response to methods used to help to alleviate the pain. Although one might argue that this may be encouraging the patient to focus on his pain, if used in a sensible way it is of help rather than hindrance. Research has shown that information given to the patient can help to reduce pain and improve recovery (Hayward, 1975).

A good nurse-patient relationship is essential when dealing with patients in pain. Listening skills are important, and the patient's wishes should be respected. Whatever the nurse's views, the pain is real to the patient and he has the right to be believed. Pain can interfere with rational thought and produce problems in relation to normal activities. The patient's dignity must be maintained at all times.

Examples of pain assessment/observation charts

1. **Simple linear chart** (Fig. 21.2). Using a cross on the linear scale the patient is

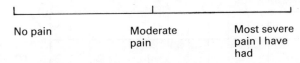

No pain   Moderate   Most severe
              pain   pain I have
                              had

Fig. 21.2 Linear scale for pain assessment.

requested to mark where he thinks is most appropriate to the intensity of his pain.

2. **A creative chart**, such as one related to the weather (Fig. 21.3), may help the patient to identify his pain perception. The chart can be continued over a period of time (Irving & Sellek, 1982). The weather is often a topic of interest, and helps as a form of distraction

3. **The London Hospital pain observation chart** (Fig. 21.4), which owes a lot to neurological observation charts, is intended to help in communication between the patient and the nurse. It can also be useful in passing on information and evaluating the management of the patient's pain. This chart incorporates a body diagram, to indicate where the site of

the pain is, a scale to indicate the severity of the pain, measures taken to relieve the pain, and additional comments. Comments can be included by both staff and patients. It may be necessary, on some occasions, to have two charts — one kept by the patient and one by the staff

Assessment of the patient's pain, and his responses to it, is necessary so that the patient's needs can be identified and met. Pain relief and pain control are more likely to be effective if the care is appropriate to the individual.

MANAGEMENT OF PAIN

The main aspects to consider when dealing with patients in pain are:

— Is the pain a symptom of an underlying disease which can be treated?

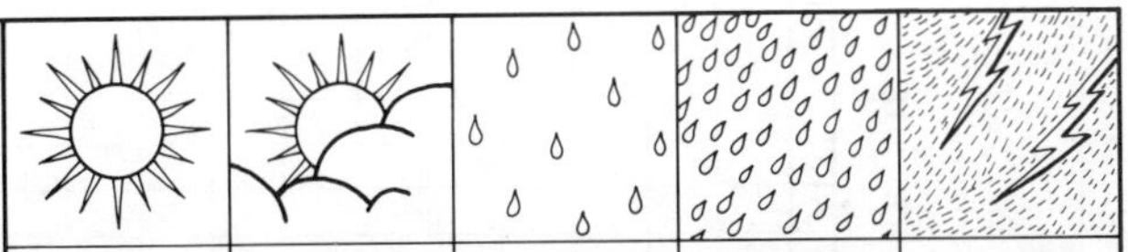

Weather outlook		Sunny	Cloudy	Drizzle	Heavy rain	Stormy
Description of pain		No pain	Slight pain	Bad pain	Severe pain	Sickening unbearable pain
Date	Time					

Fig. 21.3 Creative pain assessment chart. The date and time are written in the appropriate column, and a tick placed in the column which most accurately relates to the pain. (Reproduced by kind permission of Nursing Times where this diagram first appeared on June 9, 1982.)

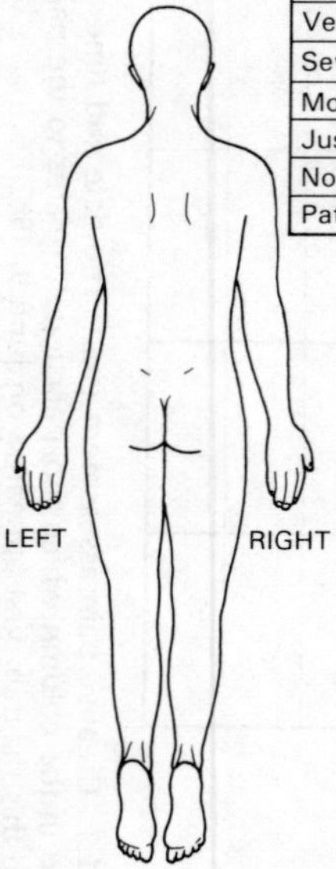

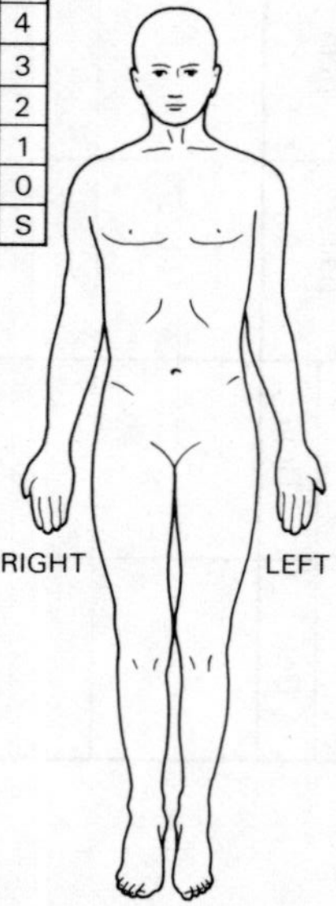

DATE _____

SHEET NUMBER _____

PATIENT IDENTIFICATION LABEL

PAIN RATING

BY SITES
A B C D E F G H

OVERALL

TIME

MEASURES TO RELIEVE PAIN   Specify where starred

ANALGESIC GIVEN (Name, dose, route, time)

Lifting
Turning
Massage
Distracting activities *
Position change *
Additional aids *
Other *

COMMENTS FROM PATIENTS AND/OR STAFF

INITIALS

Excruciating	5
Very severe	4
Severe	3
Moderate	2
Just noticeable	1
No pain at all	0
Patient sleeping	S

RIGHT   LEFT

LEFT   RIGHT

THIS CHART records where a patient's pain is and how bad it is, by the nurse asking the patient at regular intervals. If analgesics are being given regularly, make an observation with each dose and another half-way between each dose. If analgesics are given only 'as required', observe 2-hourly. When the observations are stable and the patient is comfortable, any regular time interval between observations may be chosen.

TO USE THIS CHART ask the patient to mark all his or her pains on the body diagram below. Label each site of pain with a letter (i.e. A, B, C, etc.).

Then at each observation time ask the patient to assess:

1 the pain in each separate site since the last observation. Use the scale above the body diagram, and enter the number or letter in the appropriate column.
2 the pain overall since the last observation. Use the same scale and enter in column marked OVERALL.

Next, record what has been done to relieve pain:

3 note any analgesic given since the last observation — stating name, dose, route, and time given.
4 tick any other nursing care or action taken to ease pain.

Finally, note any comment on pain from patient or nurse (use the back of the chart as well, if necessary) and initial the record.

Fig. 21.4 London Hospital Pain Observation Chart (reproduced by permission of Jennifer Raiman, Macmillan Research Associate, The London Hospital Medical College).

Pain is a wholly subjective symptom. In consequence, there is no easy way of understanding what a patient is suffering, nor of conveying information about it from one person to another, though doctors and nurses need to do so. For instance, a doctor who needs to check the effectiveness of an analgesic prescription may find it difficult to say what information should be decisive. Thus, problems of communication can result in poor control of pain.

The pain observation chart is intended to improve communication between patient, nurse and doctor by making the recording of pain more systematic; the idea owes a lot to charts for neurological observations. Secondly, it is intended to make readily available in one place the information that is useful when taking decisions about the management of pain; for this reason some information already available on the drug chart, and some in the nursing record, is inevitably duplicated in it. Thirdly, it is intended to focus attention on the mechanisms of different pains, and to provide evidence on what relieves them, by recording each site of pain separately.

You are likely to find this chart most useful when you know that a patient's pain is a problem, or you think it may be. It is a mean of communication, to be used *with* the patient, not *on* the patient. Nurses should have it available at the handover report between shifts, and doctors will need it for ward rounds. The brief comments allowed may prove unexpectedly significant, and need amplification, so it is important that each entry is initialled. Occasionally, it may be a good idea to have two separate, independent charts, one kept by the patient, the other by the staff.

— Is the pain a temporary symptom, e.g. as a result of injury or surgical intervention, and of relatively short-term duration?
— Is the pain related to a chronic condition, such as cancer, which is not curable?
— Is the pain psychogenic, i.e. no physiological basis for the pain can be established?

Ideally, the goal in the management of pain is to provide and maintain relief from the pain — *analgesia* (without pain). This is usually easier to achieve in acute pain than with chronic pain. There are many methods which can help to lessen the individual's perception of his pain, as well as techniques which can relieve the pain by dealing with the underlying cause (where known).

A brief description of some of the factors which are important in the management of pain are included here. As stated earlier in the text, various factors can affect the individual's perception of his pain and these should be taken into account. The intensity and severity of the pain may vary from day to day, and during the day or night, therefore, regular assessment of the patient is necessary.

Nurse-patient relationship

An effective and supportive relationship with the patient will help to build up his confidence and trust. The patient is an essential source of information on his perception of the pain and should be included in the assessment whenever possible. The nurse should not let her own prejudices or preconceptions interfere with the management of the patient.

Patient teaching

The nurse has a responsibility to provide information which will be of value to the patient. She must ensure that the patient understands information which is given to him so that he can co-operate in the management of his pain.

Information to others

Communication between all involved — staff, patient and patient's family/visitors (as appropriate) — is essential. The patient's family/friends may need advice, help and encouragement. Information can be passed on more easily between staff, if some form of assessment/observation chart is used.

Complementary techniques in pain relief

Adequate rest and a comfortable position and environment can help the patient, as can psychological factors. A growing awareness and interest in techniques which, in the past, have come into the sphere of 'alternative therapies' have opened up a wide range of possibilities. It is now accepted that many of these techniques have sound physiological or psychological bases. Some examples of the techniques which can be used in the management of pain are:

— relaxation and meditation, which help to decrease stress and anxiety
— imagery: recalling pleasant events/ experiences: to decrease awareness of pain
— distraction — focusing attention away from the pain, e.g. by reading or listening to music.

These techniques may be used in conjunction with psychotherapy, hypnotherapy and biofeedback.

Cutaneous stimulation

Other sensory stimuli to the skin can result in inhibition of pain impulses, e.g. pressure or changes in temperature. The act of rubbing the affected part decreases the perception of the pain, for example. There are numerous methods of cutaneous stimulation which can be used, including the following:

- ointments, sprays and other topical applications (many of which may contain a local anaesthetic agent)
- massage — either general body massage, reflexology or acupressure — which may be facilitated by the use of oils, lotions or talcum powder; aromatic oils are used in aroma therapy; massage induces a muscle relaxant and sedative effect, making the patient more relaxed and enhancing a feeling of wellbeing
- application of heat, e.g., hot water bottles, heat pads, heat lamps, short-wave diathermy may be effective; application of cold substances, e.g., cold compresses, ice packs, ethyl chloride spray, may be used also; heat and cold elevate the pain threshold and reduce muscle spasm, but they vary in effect, depending upon the underlying condition; the patient may prefer one to the other — relief may be obtained by heat rather than cold, or vice versa, in different individuals — but care must be taken if there is impaired sensation, or with patients who are unable to communicate
- acupuncture can be effective in relieving

pain, even when applied to a site remote from the area which is stimulated; the reasons for this are not fully understood, but the theories include:

a. helping the body to return to harmony, which has been disrupted (the Chinese theory of 'yin' and 'yang')
b. a similar effect to hypnosis may be produced (this theory is not widely accepted)
c. the pain impulses are modulated — which relates to the gate theory
d. acupuncture may cause the release of endorphins, which have a natural analgesic effect
- transcutaneous electrical nerve stimulation — this is discussed in more detail in a later section, as it relates to the sphere of neurosurgical techniques.

Analgesic drugs

The use of analgesic drugs may be the first thought of many people in relation to the management of pain. Although these drugs have a very important role, they should not be considered as the only method of pain relief which can be used — as is often the case. The other techniques may be as effective, or more effective, in some patients, without the risk of side-effects which there may be from drugs. Analgesic drugs can be used in combination with other drugs and/or other techniques in the control of pain. Often, a milder analgesic is effective if used in this way.

The important points to remember in relation to the use of analgesic drugs are:

1. efficacy of the medication — i.e., the maximum effect of a given dose; in severe pain, for example, only the opiates and synthetically related drugs are effective
2. individual response — this can vary in different individuals, particularly in the very young and the elderly
3. duration of action — how long the drug takes to become effective and how long the effect lasts; this is related to plasma levels of drug concentration

4. toxicity — the level at which unwanted or dangerous side-effects occur
5. cumulation — some drugs are stored in the body and acumulative effect can arise
6. tolerance — some drugs lose their effectiveness as the body becomes used to the drug
7. dependence — physical dependence may develop, but the patient can be 'weaned off' the drug, without adverse effects
8. addiction — this is linked with psychological, as well as with physical, dependence and is usually related to drug abuse; the fear of patients becoming addicted is largely unjustified.

The nurse has an important role in evaluating if the drugs are given at adequate intervals of time and in suitable dosages, i.e. that they are effective in providing and in maintaining adequate pain relief. Also she must observe for side-effects and note whether these are acceptable or dangerous. The nurse has a responsibility to report to the doctor who has prescribed the medication, and also to consult with him if she has suggestions for helping to achieve better pain control.

Other drugs and substances

1. **Sedatives, tranquillisers and hypnotic drugs** may be used in conjunction with analgesic drugs. These are particularly useful in patients with chronic, prolonged pain to help with restlessness, anxiety, depression and insomnia. Some drugs potentiate the action of analgesics, e.g., a phenothiazide compound (such as chlorpromazine) enhances the effect of analgesics, and can be used with a mild or moderate analgesic. The patient is then not subjected to the stronger analgesics which have undesirable side-effects, especially those taking away the patient's independence.

2. **Alcohol**, in moderate amounts, (if not contra-indicated) can be useful, e.g., prior to sleeping.

3. **Anti-inflammatory drugs**, such as phenylbutazone and indomethacin, are particularly useful for bone pain (e.g., spinal metastases) and also for muscular aches.

4. **Muscle-relaxant drugs**, including diazepam, are effective, e.g., in lumbar disc protrusions.

5. **Hormone therapy and steroids** are useful, e.g. dexamethasone for cerebral metastases and prednisolone for bone metastases.

6. **Entonox** (oxygen and nitrous oxide) is a gas which can be used for short-term effect, e.g., when dressing painful wounds. It should not be used, however, if the patient is unconscious or has severe head injuries.

7. **Side-effects** of the patient's condition, and of the analgesic drugs being taken, can be reduced or relieved, e.g. anti-emetic drugs can be given for nausea and vomiting, laxatives and aperients can be given for constipation.

The whole range of drugs and other substances which can be used is not included here. There are many situations which can arise, and the staff should use their judgement as to what might be effective according to the patient's needs. A lot is owed to the work of those involved in hospice care, and the care of the terminally ill, in the effective management of pain and its consequences.

Placebos

A placebo is an inert preparation or form of treatment which produces a response in the patient. The response may be positive, i.e. the patient reacts favourably, or it may be negative, i.e. the patient does not benefit by the treatment. A significant aspect of the use of placebos is suggestion of the purpose of the 'drug' or treatment. About one-third of patients given a placebo for pain relief will actually report this effect, if they have previously been told to expect it. Conversely, patients given a strong analgesic drug may not feel any effect if told that the drug is not very effective.

The area of using placebos and their effects is very complex. It is important not to draw the wrong conclusions when the patient reacts in a positive way to a placebo. A positive reaction, e.g. when the patient reports that his pain has been relieved, does not necessarily mean that his pain is psychogenic in origin. Nor does it mean that he did not have any pain in the first place.

Irradiation

Pain arising from bone metastases can be relieved or reduced by irradiation therapy. The patient needs to be in a reasonably fit condition to undergo this kind of treatment, because of its severe side-effects.

Neurosurgical techniques

Pain which is not relieved by other methods, i.e., intractable pain, such as the pain related to nerve compression, may be treated by surgical intervention. Some other aspects of pain control come into the sphere of neuro-surgery, e.g. neural stimulation, nerve blocks and hypophysectomy. These are discussed in more detail in the following section.

NEUROSURGICAL ASPECTS OF PAIN CONTROL

The areas which come into the sphere of neurosurgical techniques, in a more specific way, include electrical nerve stimulation, nerve blocks and surgery to treat an under-lying condition or to interrupt pain pathways.

Electrical stimulation

Electrical nerve stimulation works by applying, or implanting, small electrodes which can be activated to supply a low electrical current. This results in stimulation of nerve fibres and reduction of pain impulses. It produces a tingling sensation, which can be modified so that it is not unpleasant. The technique does not work in all cases, but is effective in some patients with chronic pain.

The main advantages of the system are that the patient has some control over his pain and there are few or no harmful side-effects.

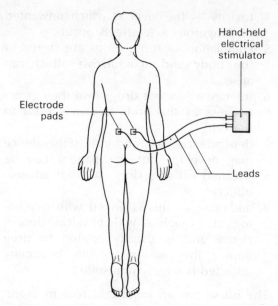

Fig. 21.5 Example of transcutaneous neural stimulation of low back pain.

Transcutaneous electrical nerve stimulation (TENS) (Fig. 21.5)

In this technique, electrodes are placed on the surface of the skin over the painful area (two electrodes are usually used). These are connected, by leads, to a battery-operated generator, which is portable and controlled by hand. The patient needs to have the electrodes placed in the optimum position, allowing for comfort, where they are taped onto the skin. He also needs to be instructed about the use of the controls, and to be seen regularly to ensure that the stimulation is effective in reducing his pain.

The main disadvantages of this system are that the electrodes may easily become dislodged and strong magnetic fields can affect the stimulator.

Direct neural stimulation

This is a similar technique to TENS, except that the electrodes are implanted, either in contact with peripheral nerves or into the epidural space, near the dorsal columns of the spinal cord. The electrodes are implanted under local anaesthetic, so that the effectiveness of the stimulation can be assessed before their final position is determined. The spinal cord electrode is implanted through a hollow needle, using a technique like lumbar puncture, and is attached to a small insulated wire. This is connected to a stimulator.

The stimulator for the electrode is usually implanted into the chest or abdominal wall. It is about 5 centimetres in diameter. The rate and intensity of stimulation can be adjusted by an external control, and this is usually performed by the surgeon. However, the patient may be able to have his own programming control if the doctor prescribes it. The stimulator can be turned on and off using a special magnet, which the patient is instructed how to use.

Batteries in the stimulator last for 2 years or more, but the patient is advised to see his doctor twice a year to check that the programming is suitable. There is a small risk of problems such as infection, leakage of cerebrospinal fluid, spinal cord damage, displacement of the leads and rejection of the implants.

The patient is advised to carry an identification card, indicating that he has this type of implant, with details of the type of stimulator and rate and intensity at which it is set. Airport screening equipment can detect the metals, and an identification card could prove helpful in this situation.

Precautions to be taken when using a neural stimulator are in pregnancy (effects not known), near strong magnetic fields (can activate or deactivate the stimulator and with ultrasonic scanning equipment (may deactivate stimulator). Also, the patient should be advised not to wear tight clothing over the stimulator, as this can cause friction of the skin, and to avoid very strenuous activity, as this could dislodge the lead. The patient can usually bathe and swim without ill effect. Movement of the lead can result in a change in intensity of the stimulation, but this is no cause for alarm unless the intensity becomes uncomfortable.

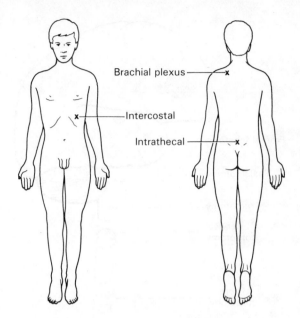

Fig. 21.6 Examples of sites for nerve blocks.

Nerve blocks (Fig. 21.6)

Peripheral nerves may be interrupted by injection of a local anaesthetic (temporary effect) or destroyed by a neurolytic agent such as phenol. In the latter, however, the treatment may have to be repeated at intervals, as regeneration of the nerve tends to occur, and the pain returns. Some of the areas which can be treated, using these methods, are the brachial plexus, intercostal nerves and injection into the subarachnoid space (intrathecal injection). Motor function will also be impaired, but is not really of significance, except in intrathecal injection. Intrathecal phenol is sometimes used to reduce spasticity. Spinal anaesthesia (an anaesthetic agent is introduced into the subarachnoid space) and epidural anaesthesia (an anaesthetic introduced into the epidural tissue) are used in surgery and in labour.

The main dangers associated with intrathecal and epidural anaesthesia are damage to the spinal cord, resulting in unintentional paralysis and loss of sensation, and side-effects such as severe headache, seizures and impaired consciousness. If performed by an

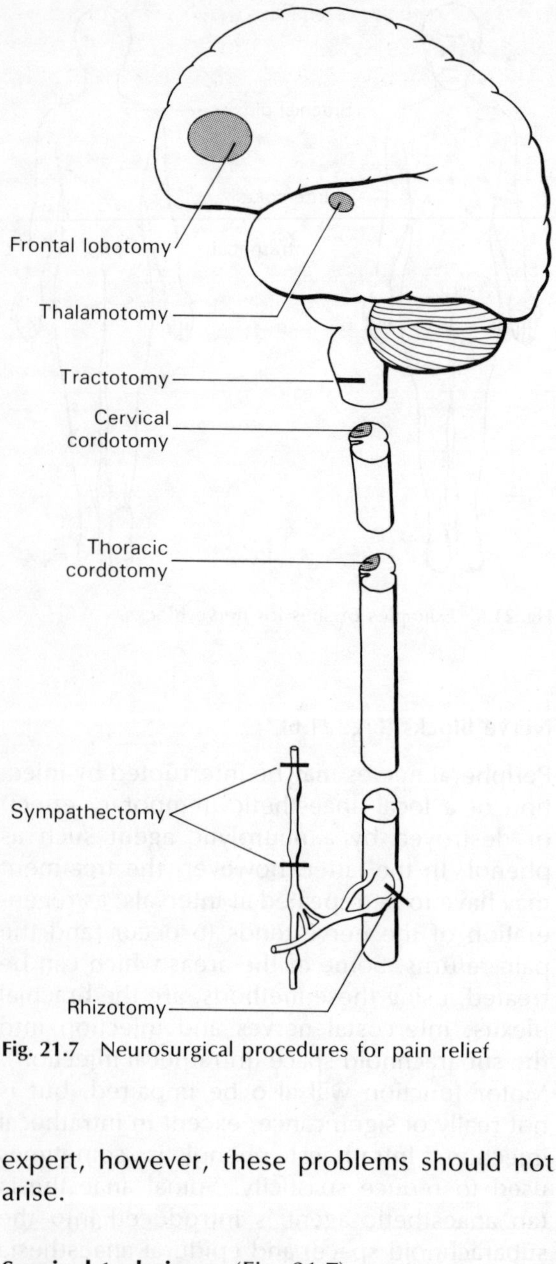
Frontal lobotomy
Thalamotomy
Tractotomy
Cervical cordotomy
Thoracic cordotomy
Sympathectomy
Rhizotomy

Fig. 21.7 Neurosurgical procedures for pain relief

expert, however, these problems should not arise.

Surgical techniques (Fig. 21.7)

Surgery to relieve pain consists of a number of techniques, which are discussed below:

Rhizotomy

This involves division of sensory nerve roots at the level of pain and the segments above and below. Motor function can be preserved but other sensations are lost. It is useful in conditions such as intractable pain, herpes zoster and neuroma pain from the stump of an amputated limb. Patients with partial spinal cord lesions, due to trauma or degenerative conditions, may also benefit from rhizotomy, because it reduces spasticity and painful reflex contractions which are associated with these.

Rhizotomy is often combined with injection of alcohol or with electrode destruction of the nerve roots to prevent regeneration of the axons.

It is important to ensure that the patient is aware of sensory loss, so that he avoids injury — e.g. trauma, burns — to the affected area.

Cordotomy

This involves division of sensory fibres in the lateral spinothalamic tract of the spinal cord. It results in a loss of pain and temperature sensation on the opposite side of the body, below the level of surgery. The cervical and thoracic areas are most commonly operated upon, to relieve pain in the arm and chest and the abdomen/lower limbs, respectively.

Cordotomy is useful in conditions such as herpes zoster, neuralgia and deep pain. However, the effect may only last up to about 18 months, as adjacent nerve tissue tends to take on the function which has been lost. If the pain is in the midline or bilateral, both sides of the cord have to be treated.

Problems which can arise, apart from loss of temperature sensation, are respiratory depression (in cervical cordotomy) and disturbances of bladder control and spasticity of the legs (in thoracic cordotomy). It is important not to give respiratory depressant drugs to patients who have had a cervical cordotomy.

Tractotomy

This involves division of nerve fibres in the medulla and midbrain. It is not as effective in relieving pain as cordotomy, and is associated with severe side-effects such as visual and auditory disturbances.

Thalamotomy

As pain fibres synapse in the thalamus, this region can be treated by stereotactic measures. However, it is usually carried out as a last resort in intractable pain, because adjacent structures may be destroyed. Patients with malignancy of the face or cranium may benefit from this procedure, but the complications often outweigh the advantages.

Frontal lobotomy

In this type of surgical intervention the patient's response to pain is altered. He is still aware of the pain but it does not bother him. It is a rather drastic form of treatment as it is accompanied by frontal lobe changes. The patient may exhibit personality changes, apathy, incontinence and socially unacceptable behaviour. Unilateral surgery is not very effective, as the relief tends to last only for a few months. Bilateral surgery results in permanent changes.

A newer technique, using cryosurgery, may reduce the problems, as a smaller area can be treated than with surgical resection.

Sympathectomy

This is resection of part of the sympathetic trunk. It is sometimes carried out for intractable pain, chronic pain and causalgia (intense, burning pain, which usually results from trauma). The results are not always good, because 'rerouting' of nerve pathways may occur or regeneration of the nerve fibres which have been severed.

The patient should be observed for disorders arising from loss of sympathetic control, following this procedure.

Hypophysectomy and pituitary ablation

Surgical removal or destruction of the pituitary gland has been used to control generalised pain. Patients with terminal cancer and hormone dependent tumours benefit from this technique. The pituitary gland may be surgically removed or destroyed by electro-coagulation, injection of alcohol or stereotaxis. The gland is usually approached by the trans-sphenoidal route.

It is not clear exactly why this is an effective method of controlling severe, generalised pain, but it is possibly related to endorphin production.

The patient undergoing this form of treatment will require similar care to any patient undergoing hypophysectomy.

Peripheral nerve section

Pain arising from tumours or trauma to peripheral nerves may be alleviated by surgery. This includes neurotomy (division of a nerve), neurectomy (excision of a nerve) and neurolysis (freeing of a nerve from adhesions or bone callus). Depending upon the underlying condition, repair of the nerve may be attempted, in order to restore normal function.

Surgery for an underlying cause of pain

This may be the obvious treatment if a cause for the pain has been identified and can be treated by surgical intervention, e.g. relief of intracranial pressure or removal of a prolapsed intravertebral disc. The pain, especially in the latter condition, may take some time to resolve following surgery, and the patient should be aware of this.

CONCLUSION

The management of patients with pain is a very challenging area, especially when dealing with patients who have chronic or intractable pain. The nurse working in a neurological or neurosurgical unit will come into contact with patients who have both acute conditions which give rise to pain and chronic or intractable pain problems. She needs to be aware of the physiological mechanisms of pain, types of pain, physical and psychological responses to pain and methods of assessment and observation. These will help in the understanding of methods of pain relief and pain control.

In recent times, there has been a growing awareness and interest in the management of pain. There is no valid reason to dismiss patients who may be regarded as 'failures' because they have not responded to conventional methods of treatment. Rather, we should seek a greater understanding of their responses to pain and try to offer as much help and support as possible.

In some areas, 'pain clinics' have been established — many of them by anaesthetists — and patients can be referred to these. The general aim of these clinics is to care for people with prolonged and chronic pain, who find that their quality of life is affected by the pain. An advantage of these clinics is that a holistic view of the patient is taken,and this is an essential part in dealing with the problems of pain. Many of the patients who are eventually referred to a pain clinic may have been passed from one doctor to another, and tried many forms of treatment without avail.

Each pain clinic differs to some extent, and there are not enough to meet the needs of all patients who could benefit from referral. However, the setting up of such clinics reflects a growing attitude of trying to meet the needs of people who might otherwise be left to cope on their own.It could well be beneficial to both professionals and patients alike, if 'conventional' practitioners were to become more open to some of the 'alternative' or 'complementary' spheres of therapy.

BIBLIOGRAPHY

Anthony C P, Thibodeau G A 1979 Text book of anatomy and physiology 10th edn. C V Mosby, St Louis

Bell G H, Emslie–Smith D, Paterson G R 1976 Textbook of physiology and biochemistry, 9th edn. Churchill Livingstone, Edinburgh

Collins S, Parker E 1983 The essential of nursing — an introduction to nursing. Macmillan, London

Conway–Rutkowski B L 1982 In: Carini and Owens Neurological and neurosurgical nursing 8th edn. C V Mosby, St Louis

Copp L A 1985 Perspectives on pain. Churchill Livingstone,Edinburgh

Cordis Corporation. Stimucord Mark 2 Programmable Neural Stimulator, Patient Manual. Cordis Corporation, USA

Gibran K 1972 The prophet. William Heinemann, London

Hayward J 1975 Information — a prescription against pain. Royal College of Nursing, London

Irving C, Selleck T 1982 Pain — the creative approach. Nursing Times 78 (23): 966

Keele C A, Armstrong D 1964 Substances producing pain and itch. Edward Arnold, London

McCaffery M 1979 Nursing the patient in pain. (Adapted for the UK by Sofaer B). Harper and Row, London

Melzack R, Wall P D 1965 Pain mechanisms — a new theory. Science 150: 971

Pemberton L 1983 The nurse's role in pain control. Proceedings of the European Association of Neurosurgical Nurses — 2nd Congress, Brussels

Pemberton L 1985 Physical and psychological effects of pain. Unpublished paper

Purchese G, Allan D 1984 Neuromedical and neurosurgical nursing, 2nd edn. Bailliere Tindall, London

Raiman J A 1981 Responding to pain. Nursing 1: 1362

Sofaer B 1984 Pain: a handbook for nurses. Harper and Row, London

Watson J E 1979 Medical-surgical nursing and related physiology, 2nd edn. W B Saunders, Philadelphia

Index